"Anyone with an interest in health should read *Total Wellness*. . . . This book helps the reader to find out specifically what he/she needs to do to maintain and optimize health. . . . Even readers who are experts in alternative health will find new insights and facts in this book. . . . This is a highly readable, well-researched, sensible (as opposed to overhyped) introduction to natural medicine for individuals who want to take responsibility for their own health—if you don't just read the first twenty pages."

—*Alain Dessaint*, Healthy & Natural Journal

"*Total Wellness* contains a wealth of information on the factors contributing to a state of disease and how a person can get well by having a healthy lifestyle."

—*Jeffrey Schiller*, Creations Magazine

"Pizzorno emphasizes ways that people can educate themselves to take control of their health and prevent problems before they occur. . . . Pizzorno provides extensive scientific research that supports the various treatments he recommends. . . . For anyone interested in natural medicine, *Total Wellness* serves as an excellent introduction to one of the most ardent advocates and his philosophy of health."

—*Rosemary Jones*, Common Ground *magazine*

TOTAL WELLNESS

Improve Your Health by
Understanding and Cooperating with
Your Body's Natural Healing Systems

Joseph Pizzorno, N.D.

Prima Publishing

PRIMA PUBLISHING and colophon are registered trademarks of Prima Communications, Inc.

Library of Congress Cataloging-in-Publication Data

Pizzorno, Joseph E.
    Total Wellness : improve your health by understanding and cooperating with your body's natural healing systems / by Joseph Pizzorno.
        p.   cm.
    Includes bibliographical references and index.
    ISBN 0-7615-0433-8
    ISBN 0-7615-1094-X
    1. Self-care, health.   2. Medicine, Popular.   3. Pathology—
Popular works.   I. Title.
RA776.95.P583   1996
613—dc20   96-224
                                                             CIP

98 99 00 01 HH 10 9 8 7 6 5 4 3 2
Printed in the United States of America

All products mentioned in this book are trademarks of their respective companies.

Warning—Disclaimer
Prima Publishing has designed this book to provide information in regard to the subject matter covered. It is sold with the understanding that the publisher and the author are not liable for the misconception or misuse of information provided. Every effort has been made to make this book as complete and as accurate as possible. The purpose of this book is to educate. The author and Prima Publishing shall have neither liability nor responsibility to any person or entity with respect to any loss, damage, or injury caused or alleged to be caused directly or indirectly by the information contained in this book. The information presented herein is in no way intended as a substitute for medical counseling.

How to Order
Single copies may be ordered from Prima Publishing, P.O. Box 1260BK, Rocklin, CA 95677; telephone (916) 632-4400. Quantity discounts are also available. On your letterhead, include information concerning the intended use of the books and the number of books you wish to purchase.

To my loving wife, Lara (who edited this book and wrote Chapter Ten), and two wonderful children, Raven and Galen. I am a lucky man. Words are not adequate to express what is in my heart for you who have made my life a joy.

Contents

Acknowledgments

I can think of no greater joy for a teacher than to become the student of one who was once his student. Michael Murray, N.D., this book is dedicated to you. I vividly remember you as a voracious student and remarkably insightful student clinician in the early 80s, always challenging me and other faculty to provide the best education we could. Now, when I want to learn about the latest research in the clinical applications of herbal medicine, I find myself looking to your books and relying on your expertise. Thank you, Michael, and all the other graduates of Bastyr Unversity, for making such an important contribution to the health and well-being of the human community.

Foreword

Have a headache? It really isn't due to an aspirin deficiency, you know. Feeling nervous? It's not because your brain isn't synthesizing enough Valium. If there's something wrong with your health, the overwhelming likelihood is that it has nothing at all to do with a lack of the latest patent drug or a genetic requirement for surgery, radiation, or chemotherapy.

And that's what this book is all about! If there's something wrong with our bodies, it's very likely that there's a problem with the molecules that make up our bodies—a lack of this, an excess of that, perhaps the presence of molecules that don't belong there at all. Germs and microorganisms don't cause disease all by their microscopic selves; they only take advantage of us when our bodies are weakened by nutrient-poor food or burdened by toxins that don't belong in our systems anyway. Healthy, vibrant plants, animals, and people don't "catch" germs very often, if at all!

Dr. Joe Pizzorno is one of the most qualified people in our country—in fact, in our world—to guide us toward a much healthier (and likely longer) life. Dr. Pizzorno never ceases to amaze me: he had a busy, successful naturopathic practice for seven years, then over the past eighteen years, he has co-founded and led from absolutely nothing—no students, no professors, no building, no supplies, no money—Bastyr University, our country's only fully accredited university of natural healing. Today, Bastyr has nearly 900 students, degree programs in naturopathic medicine, acupuncture and Oriental medicine, nutrition, and applied behavioral science. (He and his team did it all with no taxpayer dollars at all!) Despite the enormity of this job, he has kept absolutely current with the very latest in natural health care, and somehow finds the time to organize this enormous mass of data, edit it into useful form, and write it out clearly for us. And before writing *Total Wellness*, he co-authored the *Textbook of Natural Medicine*, the authority in the field, and its popular adaptation, *Encyclopedia of Natural Medicine*. In his "spare time," he serves on the Seattle–King County Board of Public Health, the first naturopathic doctor in the U.S. to hold such a position. There just isn't space or time to list all of Dr. Pizzorno's other accomplishments and activities, although it's only fair to say he couldn't have done it all without the support of his wife, Lara, his two children, and the entire Bastyr team.

So back to this book. If you're not feeling as well as you'd like, this is definitely the book for you. If you're feeling perfectly well, and want to stay that way, this is the book for you, too!

Toward your good health,

Jonathan V. Wright, M.D.
Tahoma Clinic
Kent, Washington

Preface

Total Wellness was a challenge to write, not because it was difficult (it was), but because it was hard to stop. This book was only supposed to be 75,000 words; it ended up twice as many words and took me six months past my deadline to complete. While I have used and taught the concepts in this book for 25 years, as I reviewed the scientific literature for the latest research, I experienced major insights that deepened my understanding of healing. This resulted in a constantly expanding knowledge base that I wanted to provide to you, the reader. While much more could have been written, I think Lara and I were successful in distilling the very best health promoting information.

This is not a casual book meant to be read in an evening. It is a substantive work for those seriously interested in fundamentally improving the course of their health. We have provided some unique and powerful tools to aid you in becoming your own best physician. You will experience the greatest improvement in your health by reading the entire book, since this will give you the understanding you need to shift perspective from symptomatic relief to understanding and facilitating the body's potent, innate healing systems.

Introduction

Each of us is our own best doctor.

This book is for those who are tired of the old clichés of "eat right," "exercise more," and "reduce your stress." It is for those who want to understand their own unique needs for optimizing health, where they are weak, and how to strengthen themselves.

This book teaches you how to take a laser-gun approach to your health concerns rather than the shotgun approach recommended to everyone. For example, although we are all concerned about cholesterol and are advised to decrease cholesterol intake by dietary restriction, only about 10% of us can actually decrease our serum cholesterol levels by lowering dietary cholesterol. Likewise, for hypertension, while all are recommended to decrease salt intake, salt is only an important contributing factor for about 10% of us. Some people can smoke from an early age with seeming impunity (thus the now banned ads we used to see in magazines and on television of the octogenarians claiming they've smoked since their teens without a problem), while others succumb to lung cancer within a few years.

It's all very frustrating for a health-conscious person to understand what he or she really needs, thus we chase one health fad after another, always disappointed because we really don't feel all that much better. The basic problem is we are all so different, or as Roger Williams, Ph.D. (the noted nutrition researcher who discovered the vitamin pantothenic acid) first observed in the 1960s, we each have a unique "biochemical individuality." Basically, fads and generic information fail because they aren't really for us as *individuals*—they are for "everyone" and thus are optimal for practically no one. Each of us is as unique biochemically as our fingerprints are unique physically.

Maintaining good health takes significant commitment and effort, so why hassle yourself unnecessarily or waste your effort on things that aren't for you? This book will help you to find out what *you* need to maintain and optimize your health, so you can concentrate your energies on the major health improvement efforts that will do you the most good.

Many Diseases; Few Causes

After 25 years of research, seeing thousands of patients, and teaching over a thousand naturopathic students, I have come to recognize that, although thousands of diseases have been named, relatively few causes or imbalances underlie most health problems. The actual symptoms or diseases a person manifests are determined by his or her underlying imbalances/susceptibilities, the lifestyle he or she chooses, and the environmental challenges he or she experiences.

A distillation of my thoughts as a physician, this book provides a step-by-step journey through each of the crucial systems of your body. I present, in layperson's terms, a comprehensive, but understandable, discussion of the key underlying systems of the body, which must work effectively for each of us to establish and maintain total wellness. For each of these systems, I talk about how the system works, how to recognize when it is not working properly, how it can be damaged or impaired, and how to help make it work the way it should by using natural medicines and healthful lifestyle behaviors to strengthen it. Throughout the book I provide detailed methods of self-diagnosis plus practical healing therapies for the person suffering from chronic disease or who is constantly contracting one disease after another. More important, the aim of this book is to teach the reader not merely to identify a disease or treat it with natural medicine, but to prevent it. For those who are healthy, it provides the medical insight needed to develop and maintain optimal health, not only by identifying and meeting current needs but by providing the capability to monitor and respond to changing needs in the future.

This is a unique book. While several books (such as *The Encyclopedia of Natural Medicine*, which I co-authored with Dr. Michael Murray) are available that show ways to treat disease using natural therapies and lifestyle changes, none give you the tools to *personalize* the process, and none look at the underlying susceptibilities you may have that increase your likelihood of developing specific types of diseases. Unless these underlying predispositions are recognized and rectified, just treating a disease, even with natural therapies, will not optimize your long-term health.

Natural therapies, while typically less expensive, more effective, and safer for treating the causes of specific diseases than drugs (which are usually more effective in alleviating the symptoms of disease), still usually focus on disease and pathology. Long-term optimal health and the prevention of disease depends on understanding the imbalances in your body—whether due to genetics, diet, environment, or lifestyle—that render you susceptible to specific types of disease.

It is easy to prescribe a whole-foods diet, more exercise, less pollution, and less stress for everyone, but such generic prescriptions do not recognize the unique needs of each individual. By understanding the symptom constellations that underlie most diseases, we can learn to recognize our own imbalances and, where possible, reestablish normal function and adopt the specific behaviors that will promote our own long-term optimal health.

Some Important Concepts

The Healing Power of Nature (Vis Medicatrix Naturae)

Our bodies have a tremendous ability to heal, usually without medical or drug intervention—if given a chance. In fact, 70 to 90% of all diseases are self-limiting, that is, the body will heal itself without intervention. Natural healers refer to this inherent drive as "the healing power of nature" or the *vis medicatrix naturae*. We must learn to view the signs and symptoms of disease not as inconveniences that should be eliminated as soon as possible, but as important messages to which we must listen. They tell us how our body is trying to heal and can serve as clues when our underlying healing systems are being overloaded—a situation that will result in progressively increasing susceptibility to serious disease if we don't pay attention. This book will teach you how to listen to these messages, what they mean, and how you can use them to promote your long-term health.

Functional Reserves

The functional reserves of your protective systems are like a bank savings account; everything is fine until it's depleted. For example, you can go for a few days without vitamin C, or overexpose yourself to a toxin, and nothing may appear to happen. Then you do exactly the same thing, and disease strikes and you wonder why. You are now manifesting disease because your reserves became too low, so your protective systems can't work adequately anymore.

However, susceptibility (or low reserves) doesn't usually mean immediate disease. A trigger is needed. For example, a poorly functioning immune system typically doesn't result in an immediate infection—we won't develop a recognizable disease until we are exposed to a large enough dose of a pathogenic bacteria or virus. The weaker our immune system, the lower the level of exposure that will cause disease. This is especially evident in AIDS patients, whose immune system becomes so weak that common microorganisms, which are usually easily eliminated, now become life-threatening.

Most of our organs and systems, when functioning optimally, have a reserve capacity equal to about seven times that needed at rest. For example, when resting, the average adult's heart pumps about five and a half quarts of blood a minute. When a well-conditioned adult runs a sprint, his or her heart beats harder and faster resulting in an increase in blood flow to a remarkable 30 to 35 quarts a minute.

As can be seen in Figure 1-1, our vital force, the *vis medicatrix naturae*, is always pushing us toward better health. However, as we accumulate deficiencies from a poor diet or damage from environmental insults, we drift down the health scale and become progressively more susceptible to dysfunction and disease. As our physiology becomes imbalanced, we first experience fatigue and

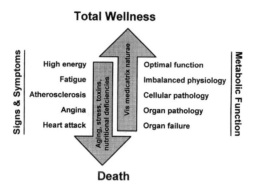

Figure 1-1 *Our Functional Reserves Work to Push Us Toward Health*

then increased susceptibility to minor health problems such as the common cold. If we allow the weaknesses in our protective systems to continue, we develop ever more serious disease.

Using the heart as our example again, as the heart becomes weaker, it is not able to increase its output as much. Most of us start life in good physical shape. As young adults we are able to enjoy a hard game of tennis, a long run over hilly terrain, or an overnight hike in the mountains. Then these activities become too demanding, but we feel fine during normal activities, such as a brisk walk to catch an airplane. Next we may notice shortness of breath when climbing several flights of stairs. Then just walking a few blocks causes pain in our legs (we have no extra reserve), and finally, we can't lie down at night because our heart can't pump enough to keep fluids out of our lungs (cardiac failure). The same gradual deterioration will happen in all the systems of our body if we don't take proper care of ourselves.

Prevention

All agree that the concept of prevention makes a lot of sense. Unfortunately, the medical profession has warped the concept of prevention to include diagnosis and treatment of disease. Table 1-1 shows the current definitions of prevention. In this book we are talking about primary prevention, and not merely early diagnosis and treatment of disease.

Functional Medicine

Functional medicine is a term coined by internationally recognized nutritional biochemist Jeffrey Bland, Ph.D., who defines it as: "The field of health care which employs assessment and early intervention to improve physiological, emotional/cognitive and physical function." According to Dr. Bland:[1]

Table 1-1 Definitions of Prevention

Definition	Description
Primary prevention	Lifestyle modification, decreased dietary fat, increased fiber intake, nutritional supplementation, smoking cessation, alcohol abuse cessation, counseling, immunization
Secondary prevention	Early detection of subclinical disease to prevent further disability; screening for hypertension, hearing impairment, visual acuity, osteoporosis, high cholesterol, malignant diseases, e.g., mammograms, prostate specific antigen testing
Tertiary prevention	Minimizing disability and handicap from established disease

> In functional medicine, the presence or absence of a disease is of secondary consideration to an understanding of the function or dysfunction which prevents or allows a disease to occur . . . Functional medicine does not focus on the isolated entity called disease, but rather on the specifics of structural and functional mechanisms which comprise the whole person at any particular point in his or her life . . .

We are indebted to Dr. Bland and his cadre of physicians, researchers, and laboratory diagnosticians across the nation who have worked so hard to develop this field. They have effectively brought rigorous science and good documentation to concepts that have been preached by practitioners of natural medicine for centuries.

How This Book Is Organized

Chapter Two presents the appalling condition of our health care system. Despite the overwhelming and ever escalating costs, we are sicker and suffer from more chronic diseases than ever.

Chapter Three presents the philosophical underpinnings of this book and describes the key systems that must function optimally for total wellness.

The remainder of this book provides a comprehensive description of these key systems: how to recognize when a system is not working properly, how it can be damaged, and how to use lifestyle and natural medicines to reestablish optimal function. I've used a lot of real-life examples to make the information more personal and understandable. The examples are all real patients from either my private practice or the student teaching clinic at Bastyr University. The names have, of course, all been changed to protect their privacy.

I've organized these chapters to allow you to investigate your health as deeply as you wish. Each chapter consists of two basic parts: a simplified overview and an in-depth study. The simplified overview presents real-life examples of what happens when the system being discussed isn't working as well as it should. It also includes a list of common symptoms and diseases that indicate when the system is not working, and a thumbnail list of recommendations on ways to help the system work better.

The in-depth portion of each chapter provides a description of how the system works and what can cause it to become dysfunctional. Naturopathic treatments to reestablish optimal function of the system are provided. In addition, I give examples of common diseases of the dysfunctional system and suggested treatments for these. Remember that although many of these problems can be resolved with self-treatment, there are times when a physician must be consulted. I provide examples of these situations as well.

Lastly, the appendices provide several useful tools: a health log to help you plot the efficacy of your efforts to improve your health, a list of common diseases and the underlying dysfunctions that allow them to develop, and finally, a list of resources so that you can study the subjects discussed more deeply or find a health care practitioner who can help you in your efforts to become healthier.

Conclusion

The intent of this book is to help you fundamentally improve your health. You will learn how well the systems of your body are working (or not working) and how to make them work better, how to identify and use the special nutrients and herbs your body needs, how to protect yourself from the things that are hurting you, and how to eliminate from your body what you don't need.

While this book contains easily understood descriptions and plans to help you take full control of your health, it also contains a fair amount of technical information because, at times, you will need to delve more deeply into difficult problems. Much of this can be done by yourself, without a doctor. However, even more can be done with the help of a doctor trained in thinking about health promotion rather than simply disease treatment. A good physician can help you make a more accurate diagnosis and develop a treatment plan that best meets your unique needs. Unfortunately, few doctors have studied this type of medicine, so if you can't find the right doctor, you are going to have to educate the one you have. This is one reason why all the information in this book is fully referenced to the scientific research literature. If your doctor is unwilling to listen to you, despite a well-referenced presentation, find a better doctor—one who is more concerned about *your* health than blindly following a health care philosophy that is reaching its limits. The kinds of physicians most likely to understand this book's approach are naturopathic doctors, holistic medical doctors, broad-scope chiropractors, or any physician who has studied "functional medicine."

You may have many health problems and dealing with them all at once may be overwhelming. If this is your starting point, prioritize by focusing first on the problems that are bothering you the most. As the functioning of each of your body's systems improves, your growing feeling of wellness will make it progressively easier to take on the rest.

Chapter Two

The Crisis in Health Care

We can't afford to only treat disease, we must learn how to stay well.

In 1994, we spent $1 trillion on health care in the U.S., or, more accurately, we spent most of this astounding sum on disease treatment. This represents an increase of 300% in the last 15 years.[1] Health care costs now consume 15% of the gross national product (GNP), with the percentage of GNP spent on health care continuing to increase at twice the rate of inflation (see Figure 2-1). If the rate of increase continues, health care costs will consume the entire GNP within 50 years!

Corporations now spend an incredible 48% of their after-tax profits on health care, and it is projected that by the year 2000, health care costs will equal 60% of after-tax profit at the average Fortune 500 company.[2] Even now in the U.S., it costs more in health care to build a car than it does in steel! In the U.S., we spend 40% more per person on health care than the next closest country, Japan. The difference in cost between an American car and a Japanese car of comparable quality is asserted by some economists to be due entirely to the higher costs to industry of health care for American workers.

Why Health Care Costs Have Increased

Why have health care costs escalated so dramatically? As might be expected, there are many opinions. While I believe the real underlying cause is that we have a *disease-treatment* rather than a *health-promotion* system, much can be learned by looking at problems with our current system. As discussed in detail below, we use doctors too much (especially specialists), use too many expensive hospital-based procedures, use too many expensive drugs, use many expensive medical procedures inappropriately, experience a lot of side effects from drugs and medical procedures, and spend too much money subsidizing medical education and administrative inefficiency.

7

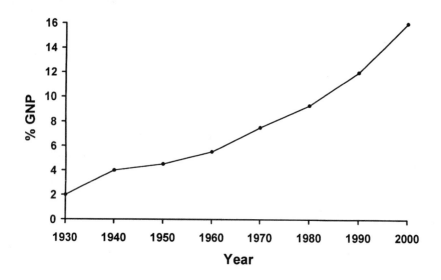

Figure 2-1 Health Care Costs as a Percentage of GNP

Excessive Use of Doctors, Especially Specialists

Due to the massive influx of federal and state subsidies, the number of graduating medical doctors doubled from 1965 to 1980, a much greater rate of increase than in the population. The number of practicing doctors in the U.S. has increased from 308,487 in 1970 to 627,723 in 1992. The ratio of medical doctors to the population went from 151 doctors per 100,000 people in 1970 to 245 per 100,000 in 1992, an increase in ratio of 62%. More of a problem, however, is the dramatic shift from family practice doctors to specialists. From 1950 to 1990, we moved from specialists comprising 30% of the physician work force to specialists accounting for 70 to 80% (depending on how one categorizes medical practitioners).[3] This has had a huge impact on the cost of health care because specialists charge far more for their services (they earn two to three times as much as generalists) and tend to prescribe and utilize the most expensive procedures. This imbalance in specialists is not likely to change soon; the number of medical students choosing general practice has dropped from 22.7% in 1989 to 14.6% in 1992.

Most medical apologists say, "Don't blame doctors for the escalating costs of health care—their fees are only a small percentage of the total." This is an accurate statement, but it ignores the fact that doctors are the ones who order the drugs, hospital stays, and surgeries—80% of medical services are prescribed by medical doctors. Currently, medical analysts estimate that 36% of physician visits are unnecessary (I believe the number is actually greater), 56% of surgeries are unnecessary, 15% of hospital outpatient visits are unnecessary, and half of all time spent in hospitals is not medically indicated.

A direct correlation exists between the ratio of surgeons in an area and the percentage of that population receiving surgeries. One research study found that an area with 4.5 surgeons per 10,000 population experienced 940 operations per 10,000 while an area with 2.5 surgeons per 10,000 experienced 590 operations per 10,000.[4] In other words, when the concentration of surgeons doubles, so does the rate of surgeries—every doctor needs to perform about 200 operations a year to cover overhead and maintain his or her desired income.

The problem is apparently worse for the especially expensive surgeries. A recent study of 168 patients either scheduled for coronary artery bypass or strongly recommended to undergo the procedure found such a procedure inappropriate in 80% of the cases.[5] This may explain why from 1983 to 1990, these operations have more than doubled—to 380,000 a year (at an average of $40,000 an operation). Of even greater concern is that the majority of patients receiving these operations reclog their arteries within five years.

The rise in expensive hospital-based procedures prescribed by highly specialized physicians is considered by health economists to be the primary cause of our escalating health care costs. The more doctors there are, the more the use of the health care services increases, and the more specialized the doctors, the more expensive the procedures they utilize. Unfortunately, as I discuss below, this has not led to improved health, quite the contrary.

Excessive Use and Expense of Drugs

According to health care insurance sources, in 1979, the average person was prescribed an average of one drug per year, which cost an average of $5.50. In 1991, the average person was prescribed six and a half drugs per year, and the drugs cost an average of $22.50 *each*, an increase of three times the rate of inflation![6,7] Although drug companies say this rise is due to the high cost of research, the hard facts are that drug companies spend one to three times as much on advertising as on research, and their profit margins run as high as 29%. Four of the largest drug companies spend an average of 8% on research and 12% on advertising and make a 24% profit.[8] The drug industry has been the most profitable business in America since 1950. Over 50% of the world's total supply of drugs are used in the U.S. alone.

Not only are drugs far more expensive than they used to be, they also are greatly overused, a situation that leads to further illness and expense. According to recent research, preventable prescription-drug related diseases and deaths cost us $77 billion a year.[9] This is not only the fault of doctors, but also of their patients, for the public now equates receiving a prescription with health care. The misuse and overuse of medications is even worse for the elderly, especially those in nursing homes. Although those over 60 make up only one-sixth of the population, they take 40% of all prescription drugs. The typical elderly patient takes 13 different medications each year, resulting in a 10% incidence of adverse drug reactions.[10] A study of 1,106 nursing home residents revealed that the average resident took seven drugs, at least one of which was inappropriate in 40% of the patients, and two or more of which were inappropriate in 10% of the patients.[11]

Side Effects of Drugs and Medical Procedures

While medical interventions are usually effective, they also often cause undesirable side effects. According to some researchers, 36% of hospital admissions are caused by side effects from medical treatments, and 17% of hospital admissions are for adverse drug reactions. Other research has found that 8 million people are hospitalized per year—28% of all admissions—for diseases brought on by prescription drugs. Adverse drug effects are thought to be responsible for 100,000 deaths a year—more than double the 45,000 caused annually by automobile accidents. In 1990, the U.S. Government Accounting Office (GAO), after reviewing the 198 drugs that were approved from 1976 to 1985, found that 102 of them had side effects serious enough to warrant either withdrawal from the market or marked changes in labeling to warn of their serious dangers.

Once hospitalized, patients' problems can sometimes increase. Infections acquired in the hospital (nosocomial infections) strike up to one in every ten patients, or almost 2.5 million people a year. On average, nosocomial infections add a minimum of four days and $1,800 to a hospital stay, for a total cost of well over $4 billion nationwide. Hospital-induced infections cause 20,000 deaths each year and contribute to 60,000 more, giving them a place among the top ten leading causes of death in the U.S.[12]

How Subsidies Produce Expensive Doctors

In 1992, the federal subsidy for medical schools was a staggering $15.2 billion.[13] In addition, 76 of the 126 medical schools are state supported. In other words, we invest a huge amount of public resources to subsidize the education of medical doctors, of which there are already too many, who then go out and make incomes four times that of the average American (and three times that of a college professor with comparable education).[14] These physicians prescribe excessive utilization of medical services and, through their paid lobbyists, resist efforts to reform the system.

Excessive Bureaucratic Growth

Aggravating the crisis in health care costs is the growing inefficiency of the bureaucracy that has grown to manage (and profit from) this huge medical system: we now spend almost one quarter of every health care dollar just paying for administration![15] This proportion is 117% higher than in Canada and 97% higher than in Britain. While the number of U.S. physicians increased about 60% from 1970 to 1987, the number of health care administrators increased a whopping 375%!

What Do We Get for $1 Trillion?

Are we getting healthier or living longer after seeing specialists more, using more drugs, adding more administrators, and spending all this money? No. Most chronic diseases are *more* common, the incidence of most cancers continues to increase, and the real longevity of adults has changed little this century. The only serious disease that has become less common is coronary artery disease, but this improvement is due more to people reducing cholesterol and getting more exercise than to medical intervention, even though we spent $109 billion in 1992 on cardiovascular disease care.[16] Currently, we spend 70% of our health care dollars treating chronic disease.

The Health Status of Americans

How healthy are Americans? Table 2-1 shows the appalling statistics—almost half of working Americans have either a serious chronic disease (arthritis, heart disease, high blood pressure, cancer, gall bladder disease, diabetes, rheumatism, emphysema, serious arteriosclerosis, and so on) or are in ill health. But the health of their non-working dependents is even worse. As shown in Table 2-2, half to two-thirds of these dependents suffer from chronic disease (such as cancer, diabetes, and heart disease) and ill health. What's especially alarming about these statistics is that these are adults supposedly in their prime. It gets worse for the elderly, virtually all of whom suffer from one or more chronic degenerative diseases.

Table 2-3 lists alphabetically the shocking incidence of America's most common chronic diseases. What's especially distressing is that as high as these numbers are, they don't include the incidence of acute diseases, nor the fact that many people suffer from more than one chronic disease. In the table I've added a listing of the underlying disorders that allow these conditions to

Table 2-1 Health Status of Working Americans Aged 18 to 65[17]

Insurance Status	Poor Health	Chronic Health Problems
Uninsured	17%	23%
Insured	12%	29%
Federal/state employee	21%	37%

Table 2-2 Health Status of Non-Working Dependents of Americans Aged 18 to 65[17]

Insurance Status	Poor Health	Chronic Health Problems
Uninsured	23%	27%
Insured	17%	32%
Dependent of federal/state employee	30%	33%

Table 2-3 The Percentage of Adult Americans Suffering from the Ten Most Common Chronic Diseases[18]

Condition	Men 18–44	Men 45–64	Men 65+	Women 18–44	Women 45–64	Women 65+	Underlying Disorder
Arthritis	4.1%	21.4%	38.3%	6.4%	33.9%	54.4%	Inflammation, toxicity, degeneration
Asthma, emphysema, and chronic bronchitis	5.5	8.8	16.7	9.3	11.4	12.6	Inflammation, toxicity
Cancer	0.2	2.3	5.2	0.5	2.2	3.8	Toxicity, immune dysfunction
Chronic sinusitis	13.6	16.3	14.1	18.3	19.9	17.0	Immune dysfunction
Diabetes	0.8	5.1	9.1	1.0	5.7	9.9	Metabolic dysfunction, toxicity
Hay fever	10.3	7.9	na*	12.1	9.8	na*	Inflammation
Hearing impairment	6.3	19.6	36.2	4.0	10.6	26.8	Degeneration
High blood pressure	6.6	25.4	32.7	5.7	27.4	45.6	Metabolic dysfunction
Ischemic (inadequate blood supply) heart disease	0.3	8.7	17.9	0.3	4.3	12.1	Metabolic dysfunction
Visual impairment	4.3	6.2	10.4	1.7	3.2	18.8	Degeneration

*na = not available

develop and continue. I'll talk about how to correct each of these syndromes later in the book.

Didn't the "War on Cancer" help? The grim data are presented in Figure 2-2. On December 23, 1971, President Nixon signed a bill funding the "War on Cancer," starting the federal cascade of tens of billions of dollars into medical research on cancer treatment—at which point, the rate of death from cancer immediately began to rise. And don't let anyone try to convince you it's because people are living longer. These data are age-corrected. Yes, we have made progress in the treatment of a few cancers, especially for children. However, those cancers are uncommon (although their incidence has gone up considerably the past two decades), while the common cancers, e.g., lung cancer, are increasingly worse. The incidence of prostate and brain cancers and non-Hodgkin's lymphoma (which used to be a more common cause of death in farmers), is beginning to rise in the general population, suggesting that exposure to some

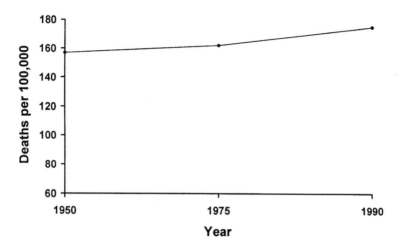

Figure 2-2 *Age-Adjusted Incidence of Cancer Deaths per 100,000 Population[20]*

common environmental factor(s), such as pesticides and herbicides may play a role in cancer etiology.[19]

Our Real Longevity Has Changed Little This Century

Most people believe we now live longer, and medical apologists attribute this supposed increase in longevity to the health care system in order to justify its cost. This is actually a very misleading statistic. At the turn of the century, many children died from infections and when their very short life spans are calculated into the total, the result, of course, is a dramatic decrease in average life expectancy. For example, if three of ten people die at the age of 1, while the other seven live to 75 years of age, the life expectancy for the ten is calculated as $(3 \times 1) + (7 \times 75)/10$, which equals 52.8 years average life expectancy. If those three children do not die, the average life expectancy suddenly jumps to 75.0 years. While the lives of some children with infections were saved by medical intervention, i.e., antibiotics, the vast majority were saved because of the intense public health movement in the early part of this century. A concerted effort by the FDA, the USDA, and the county public health departments across the country cleaned up the food and water supply and dramatically decreased the number of pathogenic bacteria they contained. (Some historians consider the introduction of home refrigerators to have been equally important.) This effort resulted in a dramatic drop in the rate of infections in children, which is the real reason they stopped dying.

A better question then is, "How long do people live *after* they survive childhood?" The answer, shown in Figure 2-3, is actually pretty discouraging. While the longevity of white men after birth increased 24.5 years from 1900 to

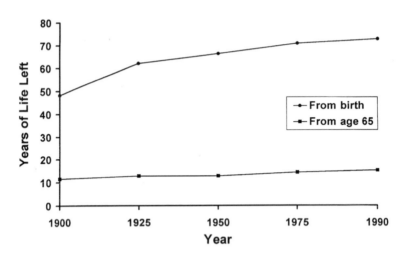

Figure 2-3 Changes in Life Expectancy at Birth and at Age 65 from 1900 to 1990

1990, the life expectancy of men 65 years of age increased only 3.7 years.[21] The numbers are slightly better for women and slightly worse for blacks. If we look at the total population and compare 1980 to 1993, a period during which excellent data is available, we find that longevity from birth increased 1.5 years, and longevity from age 65 increased 8 months. During that same time, health care costs increased from $350 billion (9% of the GNP) to $880 billion (13% of the GNP)!

However, an even better measure of health is changes in our *healthspan*, the years of life we enjoy free of disabling disease. We all know the scary stories of people being kept alive on life support, long past the time when "life" had any meaning. What we all really want is an increase in not just the number of years we live, but in our "healthy life expectancy." This is a difficult number to measure. Fortunately, a few researchers have found enough consistent data to allow them to calculate how our healthy life span changed from 1970 to 1980. Unfortunately, what they found is profoundly disturbing: although we do live slightly longer, *our healthy life span hasn't increased.*[22] In other words, we are living longer, but only as disabled invalids.

Medical Doctors' Excellent Fiscal Health

Most would agree that, in general, doctors are highly dedicated individuals genuinely concerned about their patients. However, the current system ensures that doctors maintain a very high income. In fact, as can be seen from Table 2-4, there is considerable financial incentive for physicians to specialize in the most expensive therapies and thus little reason to support change, particularly that which promotes prevention. These data also help explain why, as shown

Table 2-4 Physician's Net Annual Income (1991)[23,24,25]

Physician Class	Net Annual Income
Preventive medicine	$90,000
Family practice	$124,000
Internal medicine	$174,000
General surgery	$208,000
Orthopedic surgery	$278,000
Cardiac surgery	$500,000

in Figure 2-4, the number of doctors per capita has increased 22% in just the past 10 years and almost 100% in the past 60 years. But more important, the percentage of specialists has increased from 10% in 1930 to 70% in 1990.[1]

Prevention and Natural Medicine Promote Health and Decrease Costs

Researchers have been evaluating the health benefits and cost effectiveness of prevention and wellness programs for the past two decades. Research evaluating the cost and clinical effectiveness of utilizing natural medicine practices, replacing drugs with natural medicines, and combining natural medicine with conventional medicine has concluded that these practices promote health and decrease costs.

Wellness and Prevention Programs Work

Probably the best research has been in the area of evaluating the health benefits and cost-effectiveness of disease prevention programs at work sites. Kenneth Pelletier, Ph.D., has published two articles reviewing the results of these programs. His reports are very encouraging.[2] In the eleven years from 1980 to 1991, 24 research articles were published in this area. The rate of publication increased dramatically in the following two years, when an additional 23 studies were published. Not only did the rate of research publication increase, but so did the quality of the research design and statistical methods. All but one demonstrated an improvement in health and a decrease in costs. These studies consistently found that participants reduced their number of days of disability (43% in one study), number of days spent in a hospital (54% in one study), and amount spent on health care (a remarkable 76% in one study). The ratio of dollars saved to dollars spent ranged as high as $3.40 saved for every dollar spent on health promotion.

Several community-based health promotion programs also show that when people take better care of themselves, the results are better health and lower costs. In one study, two cities (with a total population of 122,800) that provided four or five education programs a year focusing on decreasing smoking

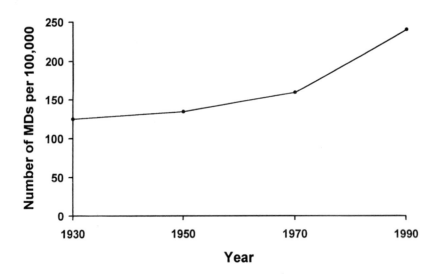

Figure 2-4 *Number of Medical Doctors in the U.S. per 100,000 Population*[26]

and improving diet were compared to two other cities that did nothing. After five years, the mortality rate of the "educated" cities dropped a remarkable 15%.[27] Another study published the results of a multi-year prevention program with workers in the city of Birmingham, Alabama. After six years, they found that, while health care costs of other cities had almost doubled, their health care costs did not increase, implying a huge savings.

An innovative insurance company, American Western Life Insurance in South San Francisco, has been offering a wellness-oriented insurance program for two years as of this writing. The voluntary program asks each enrollee to develop a personalized wellness program in consultation with a wellness counselor. When enrollees get sick, they utilize a self-help program (under the guidance of a naturopathic physician) when appropriate. American Western Life Insurance gathered data from a group enrolled in their regular program who then decided to switch to the new program. In this group of patients, they found a decrease in costs of 30% after only one year.[6] They expect that the cost savings will continue to increase over time as the health benefits accumulate.

Substituting Natural Medicines for Prescription Drugs

Many studies have shown that, for a number of conditions, natural medicines and natural medicine therapies are more effective than conventional medicines, cost less, and cause fewer side effects. For example, migraine headaches affect about 3% of the population. The current medical approach is to use a drug, sumatriptan, which, while it relieves the symptoms in about 70% of sufferers, is expensive, has several side effects, and *does not decrease the rate of recurrence*. In contrast, the natural medicine approach recognizes that 80% of patients with migraine headaches have them because they are eating foods that are not right for them. The average migraine patient will have *no more migraines* if he or she simply avoids these foods (which average about six—a different six for each person).[28] Although this has been known since 1980, it is a therapy still not used by the conventional medical doctor.

Natural medicine often substitutes herbs for more expensive drugs. For example, in benign prostatic hyperplasia (a common problem of men as they age), the typical medical drug treatment, Proscar, costs about $75 a month and can cause several unpleasant side effects, including decreased libido and impotence. Less than 50% of patients taking Proscar experience clinical improvement after taking the drug for one year, and it must be taken at least six months before any improvement can be expected. In contrast, the herb *Serenoa repens* (saw palmetto) is effective in nearly 90% of patients, usually in four to six weeks, costs only one-fourth as much, and has no negative side effects.[29]

Using Natural Medicine and Conventional Medicine Together

Several very interesting studies have looked at the impact of combining nutrition or herbal medicines with conventional therapies with encouraging results. Malnutrition has long been recognized as a common problem in hospitalized patients. As might be expected, malnutrition decreases the rate of wound healing and increases the risk of wound-related complications.

For example, vitamin C is especially important for wound healing. Even in supposedly healthy adults, vitamin-C deficiency occurs after acute injury. Tensile strength of experimental wounds in humans who had consumed a diet containing 0 to 10 mg of vitamin C per day for seven months was much weaker than that found in people eating the same diet, but supplementing it with 75 mg of vitamin C. Unfortunately, vitamin C status generally deteriorates in hospitalized patients during their stay.

Even if the patients are not deficient, supplying extra amounts of some nutrients can help wound repair. For example, supplementing with a mere 25,000 iu of vitamin A increases the collagen content and strength and improves healing of experimental skin wounds and internal surgical procedures in animal models. Supplementing with large amounts (17 to 25 gm) of the amino acid arginine has also been shown to enhance wound healing.[30]

In an interesting study, 59 hospitalized elderly patients (mean age of 82) with femoral neck fractures were divided in two groups. Twenty-seven were given a very conservative oral nutritional supplement. It contained modest amounts of protein, carbohydrate, fat, calcium, vitamins A, D_3, E, B_1, B_2, B_6, B_{12}, C, nicotinamide, folate, calcium pantothenate, biotin, and trace minerals. Even though the nutrient drink contained relatively low levels of nutrients, the clinical benefit was dramatic. The supplemented group stayed in the hospital 16 days less than the unsupplemented group (24 compared to 40 days), and complications resulting in deaths were cut in half (44% versus 87%). Even six months after stopping supplementation, the rates of complication and mortality were still lower in the supplemented group (40% versus 74%).[31]

Nutritional supplements that support the body's detoxification system are also of value for patients exposed to a lot of drugs after undergoing highly invasive medical procedures. One study evaluated the effect of glutamine supplementation (we'll talk about this important nutrient in Chapter Five) in 43 bone marrow transplant patients. The length of hospital stay was significantly shorter in the glutamine supplemented group compared to the control group (29 versus 36 days); the incidence of microbial cultures and clinical infections was significantly lower; and per patient costs were considerably lower. Hospital charges were $21,095 less, and room and board charges were reduced $10,115. Clearly, the introduction of the detoxifying nutrient glutamine results in significant cost savings and clinical benefit for the patient subjected to high levels of toxic drugs.[32]

Even with serious conditions, natural medicines can augment the effectiveness of conventional treatments. For example, some very interesting research studied patients with severe infections in their blood, a condition called *sepsis*. Sepsis is so serious that, once diagnosed, patients are immediately hospitalized and treated with intravenous antibiotics. Even with this care, 52% die. Adding a flavonoid (a vitamin-like substance) from the leaves of *Ginkgo biloba* to the patients' regime proved to be very helpful, decreasing the mortality rate to 33%—a remarkable improvement.[33]

I could go on and quote a lot more research (A *Textbook of Natural Medicine* contains approximately 10,000 citations documenting the clinical efficacy of natural medicine), but the message is clear. Prevention, wellness programs, and mixing natural medicine with conventional medicine works; people are healthier and costs drop significantly.

Satisfied Patients

As important as natural medicine's clinical- and cost-effectiveness is its increase in patient satisfaction. Studies have observed that patients utilizing the natural medicine/health promotion approach are more satisfied with the results of their treatment than they are with the results of conventional treatments. A few studies have directly compared patient satisfaction using natural medicine to patient satisfaction using conventional medicine. The largest was done in the Netherlands, where natural medicine practitioners are an integral part of the health care system. This extensive outcomes study compared satisfaction in 3,782 patients seeing either a conventional physician or a "complementary practitioner." The patients seeing the natural medicine practitioner reported better results for almost every condition (see Table 2-5). Of particular interest was the observation that the patients seeing the complementary

Table 2-5 Patient Satisfaction with Complementary Practitioners Compared to Medical Specialists[34]

Symptom	Complementary Practitioner Patients	Medical Patients
	% Improved	% Improved
Palpitations	63	59
Stiffness	67	54
Feeling very ill	75	78
Itching or burning	71	50
Tiredness or lethargy	70	60
Fever	86	100
Pain	70	58
Tension or depression	69	65
Coughing	76	50
Blood loss	100	100
Tingling, numbness	59	40
Shortness of breath	77	53
Nausea and vomiting	71	67
Diarrhea and constipation	67	50
Poor vision or hearing	31	47
Paralysis	80	67
Insomnia	58	45
Dizziness and fainting	80	53
Anxiety	65	64
Skin rash	58	50
Emotional instability	56	63
Sexual problems	57	57
Other	75	56

practitioners were somewhat sicker at the start of therapy and that in only 4 of the 23 conditions did the conventional medical patients report better results.

Conclusion

Our "health care" system has serious problems that are worsening. This disease-treatment, specialist-dominated system is very expensive. Half the costs of illness are wasted on conditions that could be prevented, the incidence of chronic disease and ill health has increased, and the small increases in longevity have been in years of disability rather than in years of health. We are spending an awful lot of resources on an ineffective system. Dramatic change is needed.

While change in the health care system seems to be on everyone's political agenda, the vested interests of the $1 trillion medical-industrial complex will probably allow very little real change to occur. We will likely still have a system oriented toward disease treatment with little attention to prevention or health promotion. Thus, if we want to be healthier and save money, it is up to us to change the system and take better care of ourselves.

According to health habit surveys, 30% of American adults smoke, 10% are alcoholic, 65% are overweight. The consumption of both sugar and caffeine have increased, and only 20% of adults consume the recommended five servings of fruits and vegetables a day (the average is 3.3 for men and 3.7 for women).[35,36] The impact of these bad habits is huge on both the medical and financial fronts. For instance, men who smoke heavily incur health care costs 47% above nonsmokers.[37] According to a U.S. Office of Technology Assessment report, the total price tag for health care, accidents, and lost productivity due to alcoholism was $120 billion in 1985 alone.

I believe the primary way out of this mess is to take better care of ourselves *and* decrease our use of conventional medical doctors. Sound crazy coming from a doctor? Perhaps, but I believe the research supports me. All of us must learn to modify our lifestyle in order to become healthier and, when health problems develop, take care of those that are self-treatable ourselves. We need to become our own best physicians; in other words, we need to master some basic skills of self diagnosis and self treatment. When a doctor is truly needed, we must become much more savvy and aware consumers. We need to use doctors that teach us *why* we become sick. When treatment is needed, we need to go to doctors who use therapies that help make us stronger rather than therapies that take over a function of our bodies, setting the stage not for improved health but for escalating dependence on doctors and drugs.

Chapter Three

A Systems Approach
to Total Wellness

Our bodies have a tremendous ability to heal, if just given a chance.

In conventional medicine, the primary function of the physician is diagnosis, i.e., identifying which disease a person is suffering from. This disease-diagnosis orientation leads to the disease-treatment, symptom-relief system that dominates health care in our country. As discussed in Chapter Two, this system is failing. We need a different kind of health care thinking and a different kind of physician. If we want to be healthy, it's up to us. We must become more aware of our bodies, learn how they function, understand what makes us healthy or sick—in short, become our own best physician.

Being Our Own Best Physician

Daunted by the prospect of self-diagnosis? Indeed, it is an almost impossible task to determine which one of several thousands of different diseases you may be suffering from. Physicians with thousands of hours of sophisticated medical training and years of practice frequently make inaccurate diagnoses where specific diseases are concerned. However, I believe the *name* of the disease is not what we need to know to get well. The necessary diagnosis is actually much simpler. In fact, our cultural obsession with complex diseases not only blinds us to the real causes of illness but disempowers us and gives over control of our health to doctors in a system that often relieves only symptoms. It's as if we spent all our time and resources hiring highly skilled specialists to repair a crack in the ceiling with spackle and paint when the root of the problem is a structural weakness in the building's foundation.

Consider the following:

1. We are often quite capable of treating ourselves without resorting to physicians. In 70 to 90% of all episodes of disease, we recover without seeing a physician.[1]
2. Our bodies have a tremendous ability to self-heal. When we go to see a physician, we, of course, expect to receive an effective therapy. The current

"gold standard" for determining the efficacy of a therapy is the double-blind, placebo-controlled clinical study, where neither the patient nor the physician knows if the patient is receiving the drug or the placebo. However, research demonstrates that 35 to 70% of the time, the patient gets better on the placebo! While a somewhat larger percentage get better on the drug, they also suffer the consequences of its side effects and expense. Even more interesting is the observation that the placebo patients in double-blind studies who comply with their therapy, that is, religiously take the placebo as directed, exhibit far more favorable results than those who do not comply with the therapy. Clearly, our beliefs profoundly affect the healing process.

3. Focusing on the pathology obscures recognition of our inherent healing power and disassociates us from understanding our body's signals. For example, in one study of the efficacy of a particular drug as compared to placebo in the treatment of endoscopy-documented stomach ulcers, 27% (12 of 45) of those whose ulcer had healed continued to have symptoms, while 55% of those whose ulcer had not healed became asymptomatic, no matter what treatment they had received.[2] In other words, the therapy focused only on the pathology, which, while recognizable, was not the only or even the primary factor causing the patients' symptoms.

Disease orientation is focused on end-stage pathology, whereas much of symptomatology, i.e., what we actually experience, is actually due to either the body's efforts to heal or messages that the healing process needs assistance. The challenge then is not to diagnose which particular end-stage pathology has developed, but rather to recognize the impediments to healing. I believe the very best physicians are those who understand the body's healing processes, recognize what the body needs to facilitate the healing processes, and encourage in each patient the belief in his or her ability to heal. I also believe each of us is capable of developing this understanding of our own body, and that ultimately, each of us can be his or her own best physician—if taught how.

After many years of extensive medical practice, I have come to believe that relatively few causes or imbalances underlie most diseases. However, recognizing these imbalances takes careful study because most people suffer from several such causes or syndromes. In addition, most diseases are caused by a combination of syndromes; sometimes the same disease can be caused by different syndromes. The actual symptoms or disease a person manifests is determined by his or her imbalances/ susceptibilities, the lifestyle he or she chooses, and the environmental challenges he or she experiences.

While this may appear complex at first, the symptoms we experience give us important, understandable messages about our susceptibilities. A step-by-step approach, starting with the most severe symptoms, allows us to recognize and focus on the susceptibilities or imbalances causing us the most trouble. Reestablishing balance in one area or syndrome may then more clearly reveal another, which can then be resolved, allowing us to progressively improve our health.

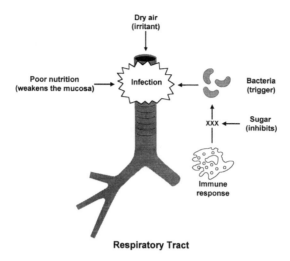

Figure 3-1 *The Manifestation of Disease*

The Manifestation of Disease

The actual disease a person manifests is determined by the balance between his or her genetic susceptibility, lifestyle, nutritional status, toxic influences, and any previous damage or abnormality. For example, at the beginning of winter, many people develop upper respiratory tract infections. Why then, why there, and why do some escape? As can be seen in Figure 3-1, a respiratory infection develops only after four factors are in place: (1) heating buildings in the winter produces dry air that irritates the mucous membranes of the respiratory tract; (2) deficiencies of vitamins A and C (crucial for production of the mucous, which protects the membranes from irritants) allows the dry air to damage the respiratory tract; (3) consumption of excess sugar suppresses the white cells' ability to fight bacteria; (4) leaving the system vulnerable to pathogenic bacteria.

The signs and symptoms of the above syndromes are fairly easy to understand, and most of the causes can be recognized and taken care of. The process is often complicated by the unfortunate fact that most of us suffer from more than one imbalance, and some of the signs and symptoms overlap. Clearing one underlying syndrome may therefore reveal another, which must then be resolved.

It is relatively easy to utilize drugs (and sometimes herbs and nutrients) to clear up the symptoms of disease, but as long as the underlying imbalances or impairments to healing continue, ill health will simply resurface again and again as either the same disease or as another disease that shares the same underlying syndrome(s). A far more effective approach, and the only one that will control health care costs and lead to improved health, is to recognize and control the underlying syndromes. Rather than focus on the disease, we need instead to focus on the individual and what is needed to improve his or her health, through dietary and lifestyle changes and the use of supplemental health-supporting nutrients and herbs that take into account our own unique biochemistry.

Many diseases have multiple causes. This highlights another reason why our current disease orientation is ineffective; it leads to the belief that each disease is an isolated problem rather than the end result of multiple insults to the body.

Finally, for a disease to actually manifest, there needs to be not only susceptibility but also a trigger. For example, in the case of an infection, the trigger (a bacteria or virus) is easy to recognize. But while removal of the trigger (e.g., with antibiotics) is easy (and the basis of our current disease-treatment system), resolving the susceptibility, i.e., improving the weakened immune system, is far more important and virtually always ignored.

The Routes to Total Wellness

Seven underlying, health-sustaining systems of our body must function effectively to ensure our well-being, prevent disease, and allow a full life: the immune system, the detoxification system, the inflammatory system, the metabolic system, the regulatory system, the regeneration system, and our life-force (or spirit). Weakness in any of these seven systems results in susceptibilities that allow most common diseases to develop. Follow the recommendations below, strengthen all of these seven systems, and total wellness is yours.

Strengthen the Immune System

Pathogenic bacteria are always on our skins and in our throats and intestines. We are exposed to new pathogens every time we contact others, eat, or breathe, and every day, our bodies produce about 300 cancer cells (more if we are exposed to carcinogens). The healthy immune system quickly and effectively recognizes and destroys invaders (viruses, bacteria, fungi) and abnormal cells (cancer). When the immune system is not working well, however, the result is frequent or chronic infections, chronic fatigue, and, eventually, cancer. Optimal immune function can be attained by recognizing and eliminating those factors that damage the immune system and by strengthening it with specific nutrients and herbs. If an infection does become established, many natural therapies are available to help fight the infection. Chapter Four discusses the immune system in detail.

Decrease Toxicity

Not only are we exposed to a large amount and wide variety of pollutants in our environment (especially in cities), but our regular metabolic processes produce toxic metabolites as well. Normally, the liver and other detoxification processes efficiently neutralize and remove these poisons before they can cause damage.

However, excessive exposure, incomplete metabolism, and a dysfunctional detoxification system result in toxicity. When toxic, our bodies build up inappropriate or excessive levels of chemical poisons or incompletely processed metabolites, microbial toxins, heavy metals, and other adverse influences (e.g., electromagnetic radiation, radon, and so on) in cells, tissues, and fluids. The build-up of such toxins manifests as toxic headaches, chemical sensitivity, chronic fatigue syndrome, and acne, and contributes to most chronic diseases. Lifestyle changes, special detoxification diets, hydrotherapy, and other detoxification procedures combined with herbs that strengthen the liver will progressively eliminate the toxic burden. In addition, some nutrients directly neutralize toxins before they can cause harm. Chapter Five explores toxicity in depth.

Normalize Inflammatory Function

Inflammation is a crucial part of the process by which the body removes damaged cells and tissues and begins the repair process. In addition, inflammation is used by the immune system to attack pathogens and cancer cells. For most Americans this system is out of balance with a tendency to an excessive inflammatory reaction to damage whether that damage is physical, immunological, or chemical. This can be due to overly sensitive inflammatory mechanisms, inadequate inflammatory controls, or excessive inflammatory stimulation. Problems with the inflammatory response commonly manifest as allergies and chronic inflammatory diseases such as arthritis and eczema. Dietary changes and key nutrients will normalize the inflammatory response. In addition, once an inflammatory process is well-established, several herbs can be used to quell the inflammation and help the body restore normal balance (see Chapter Six).

Optimize Metabolic Function

All the metabolic processes of the body are run by enzyme systems that are determined by our genes. Enzymes require micronutrients (vitamins and minerals) to function. Maldigestion, malnutrition, and weak enzymes all contribute to the other imbalances and directly cause many chronic diseases. Maldigestion can manifest as bad breath, foul-smelling stools, diarrhea, constipation, and food intolerance. Common metabolic diseases include asthma, diabetes, atherosclerosis, and eczema. Enzyme and herbal aids can improve digestion, and high dosages of specific nutrients will improve the function of enzymes that are weak due to genetics. These treatments are discussed extensively in Chapter Seven.

Balance Your Regulatory Systems

Our hormonal systems maintain a delicate metabolic balance throughout the body. Both under- and over-activity of any of the hormonal systems cause widespread dysfunction. Hypothyroidism, hypogonadism, and hypoadrenalism manifest as chronic tiredness, obesity, loss of sex drive, excessive muscle wasting, and so on. Even a normal process such as menopause can cause unpleasant symptoms. Special foods, nutrients, herbs, and hormone precursors can be used to reestablish balance, which is the topic of Chapter Eight.

Enhance Regeneration

Almost from birth, our bodies are replacing cells and tissues as they wear out. However, when damage is excessive, or the normal repair and regeneration processes are impaired, degeneration results. Imbalance between "wear and tear" and the ability of the body to repair and regenerate manifests in such diseases as receding gums, osteoarthritis, chronic fatigue, depression, and premature aging. Anti-aging nutrients, improving blood supply to the heart and brain, and herbal regenerators all help slow, and in some cases, reverse the aging process. In addition, some herbs (called adaptogens), through mechanisms we do not yet understand, appear to strengthen virtually all of our functions and increase our ability to maintain health through stress and environmental challenges. Chapter Nine explains in detail how to enhance regeneration.

Live in Harmony with Your Life-Force

Our beliefs, spiritual values, and family life have a profound impact on our health. Our society has trained us to suppress many mind/body signals. Emotional imbalances, stress, unhealthy beliefs, lack of meaning in life, and dysfunctional family life fundamentally impair our body's healing mechanisms, significantly decrease the quality of our life and the lives of our loved ones, and contribute to chronic disease. Each of us needs to become more aware of the activity of the *vis medicatrix naturae* (life-force) deep within us. There are many aids to developing this awareness. Chapter Ten reviews those with the strongest historic and research support, a surprising amount of which documents the powerful impact of prayer, meditation, beliefs, and family and friends on health.

Conclusion

Each of us is our own best physician, we just need to learn how. By understanding how our own body works and how to listen to our symptoms, we can fundamentally improve our health. When disease does occur, we can use self help and natural therapies to reestablish our health. By taking personal control over our own health, we can utilize licensed health care practitioners as resources rather than giving them complete control over our bodies.

The goal of improving all of our health-maintaining pathways is to improve our resilience, making us able to both improve our health and increase our ability to function well in our increasingly stressful environment.

The two bodily systems of the utmost importance are the immune and detoxification systems. Maintaining an active, even aggressive, immune system and ensuring that toxins are eliminated from our bodies as efficiently and quickly as possible are discussed in the two largest and most detailed chapters and should be studied first.

Finally, please be patient. Real change, as opposed to alleviating symptoms, takes time. We are not talking here about eliminating symptoms as quickly as possible. We are talking about changing the fundamental course of your health, about establishing total wellness. This will take time and perseverance. Once a system gets way out of balance, reestablishing full function requires careful and rigorous control initially. Once full function is established, maintenance is much easier.

Chapter Four

Strengthen Your Immune System

You need to study this chapter if you suffer from any of the following:
- Current acute infection, e.g., common cold, flu
- History of frequent acute infections, e.g., frequent ear infections in children, frequent colds in adults
- Chronic infections, e.g., candidiasis (candida infection), parasites, fungal skin infections (e.g., athlete's foot, fungal nail infection)
- Persistent chronic viral activity, e.g., cytomegalovirus, Epstein-Barr virus, rhinovirus (cold viruses), herpes, warts
- Slow wound healing
- Unexplained fatigue
- Cancer, or a strong family history of cancer

Behaviors that increase risk:
- Excessive sugar consumption
- Eating foods to which you are allergic
- Alcohol (drinking enough to cause intoxication)
- Diet deficient in vitamins A or C (fruits and vegetables), or the mineral zinc (lamb, beef, and eggs)
- Excessive stress
- Severe trauma, such as from surgery or an accident
- Frequent exposure to infectious agents, e.g., working in a daycare center

Thumbnail: Quick Help for Your Immune System
- *To strengthen the immune response:*
  Vitamin A: 50,000 iu per day for one week
  Beta-carotene: 50 mg per day for one week

Vitamin C: 1,000 mg every three hours
Echinacea angustifolia (*Echinacea*): 1 tsp fluid extract four times a day
Lentinus edodes (shiitake mushroom): 2 (500 mg each) capsules four
   times a day

- *To treat specific infections:*
  Bacterial infections
     Hydrastis canadensis (goldenseal root): 4 (500 mg each) capsules four
        times a day
  Viral infections
     Glycyrrhiza glabra (licorice root): 3 (500 mg each) capsules four
        times a day
  Fungal infections
     Melaleuca alternafolia (tea tree oil): apply locally (dilute with sesame
        oil if sensitive)

All of these dosages are for adults. For children, modify the dose according to weight.

Are you dragged down by constant fatigue, frequent colds, flus, or infections? While the symptoms vary from person to person, as the following stories show, the underlying cause is the same: an overworked, improperly nourished immune system. This chapter shows you how to identify the source of your problems and design a program to rebuild your immune system to knock these infections out.

Real-Life Messages from the Immune System

Chronic Ear Infections

Maryann brought in her three-year-old daughter Emily for help with her chronic ear infections. Emily's story was like that of so many young children I've seen. Every six to eight weeks, Emily would develop a cold, usually after being exposed to a sick child at daycare. Almost every time, the cold would progress to an ear infection. After eight ear infections in 18 months, and 11 treatments with antibiotics, Emily's pediatrician, fearing her hearing would be permanently impaired, had recommended myringotomy—a surgical procedure that cuts a small hole in the eardrum and inserts tubes to allow drainage. Her mother wanted a less radical solution. While the standard treatments of antibiotics and myringotomy speed recovery from the acute infections, they don't decrease the frequency of recurrence of children's ear infections.[1] In fact, some research even suggests that antibiotics actually increase the frequency of children's ear infections![2] Ear infections in children are extremely common—we spend $3 billion each year in the U.S. (and perform 1 million myringotomies) on children's recurrent ear infections using therapies that don't deal with the underlying cause of the problem. Clearly our children would benefit from a better solution.

Looking at Emily, I saw a pudgy child with dark circles under her eyes, a runny nose, and red eyes. Her ears were normal when I examined her, but I knew this would only be temporary unless we made some major changes. Emily ate a standard American diet (what has been appropriately termed the SAD diet): high in sugar and fat; low in fresh fruits, vegetables, and whole grains; low in vitamins and minerals; and limited to a few favorite foods day in and day out. Unfortunately, the situation was further aggravated by Maryann's habit of giving Emily ice cream whenever she was sick because she couldn't bear to see her daughter so miserable.

Emily's real problem was not the bacteria that kept growing in her ears. It was that her normal mechanisms for resisting infection and maintaining proper ear function were overwhelmed. Her immune system was being weakened by a diet of foods containing too much sugar and too little of the vitamins A and C, and the mineral zinc.

In addition, Emily was allergic to dairy products (dark circles under the eyes and a chronic runny nose almost always indicate food allergies, with dairy products being the most common culprit). Although Emily was breast fed for four months, by two months of age she had also been given cow's milk. A child's immature digestive system cannot tolerate cow's milk for the first six months to a year, so she became allergic to it. Unfortunately, only 11% of women nurse exclusively for the six months needed to give a baby's digestive system time to mature. Emily's milk allergy was causing her Eustachian tubes (the little tubes that connect the ear to the throat—what you pop when changing elevation in an airplane) to swell closed. This blocked the ear's normal drainage route and turned her ear canal into a breeding ground for bacteria. Emily's allergic reaction to dairy products also directly inhibited the proper function of her immune system.

The treatment I prescribed for her was simple. She was to stop eating all dairy products, limit sugar intake, eat foods rich in vitamins C and A, and, for a short while, take supplements of vitamins A (10,000 iu per day) and C (1,000 mg per day) and zinc (15 mg per day). Her results were excellent. She had only one more ear infection (which we treated with the herbs *Echinacea* and goldenseal, along with hot packs on her ear), her colds dropped to one or two a year. After four months, the dark circles under her eyes cleared, and her weight normalized for her height. The key here is that not only was Emily's immediate disease treated, but because the underlying causes were addressed, further ear infections were prevented and, most important, Emily became significantly healthier.

- *The message:* Too much sugar and/or eating foods to which you are allergic suppress the immune system. Vitamins A and C, the mineral zinc, and the herbs *Echinacea* and goldenseal are very helpful for strengthening the immune system.

AIDS

Gerald was infected with the HIV virus. He was very anxious because his disease was progressing unusually rapidly. Over the past year, he had become infected with genital herpes, suffered from viral hepatitis, and had been treated with penicillin for syphilis. While he had not yet progressed to full-blown AIDS, his helper T cell counts were dropping rapidly. When questioned, he revealed a highly self-destructive lifestyle: heavy recreational drug use, multiple unprotected sexual encounters, high stress (he would go for days without sleep, using stimulants to keep awake), and a poor diet (while the foods he ate were generally healthful, he would alternate a few days of fasting with periods of gorging). One of the unfortunate aspects of the HIV virus is that it grows more rapidly when the immune system is activated by infections.

While no cure is yet known for this serious disease, several natural medicine therapies help slow its progression. I helped Gerald establish a healthier lifestyle (especially to get regular rest because the immune system regenerates during sleep), used herbs (such as licorice root) that inhibit the growth of the virus, and special nutrients (such as N-acetyl-L-cysteine) to help protect his white cells from the damage caused by the HIV virus. His rate of loss of T cells decreased, he had far fewer infections, and he felt considerably healthier. As important as the natural medicine therapies were, I believe we achieved our greatest success simply helping him learn how to avoid excessive exposure to infectious agents and to get adequate rest.

- *The message:* Excessive infectious exposure and inadequate rest overtax the immune system.

Asymptomatic Infection

I have an interesting personal story of immune suppression. Several years ago I began to develop large warts on several of my fingers. Warts are an interesting phenomenon; they tend to grow or recede according to how well the immune system is functioning. Although I treated them several times with thuja oil (a standard naturopathic treatment for warts), they had not responded very well. I was perplexed because I was living a pretty healthful lifestyle and using a therapy I'd used successfully for a lot of patients.

Then I visited the dentist. As I've only had one cavity, I hadn't been to the dentist for several years. Surprisingly, X-rays revealed an abscess in that one tooth—the filling had not been sealed properly. A week of antibiotics cleared the infection, and within three months all my warts were gone. Even though I had had no other symptoms, the abscess was continually draining my immune system.

- *The message:* Asymptomatic chronic infections can even deplete the immune system of a healthy person.

Chronic Fungal Infection

Richard came to see us at the Bastyr University teaching clinic for a very uncomfortable condition: Ever since a tour of duty in Vietnam, he had suffered from a fungal infection on his genitals. He had gone to numerous medical doctors, each prescribing the latest anti-fungal drug. Yet the inflammation, itching, oozing, and embarrassment continued.

Examination revealed that this poor man had a moist, red rash beginning almost at mid-thigh and extending up almost to his waist. We realized a most aggressive approach would be needed to help him overcome this well-established infection. We prescribed for him large amounts of the herb *Echinacea* and shiitake mushroom to provide a strong boost to his depleted immune system. In addition, we had him apply tea tree oil, the most effective anti-fungal herb, to the infected area. This combination worked well, and within a few months his decades-old infection totally cleared. As might be expected, he was very pleased with our help!

- *The message:* When properly used, herbal medicines can be effective in treating even infections that don't respond to conventional medical treatments.

Introduction to the Immune System

For many, especially children whose immune systems are still maturing, the most troublesome symptoms typically experienced are due to an overworked, undernourished immune system. A nutrient-poor diet, excessive exposure to infectious agents, immune-damaging toxins in the environment, the emergence of new viruses and antibiotic-resistant bacteria—all add up to a significant, continuous challenge to our immune systems.

Establishing and maintaining an effective immune system has never been more important. With the increasing levels of carcinogens in our environment, our bodies' demand for effective immune elimination of newly formed cancer cells is at an all-time high, and, based on the increasing incidence of cancer, more and more of us are failing to meet the challenge.

Another 20th century problem is the growing number of bacteria that have become resistant or immune to the available antibiotics. The majority of infections acquired in hospitals are due to these strains, which have developed immunity to most common antibiotics. For example, it is increasingly difficult to find antibiotics effective for treating pneumococcal infections of the ear and respiratory tract, staphylococcal infections of the skin, and gonococcal infections of the genitals.[3] Even tuberculosis, once thought to be under control, is again becoming difficult to overcome. Overuse of prescribed antibiotics plus the use of antibiotics in livestock (which are passed up the food chain to humans when the meat is eaten) appear to be the primary causes of this growing problem. Previously controlled infectious diseases are experiencing a global resurgence. Increased stress resulting from environmental changes and pollution is thought to be one reason for the increasing reappearance of cholera and the newly recognized hantavirus.[4]

One of the most disturbing pieces of research I've ever read dramatizes the crucial importance of maintaining a well-functioning immune system and optimal nutritional status. The research involved the coxsackievirus, a type of virus that infects people through the intestines, usually during the summer. It infects more than 20 million people every year in the U.S. Most coxsackievirus infections are readily handled by the immune system; many of the viruses are so weak they are considered "benign." However, 10,000 of those infected become ill, some of them seriously as the virus attacks their heart.

Researchers have known for several decades that people deficient in selenium tend to develop Keshan disease, an inflammatory heart disease. Other researchers have found that these patients are also infected with coxsackievirus. The researchers wondered if there was a link between coxsackievirus-induced heart damage and insufficient intake of the mineral selenium. They tested this by feeding mice a diet low in selenium and then infecting them with a weak strain of coxsackievirus known to be easily eliminated by the normal mouse immune system. The mice with a selenium-deficient diet developed heart damage from this supposedly benign organism. Even more disturbing, the researchers found that when they extracted the virus from the infected mice and then injected it into selenium-normal mice, these previously benign viruses now caused disease even in the normal mice! Careful research revealed that the virus was able to mutate in the selenium-deficient mice and, after six mutations, became pathogenic (capable of causing disease).[5] *This shows that poor nutrition allows normally benign microorganisms to not only become damaging to their host but to become capable of causing disease even in those who are healthy.*

This research raises a disturbing question: Are we, through unhealthful lifestyles and poor nutrition, encouraging the growth of more and progressively stronger disease-producing organisms? The researchers who conducted these studies believe the results have global implications, and state that their findings: "Help explain the steady emergence of new strains of influenza virus in China, which has widespread selenium-deficient areas . . . and might even help to explain the crossing over of certain viruses [such as HIV] to a new host species. It is alarming to note that HIV apparently first infected monkeys and then moved to humans living in selenium-poor regions of Africa."[6]

As HIV, the virus that causes AIDS, most vividly demonstrates, an effective immune system is essential to survival. This chapter explains how the immune system works, how to determine when it's not working, what damages the immune system, and how to help it work—optimally.

How the Immune System Works

The immune system is like the defensive backfield of a football team: It keeps invaders from scoring (infecting you) when they get past the defensive line—

the skin and mucous membranes. This defensive team also protects the body from fumbles, i.e., cells in our bodies that become cancerous. One of the most complex systems of the human body, the immune system has special cells in the blood called white cells, unique proteins in the blood called antibodies, chemicals that activate immune reactions, and special organs that, like special team coaches, supervise, replenish, and integrate the whole immune process. It even has its own complex of vessels called the lymphatic system.

Disease-producing microorganisms (pathogens) are always present in our environment. They are in the air we breathe, the food and water we drink, and on most of the surfaces we touch. In fact, if our skin, throat, or other mucous membranes were cultured, many of us would be found to contain pathogens. For example, 5 to 40% of us have pneumococcus bacteria in our nose and throat, yet we rarely develop pneumonia because our immune system keeps these pathogens under control.[7]

When a foreign invader enters the body or a cell becomes cancerous, the immune system handles it with two types of defenses: non-specific and specific defenses.

Non-specific defenses, called cell-mediated immunity, are our first strike forces. Cell-mediated immunity involves special white cells (typically T cell lymphocytes and neutrophils), which immediately attack the invader and either prevent its entry into the body, or if the invader manages to gain a foothold, quickly destroy it. Cell-mediated immunity is especially important to the body's ability to resist infection by yeasts (such as *Candida albicans*), fungi (such as athlete's foot), parasites (worms), and viruses (such as *Herpes simplex* and Epstein-Barr). Cell-mediated immunity is also critical in protecting against the development of cancer and is commonly involved in allergic reactions.

Specific defenses (humoral immunity) involve sensitized white cells and antibodies. These special proteins are the invaders' deadly dopplegangers. Formed to uniquely match the surface of invaders, the humoral immunity team either damages them directly (sometimes by making them clump together) or alerts other white cells to come help. Although powerful, since these sensitized white cells and antibodies are tailored to suit a specific invader, they take several days to develop.

The Body's Response to a Typical Infection

The components of the immune system are defined thoroughly below, but the following brief overview should help you get your bearings. Figure 4-1 shows the stages of the body's response to the typical infection. The first line of defense (1) is the surfaces of the body, which work to prevent pathogens from entering. This line of defense is composed of three parts: mucus, antibodies, and the cells themselves. Mucus is a sticky substance secreted by the cells of the mucous membranes. It traps the pathogens and moves them off the membranes, e.g., out the nose or into the intestines where they are destroyed

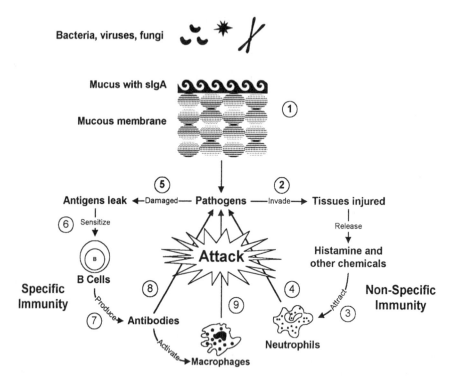

Figure 4-1 The Body's Response to a Typical Infection

by stomach acid. Mixed with the mucus is an antibody called secretory immunoglobulin A (sIgA). sIgA binds to the pathogens, blocking their penetration of the mucous membranes. Finally, the mucous membrane cells themselves form a mechanical barrier to the invader. Over-the-counter drugs that stop your runny nose may provide some symptomatic relief but, by suppressing mucus formation, they hinder rather than help your immune system to eliminate the cold-causing pathogens. The end result? A cold that lasts even longer.

Once a pathogen gets past the surface defenses, it invades (2) the tissues where it injures the cells (basically using them for food) and proliferates. When this happens, the cells secrete a wide range of special chemicals, such as histamine, which alert the immune system (3) that the body is under attack and increase blood supply to the area (which is why it gets hot). Now, the non-specific immune response—the cell-mediated defense team—is activated. Various classes of white cells, especially the neutrophils, migrate to the area (4) and attack the invaders. As the pathogen is damaged (5) by the white cells, parts of the pathogen (such as proteins and cell-wall components) leak out of the cell.

These foreign parts (antigens) activate the specific immune response—the humoral defense team. The antigens (6) come in contact with special white cells called B lymphocytes, which then produce (7) specific antibodies that are doppelgangers to the invader. These antibodies directly attack (8) the invaders and make them more recognizable by the powerful macrophages, which also attack (9) the invading pathogens.

As the figure shows, this is a complex, yet effective team effort. Unfortunately, your immune teams are very susceptible to damage and extremely dependent on adequate nutrition.

When Your Immune System Isn't Working Adequately

Do you seem to get every cold or flu that comes along? Do your children get sick every fall when they start a new school year or go to daycare? Do you have a chronic infection that keeps coming back even though it goes away when you use antibiotics? These and other common signs of a poorly functioning immune system are listed in Table 4-1.

Current symptoms and disease history are quite effective for recognizing immune deficiency. Basically, if you frequently get infections, have persistent low level infections, or suffer from cancer, your immune system isn't doing its job. While objective evaluation of how well the immune system is working would be quite useful, few such tests are available. The laboratory tests that most doctors use measure only such aspects as the number and types of white cells. This is only useful in severe immune failure and doesn't measure immune function, i.e., how well the immune system is fighting infections. Therefore, I rely primarily on clinical symptoms.

One test that I wish were more available is the phagocytic index. This useful test evaluates how effectively the non-specific defense system is working. This procedure measures how rapidly phagocytes ingest foreign materials (in

Table 4-1 Signs of a Dysfunctional Immune System

Current acute infection, e.g., common cold, flu, ear infection, sinus infection

History of frequent acute infections, e.g., frequent ear infections in children, frequent colds in adults

Chronic infections, e.g., candidiasis (candida infection), parasites, fungal skin infections (e.g., athlete's foot, fungal nail infection)

Persistent chronic viral activity, e.g., cytomegalovirus, Epstein-Barr virus, rhinovirus (cold viruses), herpes, warts

Slow wound healing

Unexplained fatigue

Cancer, or a strong family history of cancer

the test they use latex particles). The phagocytic index is particularly helpful in evaluating the body's day-to-day resistance to infection, because these white cells are our first line of defense against infections. (This test is used to measure the effects of sugar on the immune system, discussed below.)

How the Immune System Can Be Damaged

Unfortunately, many factors in our modern lifestyle damage the immune system. Table 4-2 lists, in the approximate order of importance, the common factors that cripple the immune system and notes the ways in which they do their dirty work. Most of us will recognize several of these in our lives. Figure 4-2 diagrams the effects of these factors.

Sugar

Consumption of simple carbohydrates, i.e., sugars, seriously inhibits immune function. The ingestion of 100 grams (3 ounces) of sugar at one sitting significantly

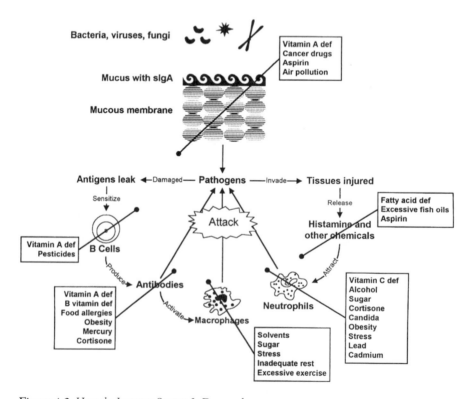

Figure 4-2 How the Immune System Is Damaged

Table 4-2 Common Causes of Immune Dysfunction

Cause	How It Affects the Immune System
Sugar and other concentrated carbohydrates	Three ounces of sugar in any form (sucrose, honey, fruit juice) results in a 50% reduction in white cell activity for one to five hours
Food allergy	Uses up immune defenses on food particles rather than invading microbes; damages intestines, allowing immune-damaging toxins to enter the body
Obesity	Decreases bacteria killing activity of white cells and production of antibodies
Alcohol sufficient to cause intoxication	Depresses white cell mobilization; significantly inhibits neutrophils
Nutritional deficiency (especially of folic acid, pantothenic acid, pyridoxine, riboflavin, vitamins A, B_{12}, C, copper, zinc)	Decreases function of all aspects of immune system
Heavy metals (cadmium, lead, mercury)	Inhibit the formation of antibodies and reduce the bacteria-killing ability of white cells
Pesticides	Depress T and B lymphocytes; cause aging of thymus
Drugs, e.g., aspirin, acetaminophen, ibuprofen, and corticosteroids	Decrease antibody production; broad immune suppression
Toxic chemicals, e.g., silicone implants, organic solvents	Decrease natural killer cell activity
Excessive exercise	Uses up immune defenses on increased free radicals generated
Stress	Directly inhibits many aspects of immune function
Inadequate rest	Suppresses natural killer cell activity
Frequent exposure to infectious agents	Overloads the immune system
Bowel candida overgrowth	Immune complexes formed by the yeast are directly immunosuppressive
Excessive fish oil supplementation	Reduces neutrophil movement to the site of inflammation
Air pollution (sulfur oxides, nitrogen oxides, ozone), dry air in heated buildings	Damages protective mucous membranes
Vaccinations	Cause a one to two week suppression of the immune response
Excessive stress and premature aging	Damage thymus resulting in decreased T-cell production and activation
Severe trauma, e.g., accident, major surgery	Inflammatory response overloads immune system
Chronic antibiotic use	General immune impairment; increases overgrowth of candida; makes bacteria stronger and more resistant to immune system
Perimenopausal hormone imbalances	Suppress immune response to invading pathogens

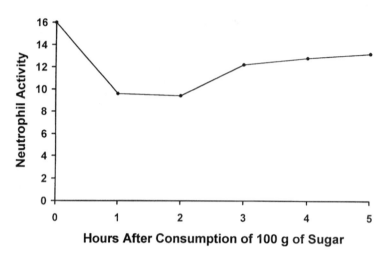

Figure 4-3 *Sugar's Inhibition of White Cell Phagocytic Activity*

reduces the ability of neutrophils to engulf and destroy bacteria (see Figure 4-3). Unfortunately, this applies to all forms of sugar, not just sucrose (table sugar). That is, glucose, fructose, sucrose (table sugar), honey, and even three glassfuls of orange juice all depress the immune system. In contrast, the ingestion of 100 grams of starch (a complex carbohydrate) has no effect on immune function. The suppressive effect of sugar consumption starts less than 30 minutes after ingestion and lasts for over five hours. Typically, at least a 40% reduction in neutrophil activity occurs two hours after ingestion. Since neutrophils constitute 60 to 70% of the total circulating white blood cells, shutting down their activity can seriously impair the immune system.[8,9] Even ingestion of only 75 grams (a bit over 2 ounces) of glucose has been shown to depress lymphocyte activity.[10]

The average American consumes a surprising 150 grams of sucrose every day. This does not include other refined simple sugars, such as fruit juice and honey. Given this data, it seems likely that most Americans are chronically suppressing their immune system with sugar.

Food Sensitivity or Allergy

A large amount of research has documented the association between food allergy and chronic infections (discussed thoroughly in Chapter Five). I consider allergic reactions to foods to be one of the most important (and generally unrecognized) immune-suppressing problems facing us today. When a person eats a food to which he or she is allergic, the immune system reacts as if it has been attacked by a foreign invader. This results in white cells being activated and migrating to the mucous membranes and the cells lining the intestines. If immune-stimulating foods are eaten frequently, the immune system's resources are continually focused on the intestines. Viruses, bacteria, fungi, and cancer cells elsewhere in the body have a great opportunity to invade and grow unchecked.

A few decades ago, a very interesting test was developed by Drs. Rinkle and Dickey.[11] After observing that patients with food allergies tended to have low white blood cell counts, they developed a test (the leukopenic index) to determine if a patient was allergic to a food by measuring the white cell count after the patient ate the food. The basic procedure was to have a patient avoid the suspected food for four days. Then, after eating the suspected food, a sample of the patient's blood was taken every fifteen minutes and the number of white cells counted. They found dramatic drops in the white count—to as little as 50% below normal! Although this interesting procedure lost favor because it is expensive, time-consuming, and inconvenient, it effectively demonstrated the harm food allergies can wreak on the immune system.

Not only does the white cell count drop as the white cells migrate to the intestines, but they are also destroyed by coming in contact with the food allergen. This destruction formed the basis of another test for food allergies, the "cytotoxic test." It tests for food sensitivity and allergy by mixing some of a person's white cells with the extracts of suspected foods. The technician then looks at the white cells under a microscope. The white cells sensitized to specific foods are destroyed by the digestive enzymes released when the white cells engulf the extracts of those foods. Highly sensitized white cells can have such powerful reactions to the allergens that even the red cells in the mixture are destroyed. Imagine what's happening in your body when you eat a food to which you are allergic!

When the white cells die, they spew digestive enzymes into the surrounding tissues, damaging them. Thus, eating allergic foods causes serious injury to the intestinal lining, which makes it leak (see Leaky Bowel Syndrome in Chapter Five). This, in turn, allows toxins from the intestines to enter the body. Several of these, such as those from yeasts in the intestine, are especially immunosuppressive.

All these destructive impacts on the immune system explain why controlling food allergies is so critical for helping with chronic infections. For example, in a recent study of 104 children with chronic ear infections, 81 were found to have food allergies, typically to milk and wheat. The ear problems were resolved when the offending foods were removed from their diet and returned when the foods were reintroduced.[12]

Alcohol

Alcoholics are known to be more susceptible to pneumonia and other infections. In fact, infectious diseases are the major causes of disease and death among alcoholics. Studies of neutrophils show a profound decrease after alcohol ingestion, even in nutritionally normal people.

Alcohol also increases the susceptibility to infections in animals. For example, in experiments with rats, chronic ethanol ingestion significantly increased the susceptibility of rats to fatal pneumococcal pneumonia by impairing the defense mechanism of neutrophils recruited to protect their infected lungs. Researchers taking white cells from the lungs of alcohol-fed rats found that three of ten totally lost their bactericidal activity against the pneumonia bacteria.[13]

Nutritional Deficiencies

Nutrition plays an integral role in immune function and thus a deficiency of virtually any nutrient can result in immune dysfunction. Unfortunately, deficiencies of the key nutrients needed by the immune system are common. Table 4-3 lists the typical signs and symptoms (in addition to frequent or chronic infections) when a nutrient is low and the foods which have high levels of these nutrients. In general, if your diet is low in the foods with high levels of a specific nutrient (or the foods are highly cooked or stored for long periods of time), you are likely to be deficient in that nutrient.

Vitamin A

Vitamin A plays several essential roles in protecting us from infections. First, it is required for maintaining the integrity of the epithelial and mucosal surfaces and their secretions. These systems constitute our first line of defense against infection. Second, vitamin A is necessary for the production and activity of several types of white cells. Deficiency can result in atrophy of the lymph glands, a decreased number of lymphocytes, and reduced B and T cell functioning.[14]

Vitamin A deficiency is very common in developing countries. For example, in Indonesia, 236 children who received the diphtheria-pertussis-tetanus vaccination were evaluated after they received either 60,000 mcg of vitamin A or placebo. It was found that both the vitamin-A deficient and the supposedly vitamin-A adequate (healthy) children who received the vitamin A supplement showed significantly greater antibody response to the vaccine than the children who received the placebo.[15] So much evidence now supports the importance of adequate levels of vitamin A for proper immune response that the World Health Organization's expanded Program for Immunization recommends that children in vitamin A-deficient communities be given vitamin A at the time of immunization.

Unfortunately, vitamin A deficiency is not unusual in the U.S. either, especially in children with significant infections. For example, in one study, when 180 children with rubeola (hard measles) were tested for vitamin A levels, 91% were found to have levels far below normal. Supplementation with 200,000 iu per day for two consecutive days resulted in an 87% decrease in death rate in the children under two years of age.[16] In another study of 123 children, those with low serum levels of vitamin A had significantly decreased

Table 4-3 Typical Signs of Specific Nutrient Deficiencies

Nutrient	Typical Signs and Symptoms When Deficient	Good Dietary Sources
Vitamin A	Night blindness, dry hair, fatigue, poor growth, insomnia, acne, poor nails, skin thickening (hyperkeratosis), lack of response to vaccinations	Liver, Cod liver oil, carrots, mint, kohlrabi, parsley, spinach, turnip greens
Vitamin B complex	Depression, dark red tongue, nervousness and irritability, poor memory, insomnia, fatigue, tongue and mouth lesions, poor wound healing	Liver, yeast, whole grains, avocados, blackstrap molasses, raw nuts and seeds, wheat germ
Vitamin C	Easy bruisability, bleeding gums, receding gums, loose teeth, depression, irritability, joint pain, tiredness, poor wound healing	Broccoli, brussels sprouts, kale, peppers, turnip greens, currants, guava, beet greens, cabbage, kohlrabi, watercress, spinach, lemons, oranges, papayas, strawberries
Vitamin E	Premature aging, excessive skin wrinkling, muscle weakness, loss of sensory function (especially sense of vibration)	Wheat germ, raw nuts and seeds, alfalfa, yeast, cabbage, spinach, asparagus
Essential fatty acids	Dry skin, acne, hair loss, chronic diarrhea, dry hair, gallstones, poor wound healing	Fresh nut and seed oils, cold water fish
Selenium	Premature aging, poor growth, high cholesterol levels, male sterility	Brazil nuts, seafood, liver, eggs
Zinc	Loss of sense of smell or taste, poor night vision, acne, poor wound healing, brittle nails, hair loss, depression, irritability, poor memory, impotence, infertility, white spots on nails, eczema	Oysters, whole grains, nuts, liver, leafy vegetables

T cell counts. Administration of vitamin A restored their T cell counts to normal.[17] Not only does vitamin A deficiency decrease the number of T cells, it also decreases T cells' ability to respond to pathogens.[18] Severe deficiency also leads to atrophy of the thymus and spleen and a marked decrease in the number of all white cells in the blood.[19]

In a recent study in New York City, vitamin A levels were evaluated in 89 children younger than two years of age with measles. In 22%, they were found to be low. Children with low levels were more likely to have fevers of 40° C or higher (68% versus 44%), to have fever for seven days or more (54% versus 23%), and to be hospitalized (55% versus 30%). Children with low vitamin A levels also had lower measles-specific antibody levels. No child in the control group of children without measles had low vitamin A levels.[20]

Worldwide, 1.5 million children die of measles each year. The children with the severest forms of measles have the lowest serum levels of vitamin A.[21] Even children from communities that are not normally deficient in vitamins are still at high risk of low vitamin A levels during infection with measles. Providing as little as a single large dose (400,000 iu) of vitamin A has resulted in a remarkable reduction in morbidity and mortality in children infected with measles. Regular vitamin A supplementation of children hospitalized with measles in Capetown, Africa resulted in reductions in hospital stay, intensive care admissions, and death rates.

Research shows that not only are children with low vitamin A levels more likely to get measles, they also get a worse case and suffer an increased rate of side effects and death. Supplementation with even modest amounts of this cheap nutrient results in a very significant improvement in immune function.

Vitamin C

Many claims, especially by two-time Nobel Laureate Linus Pauling, have been made about the role of vitamin C in supporting and enhancing the immune system. However, despite numerous positive clinical and experimental studies, this effect is still hotly debated in the medical community. Considerable evidence shows that vitamin C plays a vital role in many immunological mechanisms. Its high concentration in white blood cells (10 to 80 times greater than plasma levels), particularly lymphocytes, is rapidly expended during infection, and a local scurvy-like condition may ensue if vitamin C is not regularly replenished. Vitamin C is used in protecting the white cells from the enzymes they release to digest the ingested microbes.

When animals get an infection, their blood, urine, and tissue levels of vitamin C drop dramatically as their vitamin C goes to the site of the infection for use by white cells. Most animals then begin to rapidly synthesize in their livers large amounts of vitamin C to restore normal levels. Unfortunately, humans (along with pigs and some monkeys) lack a key enzyme for the production of vitamin C. Unless large amounts of vitamin C are in our diet, every time we get an infection, a deficiency develops. Even using the recommended daily allowance (RDA—a better choice would be the Optimal Nutritional Allowances as defined in Chapter Seven), most of us consume inadequate amounts of vitamin C. Not surprisingly then, supplementation with vitamin C helps us fight many infections.

Vitamin C deficiency seriously impairs white cell function and cellular immunity (the non-specific defense system), and limits the normal local inflammatory response necessary to activate humoral immunity (the specific defense system).[18] When levels are adequate, vitamin C stimulates the movement of phagocytic white cells, particularly neutrophils, to the site of inflammation, and also enhances the transformation of lymphocytes into T cells, B cells, and natural killer cells. An antioxidant, vitamin C protects white cells against free radicals and other toxic substances released from activated phagocytes.

Frequent Infections, Easy Solution

Gerald's first recollection of health problems was getting large boils at age seven. They were so bad that he had to regularly visit his family doctor to have them lanced. They finally went away when he became a teenager, but then he started getting colds every few weeks. Now 24, he was becoming frightened; for the past three years the colds had turned into pneumonia every fall and spring. Usually they were of the viral form (walking pneumonia), but the last one had been bacterial, which is far more dangerous, and he had become very ill. Obviously, his immune system wasn't working very well, and it was getting weaker.

A careful dietary history revealed that he was eating pretty well, with little consumption of refined foods (such as sugar). However, I noticed he was not eating many foods rich in vitamin C, and the few vitamin-C rich foods he ate were so heavily cooked, the vitamin C was essentially destroyed. I asked if he had any problems with bruising, and when he answered yes, I knew I was on to something. His physical examination was normal, except for receding gums, a problem not usually seen in one so young. This confirmed my suspicion of vitamin C deficiency, because the gums are one of the most traumatized tissues in the body (from chewing and bacteria in the mouth) and if they are lacking in any essential nutrient, they are unable to regenerate as rapidly as they are damaged.

His treatment was to simply increase his consumption of vitamin-C rich foods and supplement this with 2,000 mg of vitamin C every day. His response was remarkable: When he came back a month later, he reported that he thought he was bruising less and had not had another cold. Six months later, he had had only one cold and threw it off easily. Three years later, he was averaging only one cold a year and had had no further bouts with pneumonia. I wish all patients could be cured so easily!

■ *The message:* Even simple nutritional deficiencies can seriously impair immune function.

Vitamin C's immune-potentiating effects are reached within two weeks of supplementation. Heavy smoking decreases plasma vitamin C by about 30% compared with nonsmokers.

Vitamin E

Although normally thought of only as an antioxidant with protective effects against heart disease, vitamin E is actually quite important for the immune system, which it both enhances and protects. A deficiency in vitamin E lowers general host resistance by depressing the proliferation of lymphocytes and the antibody response to pathogens. Insufficient vitamin E also lowers delayed hypersensitivity reactions, a crucial immunological response to cancer, worms, and chronic infections.[22] A potent intracellular antioxidant, vitamin E protects lymphocytes and monocytes from dismemberment by free radicals and therefore significantly increases both the life expectancy and effectiveness of these immune defenders. Although vitamin E supplementation appears to enhance immune function, large doses (over 600 iu) may inhibit the immune response.[14]

Zinc

Zinc is a critical trace element for immune function. It plays an important role in many immune mechanisms, including thymus gland function, thymus hormone action, T-cell production, and cell-mediated and antibody immune system defenses. When zinc levels are low, the number of T cells plummets. Reduced zinc levels are associated with decreased cell-mediated immunity (non-specific defenses), depressed levels of natural killer cell activity, depressed levels of thymic hormones, shrinkage of the thymus, atrophy of the lymph glands, impaired delayed hypersensitivity, decreased lymphocyte response to pathogens, and decreased ability of white cells to engulf and dispose of pathogens and cell debris.[23,14] As might be expected with such a wide-ranging impact, children and adults deficient in zinc show an increased susceptibility to bacterial, viral, and fungal infections.

The hereditary zinc-deficiency disease, acrodermatitis enteropathica (AE), offers an excellent model for understanding the key role of zinc in immunity. In AE, the number of T cells is reduced; lymphocytes do not proliferate when needed; thymic hormone levels are lower; and delayed hypersensitivity is decreased. The movement of neutrophils to the site of inflammation, white cell phagocytosis, and the destruction of pathogenic cells are impaired. All of these effects are reversed when zinc levels are normalized.[24]

When trace mineral status was measured in 28 children ten months to ten years of age who were very susceptible to infections of the respiratory tract or middle ear (otitis media), none had any classic immunological defect. Compared to 13 healthy controls, however, these children had significantly lower levels of zinc.[25] This is not surprising since macrophages from zinc-deficient animals showed reduced ability to attach to and destroy pathogens compared with the macrophages of animals with adequate amounts of zinc. Supplying zinc to the macrophages in solution for 30 minutes completely restored normal function.[26] This may explain why zinc lozenges are effective for some people in stopping the onset of a cold.

Selenium

As noted in the discussion of vitamin E, antioxidant nutrients and enzymes are essential for protection of the immune system from environmental toxins and the chemicals released when the immune system is activated. Macrophages and cytotoxic lymphocytes (lymphocytes that destroy invading cells) produce highly reactive free radicals (a form of reactive oxygen) as a means of destroying pathogenic organisms. Unless neutralized by antioxidants after they do their job, these chemicals will damage both the cells secreting them as well as the tissues in the area. Selenium is necessary for proper functioning of one of the body's most important internally produced antioxidants, glutathione peroxidase, an enzyme that neutralizes free radicals. Selenium also neutralizes toxic metals that can be immunosuppressive.

Selenium deficiency significantly impairs antioxidant activity and is associated with depression of both the specific and non-specific immune defense systems, lower antibody levels, and decreased intracellular killing activity. Selenium-deficient macrophages develop defective membranes due to damage from free radicals. Providing these macrophages with adequate amounts of selenium results in enhanced phagocytic activity and prolonged survival. Selenium is also needed to protect the thymus from stress and free radicals; deficiency results in a reduction in thymic hormones.[25] Selenium deficiency is common in the U.S.

Selenium supplements stimulate the activation and proliferation of lymphocytes, the activation of natural killer cells, antibody production, and the destruction of tumor cells by cytotoxic lymphocytes and macrophages.[27]

Essential fatty acids

Certain fatty acids (labeled "essential" because the body can't synthesize them) are required for the production of prostaglandins—hormone-like chemicals that help activate the immune system. A deficiency will cause immune dysfunction. It is well-documented that many elderly subjects have a reduced immune response due to insufficient dietary intake of fatty acids, which is compounded by less effective absorption. In AIDS patients, malabsorption of essential fatty acids, as well as fat-soluble nutrients such as vitamin A, beta-carotene, and vitamin E, is a significant contributor to immune dysfunction.[23] These fatty acids are also necessary for protection from breast cancer.[28]

Other nutrients

Deficiencies of vitamins B_1, B_2, pantothenic acid, and biotin can lead to reduced production of antibodies. Vitamin B_6 deficiency appears to have a broad inhibitory effect on immune function because it plays an important role in nucleic acids and protein synthesis, both of which are essential for the development and continued functioning of all immune cells. Vitamin B_6 deficiency can result in atrophy of lymphoid tissue and decreased immune response to invaders. Deficiencies of folic acid and B_{12} also depress both cellular (non-specific) and humoral (specific) immune defenses.[14]

Toxins That Damage the Immune System

Heavy metals

Heavy metals cause widespread metabolic damage (discussed in Chapter Five), especially to the immune system. Exposure to mercury, lead, cadmium, and arsenic all cause immunological disorders.[29] Lead (from such sources as old paint and copper water pipes) and cadmium (from cigarette smoke) both cause immune suppression by inhibiting the formation of antibodies and reducing the bactericidal activity of white cells. Mercury (from dental amalgams and consumption of contaminated fish) inhibits antibody production.

Pesticides

Pesticides are very potent immune suppressants. Dr. William Rae, a leading researcher and clinician in environmental medicine, has reported that 81% of 107 patients with initial exposure to pesticides had depressed levels of T and B cells. He also found a significantly greater frequency of abnormal immune parameters in 40 patients with proven chemical sensitivities. As the pesticides were cleared from their bodies, 6 of the 40 patients improved their T and B cell functions. Unfortunately, pesticides are now present in most populations around the world.[30]

Dioxin is a well-known, highly toxic environmental pollutant found in pesticides. Even at low doses, it causes thymus atrophy and generalized suppression of the immune system. Dioxin also inhibits lymphocytes and other components of the immune system.[31]

We are exposed to pesticides in many ways: in foods that are conventionally grown, from spraying shrubbery and houses for insect control, from airplanes that are fumigated—even a simple act such as spraying an insect with an insecticide exposes us to these toxins.

Drugs

While many take aspirin, acetaminophen, and ibuprofen for conditions such as the common cold with little thought about toxicity or the impact on their immune system, there is real reason for concern about these over-the-counter drugs. For example, researchers performed a double-blind, placebo-controlled trial on the effects of over-the-counter analgesics/antipyretic medications on virus shedding, immune response, and clinical status in the common cold. Sixty healthy volunteers were sprayed intranasally with a common cold virus (rhinovirus type II) and placed in one of four treatment groups: aspirin, acetaminophen, ibuprofen, or a placebo. Fifty-six of the volunteers were successfully infected with the virus. The subjects who used aspirin and acetaminophen had lowered production of antibodies and increased nasal symptoms and signs. While there was no statistically significant difference in viral shedding (the expulsion of viruses from the skin) among the four groups, a trend toward longer duration of virus shedding was observed in the aspirin and acetaminophen groups.[32]

One of the most damaging classes of drugs to the immune system are the glucocorticoids (e.g., cortisone), commonly used to suppress inflammatory reactions. Unfortunately, they also suppress the immune system. They reduce the number of lymphocytes, decrease monocyte reaction to pathogens, impair neutrophil movement to the site of infection and their ability to kill bacteria, and inhibit interferon production.[33] They can be extremely dangerous in some situations, such as herpes infections on or near the eye. Use of corticosteroids in this situation can allow the infection to grow so much that the eyeball can become scarred.

Cytotoxic agents (i.e., the drugs used to treat cancer) have similar broad immunosuppressive effects. They can impair antibody synthesis, inhibit cell-mediated immunity, and decrease the number of neutrophils and their ability to function. They also damage the mucous membranes, the body's first line of defense against pathogens and the environment.[33] The end result is that the person being treated for cancer is rendered more susceptible to the development of additional cancers as well as infections.

Silicone implants

Silicone implants have been widely used by women to increase breast size and shape and men to increase muscle size and shape. Unfortunately, this procedure has now been found to have some unexpected side effects. Silicone implants have been found to suppress natural killer cell activity in 50% of patients complaining of symptoms that developed after the implants were inserted. Fortunately, their symptoms and natural killer cell abnormalities reversed when the implants were removed. More disconcerting is the apparent increased incidence of autoimmune diseases, such as lupus erythematosis, in people with silicone implants.[34]

Organic solvents

Exposure to organic solvents (such as paint thinner, petroleum distillates, and carpet cleaners) causes depression in natural killer cell activity as well as an increase in auto-antibodies, i.e., antibodies that the body mistakenly develops to its own tissues, a very serious condition.[35]

Other Damagers of the Immune System

Excessive exercise

Regular exercise is a necessary component of optimal health and supports the immune system by causing short-term increases in white cell count and decreasing the incidence of common infections. *Excessive* exercise (exercise to the point of painful exhaustion two or more times a week), however, depresses the immune system and increases the risk of infection. Exhausting activity temporarily reduces the immune system's defense capacities for several hours after the exertion. This presents a window of opportunity for pathogens. Within this time frame, intense exercisers should try to avoid contact with individuals suffering from infections.[36]

For example, in a recent study of 2,300 marathon runners, the incidence of upper respiratory infections (URI) increased during heavy training and after running in a marathon. The researchers found that runners who trained 60 or more miles a week suffer twice as many URIs as those who trained less than 20 miles a week. They also found that in the week after the marathon, those who completed the race were six times more likely to develop a URI than those who registered and trained for it, but did not run.[37] Intense exercise appears to damage the immune system through the production of high levels of free radicals. This is largely preventable by supplementation with large amounts of antioxidants (see the section on free radicals in Chapter Five), especially vitamin E.

Stress

Stress is one of the great damagers of the immune system.[38,39] Many research studies have clearly demonstrated that stress-induced illness is a real phenomenon and that stress contributes to many diseases (see discussion in Chapter Ten). Stress takes many forms for humans, e.g., tests, sleep deprivation, divorce, taking care of chronically ill family members, fighting with your spouse. The level of immune suppression is usually proportional to the level of stress. However, it is not only stress per se that causes the problem, but also how each individual reacts to the stress. The level of stress your body experiences is a combination of both the amount of stressful stimuli and how you react to it.[40] The variations in personal response help account for the wide diversity of stress-induced illnesses.

Basically, stress results in stimulation of the sympathetic nervous system, the part of the nervous system responsible for the fight-or-flight response. Stress also results in suppression of the parasympathetic nervous system, the portion responsible for bodily functions during periods of rest, relaxation, visualization, meditation, and sleep. Not surprisingly, the immune system functions better when the parasympathetic nervous system is uppermost since, when the body is mobilizing to fight or flee, dealing with an invading microorganism is not a top priority. Normally, the sympathetic and parasympathetic systems balance each other, but under continued stress, the balance is lost and the immune system suffers.

The increased activation of the sympathetic nervous system results in increased secretion of adrenal gland hormones, especially the corticosteroids and catecholamines. These hormones inhibit white blood cell function, decrease the production of lymphocytes, and cause the thymus gland, the master gland of the immune system, to shrink. The result is a significant reduction in immune function. Only recently have researchers discovered that T and B cells contain receptors on their cell membranes for these stress-induced hormones, which helps explain the immune system's sensitivity to stress.

A stress-induced immunosuppressed state leaves us susceptible to infections and allows cancerous cells to escape immune surveillance. In general, the degree of immunosuppression is proportional to the level of stress. In studies of monkeys, stress even appears to cause accelerated destruction and premature aging of brain cells!

Stress Adds Up

Jonathan came to see me for his chronic flus and colds. While this had been a problem for him for several years, it had gotten much worse the past six months. He was suffering one or the other every month and was in danger of losing his job due to excessive absences. His diet and lifestyle seemed pretty healthful, until I delved deeper. Jonathan worked as an air traffic controller, known to be one of the most stressful jobs a person can have. Added to that was the fact that his male partner had been diagnosed almost a year before as having AIDS, and his health was now deteriorating rapidly. Jonathan's HIV tests were negative, so he doubted that was the problem (although there is about a six-month lag time between infection and the HIV test turning positive, their sexual practices were low risk). It seemed to me that the combined stress of his intense job, caring for his very sick partner, and his growing sense of impending loss were suppressing his immune system.

This was tough to address since he was dependent on his high-income job and deeply committed to his partner. Together, we worked out a program for him. He lowered his stress by having his supervisor reassign him to a less intense shift, reinstituting meditation practices he had abandoned several years earlier, going to sleep earlier every night, and hiring a home-care professional to help provide some of the care for his partner. In addition, I coaxed him into taking a week-long vacation by himself. We boosted his immune system by having him take thymus extract and zinc (to try to rebuild his thymus, which was being devastated by the stress) and *Echinacea* (which boosts most parameters of immune function). Finally, he took ginseng, which both improves stress tolerance and strengthens the immune system.

The results weren't dramatic. Jonathan did slowly improve over the ensuing months, but it wasn't until his partner died and he changed jobs that his immune system returned to normal.

■ *The message:* Stress really does impair immune function.

While most of us think of stress in terms of Type A behaviors (driven, aggressive, hostile, perfectionistic tendencies), serious depression is also a form of stress that inhibits the immune system. For example, to evaluate the impact of personal loss, researchers studied 21 middle-aged widowed females who lost their spouses 2 months before their initial evaluation and compared them to 21 married women at 6-month intervals for 13 months. The subset of widows who met the criteria for major depression showed impaired immune function indicated by lower natural killer cell activity and lower lymphocyte reactivity. The results suggest a relationship between impaired immune function and depression in women experiencing the stress of bereavement.[41]

Even anxiety appears to have an adverse effect on immune function. For example, one group of researchers studied the immune systems of people who cared for loved ones suffering from Alzheimer's disease. The stress of caring for the person with Alzheimer's disease suppressed the caregiver's immune system even two years after the patient had died! In both the current and ex-caregivers, natural killer cell activity and T cell counts were significantly lower compared to controls.

Fortunately, these effects are reversible. In one study, patients who had surgery for cancer were divided into two groups—one group receiving 90-minute psychological interventions weekly for six months and the other group receiving no formal psychological help. The interventions included educating the patients about cancer, discussing their fears, teaching stress management techniques and coping skills, and promoting interaction between patients and health care professionals.

After six months of therapy, the intervention group had higher overall counts of the natural killer cells and lymphocytes that kill tumor cells. This translated over the following six years to extremely important results: the intervention group experienced half the rate of recurrence and significantly fewer deaths than the non-intervention group.[42]

Inadequate rest
The research on stress emphasizes the paramount importance of adequate rest and elimination of stressful activity when the immune system is engaged, which, in modern life, seems to be seven days a week. Even a modest loss of sleep over one night can impair the immune system. In one research study, 23 healthy men aged 22 to 61 were deprived of four hours of sleep for one night. The next day, their natural killer cell activity fell a remarkable 30%. Fortunately, a good night's sleep restored the cells to their normal function.[43]

Obesity and lipid abnormalities
Obesity is associated with poor immune system function, as evidenced by the decreased bacteria-killing activity of neutrophils and increased incidence of disease and mortality from infections. Cholesterol and lipid levels are usually elevated in obese individuals, which may explain their impaired immune function. Increased blood levels of cholesterol, free fatty acids, triglycerides, and bile acids inhibit various immune functions, including the ability of lymphocytes to proliferate and produce antibodies and the ability of neutrophils to migrate to areas of infections and engulf and destroy infectious organisms.[44] Since 25% of adult Americans are obese (50% of black women), excess weight is a very serious contributor to immune dysfunction for many.

Candida
While the normal intestinal tract harbors small amounts of yeast, yeast overgrowth is now more common due to the widespread use of broad-spectrum

Too Many Antibiotics

Even before she related her symptoms, I had a good idea about why Jacqueline was in my office. When she walked in, I immediately noticed the scars on her face. Yes, she told me, she had had severe acne, which had lasted through adolescence into adulthood and had been treated for years with the antibiotic tetracycline. She was tired all the time, suffered from chronic vaginal yeast infections, seemed to get the flu whenever it was around, and craved sweets. She knew the frequent courses of antibiotics she was taking were destroying the normal balance of healthy bacteria in her vagina, and she had tried eating yogurt and using yogurt douches, but it didn't seem to help.

Jacqueline was correct in believing that the antibiotics had upset her normal balance of natural bacterial flora in her intestines. Equally important, however, the yeast (*Candida albicans*) that had overgrown her intestines as well as her vagina was also directly inhibiting her immune system. The yeast overgrowth causes problems in several ways, one of the most important being that chemicals released by the yeast cells depress the activity of the white cells our immune system uses to fight invaders.

Unfortunately, the commercial yogurt she was using did not have the necessary *Lactobacillus acidophilus* culture. Most yogurts do not use lactobacilli but other cultures chosen because they work better for food processing. Jacqueline learned to always check the label to determine which culture(s) had been used.

Her therapy? Jacqueline stopped the tetracycline, and we began treating her acne with natural approaches instead. To eliminate the yeast, I prescribed garlic, which has been shown to be more effective than nystatin, the drug most frequently prescribed for candida. In addition to lots (two cloves a day) of garlic (she could have used capsules high in allicin containing a comparable amount of garlic), Jacqueline also took caprylic acid, a naturally occurring fatty acid that inhibits candida and helps heal the intestines. She decreased her sugar consumption (in addition to sugar's immune-suppressing effects, sugar is candida's favorite food), and we reinoculated both her intestines and vagina with an active form of lactobacilli. We also helped her eliminate the candida in her vagina by using a tampon saturated with a 40% solution of tea tree oil. Intestinal candida are quite persistent, but, after a few months, she started to notice increased resistance to infections, fewer and shorter periods of vaginal discomfort, and a growing sense of vitality.

■ *The message:* Prolonged antibiotic use, candidal overgrowth, and excess sugar consumption equal immune dysfunction. Garlic and tea tree oil are great natural antifungal agents.

antibiotics, corticosteroids, birth control pills, and the consumption of simple carbohydrates (i.e., sugar). Intestinal overgrowth of candida causes many health problems, especially suppression of the immune system. As yeast proliferate, they penetrate the intestinal mucosa, causing localized damage. The leaky gut (see Chapter Five) that develops allows increased absorption of immune-suppressing bowel toxins and food allergens. In addition, the immune complexes formed by the yeast are directly immunosuppressive.

Candida overgrowth is an all too common result of antibiotics given to hospitalized patients. For example, in a study of 55 injured patients admitted to the trauma service of a hospital, all were given broad-spectrum antibiotic therapy during some point of their stay. Sixty-seven percent developed elevated candida antigen levels in their blood during their hospital stay, indicating that candida were overgrowing in their intestines (and the vaginas of women). The researchers also found that the white blood cells of patients with candida antigens were not able to inhibit *Candida albicans* growth as effectively as white cells from the patients who did not have candidal antigens in their blood.[45] In other words, when patients receive antibiotics, the level of candida in their intestines increases so much and the intestines become so damaged, that pieces of the candida leak into their blood and inhibit the function of their immune system.

Excessive fish oil supplementation

Some people believe that if it's natural, if it's a vitamin or an herb, it's safe, and the more used the better. Unfortunately, life just isn't that easy. Supplements do have a high degree of safety, but they can be misused. Fish oil is one supplement that, while valuable to help control excessive inflammation, is cause for concern, since high doses have been found to suppress the immune system.

For example, in one study, 12 healthy volunteers were given 5.4 gm of eicosapentaenoic acid (EPA) or 3.2 gm of docosahexaenoic acid (DHA) daily. Both of these fish oils significantly reduced neutrophils' ability to migrate to the site of inflammation. Some researchers believe that the immune suppression resulting from supplementation with fish oils is due to rancidity (oxidation of the fatty acids to produce peroxides), so half the subjects were also given vitamin E to neutralize the peroxides. Although the levels of lipid peroxides were lower in the vitamin E groups, immune function was still depressed in all groups taking these amounts of fish oil.[46] However, the amount of vitamin E used was not very high, so this question may not have been answered. One gram a day appears to be a safe level for long-term use.

Trauma

Severe trauma to the body, such as major surgery, significantly depresses immune function. This immunosuppression may be the result of the inflammatory response to the trauma. Fortunately, much of this can be reversed by supplementation with nutrients such as vitamins A and C, the essential amino acid arginine, and essential fatty acids of the omega-3 group (alpha-linolenic acid). Vitamin A supplementation has been shown to help reverse the immune suppression induced by surgery. In one study, lymphocytes were counted on the first and seventh day after surgery. In the untreated placebo group, the lymphocyte count dropped significantly, while in the group treated with 300,000 to 450,000 iu of vitamin A, the number of lymphocytes remained normal.[47] Omega-3 fatty acids probably help by decreasing the number of inflammatory chemicals released at the site of injury while stimulating T cell proliferative responses. Arginine helps by stimulating T cell proliferative responses.[48]

Vaccinations Are No Substitute for a Healthy Immune System

While much has been made of the beneficial impact of vaccinations on improving health and longevity, the actual benefits of many vaccinations are probably not as good as advertised, and many problems linked to vaccinations have not been disclosed to the public. This section is not meant to discourage the use of vaccinations, but rather to ensure their appropriate use and help the reader recognize that vaccinations are not a good substitute for a healthy immune system.*

Vaccinations induce a transient depression in immune function

For several decades, researchers have known that immune system dysfunction can follow vaccination. For example, in 1964, Brody reported that live-virus vaccines can induce transient suppression of tuberculin sensitivity (a measure of how well the immune system is working).[49] A possible mechanism for this vaccine-induced suppression can be found in a Viennese study of tetanus vaccination in healthy adults. Measurement of T lymphocytes from blood samples taken before and after vaccination revealed a temporary decrease in the helper-to-suppresser T cell ratio of almost 50%. The decrease was most severe between days 3 and 14 post-vaccination. The researchers pointed out that such drops in helper-to-suppresser T cell ratios are characteristic of AIDS.[50]

Some researchers are concerned about the similar drop in helper T cells that occurs in young children and infants following their receipt of multiple vaccine regimens, since this occurs during the crucial period of their lives when their immune systems are beginning to mature. Any suppression of the helper T lymphocytes during this time, even of a transient nature, is undesirable because it may impair proper maturation of their immune system.[51]

---

*I fully realize this discussion may offend some medical personnel. Most of this section is condensed from a chapter entitled "Vaccinations and Immune Malfunction" in A Textbook of Natural Medicine. The chapter was written by a medical doctor with 40 years of experience taking care of patients. All of it is fully documented in the scientific literature. The informed consumer of health care needs to consider all sides of such an important issue, and unfortunately only one side has been presented to the public.

Use of live measles virus vaccine has caused large-scale and unpublicized immunologic disorders. Up to one-half of infants 12 months of age or less who are vaccinated with live measles vaccine develop a "permanent alteration in the individual's capacity to respond to measles virus because of the initial . . . immunizing experience" and continue to be susceptible to natural measles infection despite repeated measles vaccination.[52] In another study, the activity and mobility of neutrophils was measured in 15 children seven days after they received the measles-mumps-rubella vaccination. In all the children, neutrophil functions were significantly reduced on the seventh day. In three subjects, neutrophil functions took a full month to return to normal.[53]

The possibility of immune malfunction following childhood vaccinations has become increasingly recognized, and controversial. In March 1979, some researchers suggested that an association might exist between immunization with DPT (diphtheria, tetanus toxoids, and pertussis vaccine, Wyeth Lot 64201) and ten cases of sudden infant death syndrome (SIDS) in Tennessee. An extensive investigation following this report was not able to establish or refute a causal relationship.[54] In order to clarify this issue, the Department of Pediatrics at the UCLA School of Medicine conducted a study of SIDS in Los Angeles County.[55] Parents of 145 SIDS victims who died in Los Angeles County between January 1, 1979 and August 23, 1980, were contacted and interviewed regarding their child's recent immunization history. Fifty-three had received DPT immunization. Of these 53, 27 had received a DPT immunization within 28 days of death. Six SIDS deaths occurred within 24 hours and 17 occurred within one week of immunization. It was concluded this rate of SIDS deaths "was significantly more than expected." It has been suspected that immune dysfunction plays a significant role in SIDS or, at the very least, that SIDS is a disease that involves an unusual immunologic reaction.[56]

Vaccinations may contribute to the development of other disease
One of the most extensively documented reports on the unheathful effects of vaccines can be found in the book *The Hazards of Immunization*, by Sir Graham Wilson, formerly of the Public Health Laboratory Service of England and Wales.[57] In reviewing epidemics of the past, Dr. Wilson provided a number of examples in which vaccinations against one disease seemed to provoke another. As one example, a physician in London first drew attention to the relation between inoculation against diphtheria or pertussis and attacks of poliomyelitis when he described 15 cases he had seen between 1944 and 1949. Paralysis came on, as a rule, 7 to 21 days after injection, and affected the left arm, into which the injections were given four times as often as the right. Wilson referred to these instances as "provocational disease."

There is a growing body of evidence that vaccinations may contribute to the occurrence of non-infectious diseases. For example, there is now serious suspicion that measles vaccination may be a significant cause of inflammatory bowel disease. This was brought to light in a very large retrospective study of

3,545 people who had received the measles vaccination in 1964, 11,407 matched unvaccinated controls, and the 2,541 partners of those vaccinated. Those who had been vaccinated had a three times greater risk of developing Crohn's disease and a two and a half times greater risk of ulcerative colitis.[58]

This raises the question (which has been at the heart of the arguments of many of those opposed to vaccinations): Does the measles vaccine prevent a mild, benign illness while creating a serious, chronic disease of the intestine? The conventional medical argument is that since few children experience serious side effects from measles infection, all should be vaccinated. But as documented above in the discussion on vitamin A deficiency, it is those children with a poorly functioning immune system, usually due to a deficiency in vitamin A, who experience serious effects from the measles. It might be wiser to encourage supplementation with vitamin A for those who need it, rather than use a vaccine that increases the risk of a serious, chronic degenerative disease for everyone else.

An extensive report reviewing the safety of vaccinations, "Adverse Events Associated with Childhood Vaccines: Evidence Bearing on Causality," was published by the Institute of Medicine in September 1993. It included researchers from the National Academy of Sciences, the March of Dimes Birth Defects Foundation, and Yale University School of Medicine. They reviewed all available scientific and medical data over an 18-month period, including individual case reports as well as controlled clinical trials. As a result of their study, they came to several conclusions:

1. Diphtheria and tetanus vaccinations were *not* found to increase the risk of encephalopathy (brain dysfunction), infantile spasms, or sudden death syndrome (SIDS).
2. The flu vaccine (conjugate hemophilus influenza type B [Hib] vaccine) was *not* found to increase susceptibility to the flu.
3. Diphtheria and tetanus toxoids were found to slightly increase the risk of anaphylaxis (a life-threatening allergic hypersensitivity reaction), Guillain-Barre syndrome (nerve inflammation leading to muscular weakness and paralysis), and brachial neuritis (inflammation of nerves in the arm).
4. Measles vaccine was found to slightly increase the risk of anaphylaxis and death from measles.
5. Oral polio vaccine was found to slightly increase the risk of Guillain-Barre syndrome, poliomyelitis, and death from the polio-vaccine strain.
6. Unconjugated Hib (flu) vaccine was found to slightly increase susceptibility to the flu.
7. Measles-mumps-rubella vaccine was found to slightly increase the risk of thrombocytopenia (an abnormal decrease in blood platelets).
8. Oral polio vaccine and hepatitis B vaccine were both found to slightly increase the risk of anaphylaxis.

While some of these data are disquieting, it is important to recognize that the risks of these side effects of vaccinations are small. For example, the risk of brachial neuritis after tetanus vaccine is on the order of 5 to 10 per 100,000 persons vaccinated. The incidence of thrombocytopenia occurring within two months after the measles-mumps-rubella vaccine (MMR) is on the order of 2.5 to 3 per 100,000 vaccinated children (although this is six times higher than in unvaccinated children). The incidence of paralytic poliomyelitis from the oral polio vaccine is approximately 1 case per 500,000 first doses of oral polio vaccine (OPV), and approximately 1 case per 12 million follow-up doses administered. The incidence for the Hib disease (influenza) within seven days of the vaccination is estimated to be 1.62 cases per 100,000 vaccines. The MMR vaccine has been used for 20 years, and the committee could find only two well-documented cases of anaphylaxis. However, the review notes that the committee was "distressed" over the significant number of vaccine-related adverse events for which the data was inadequate to determine causality.[59]

The Problem with Antibiotics

While antibiotics are very useful when the body's immune system is overwhelmed, their excessive use causes many problems—including damage to the immune system, overgrowth of candida in the intestines and vagina, and the development of antibiotic-resistant bacteria and new types of bacteria that can evade the immune system.

Some very interesting evidence suggests that some forms of bacteria and fungi have developed cell forms that can function without cell walls as a result of chronic exposure to antibiotics. Most antibiotics work by inhibiting the synthesis of bacterial cells' walls. This is normally quite effective and results in the death of virtually all bacteria. However, some bacteria continue to survive with either no or only partially developed cell walls. Unfortunately, by losing their cell walls, they become essentially invisible to the immune system. That is because the body recognizes an invader by the foreign proteins in its cell wall. These cell wall-deficient forms then spread throughout the body, becoming what has been designated "stealth pathogens." Instead of proliferation by the usual process of fission (splitting in two), these stealth pathogens reproduce by budding, a process normally found only in yeasts. When appropriate conditions occur, they quickly proliferate to recognizable infections. Stealth pathogens have been tentatively implicated in septicemia (infection in the blood), urinary tract infections, meningitis (infection of the membranes of the spinal cord or brain), heart valve infection, blinding inflammation of the eye, rheumatic fever, Crohn's disease (inflammation of the small intestine), ulcerative colitis, and other chronic health problems.

Lida Mattman, Ph.D., has done important work researching this controversial theory of stealth pathogens for over two decades. She has applied rigorous science to these concepts, but these bacterial variants were first recognized over 100 years ago by Bechamp, Winkler, Almquist, and others. (Those interested in further pursuing this concept are urged to read Dr. Mattman's fascinating book.[60] It is thoroughly referenced and makes a very compelling case.)

Improving Immune Function Naturally

The first step in improving the immune system is to take a careful look at your lifestyle to determine any factors that could be inhibiting or damaging your immune defenses, e.g., debilitating reactions to stress, excessive consumption of simple sugar (in all its forms), excessive consumption of alcohol, obesity, food allergies, and overgrowth of candida in the bowel. Once identified, these harmful influences need to be replaced with health-promoting equivalents. For example, problems with stress can be ameliorated by changing the stress-inducing situation or by improving one's coping skills through meditation, regular exercise, prayer, joining a support group, buying some headphones and listening to music—whatever positive action helps you release tension. Allergenic foods such as cow's milk can be replaced with fruit and vegetable juices or milks made from rice, soy, or almonds; all of which are now available in most health food stores and supermarkets.

The second step is to ensure adequate consumption of all nutrients needed for optimal immune function, especially vitamins A, C, and the mineral zinc. Much of this can be accomplished by consuming a whole-foods diet of diverse, organically grown foods—not a simple task, however, since our modern environment contains high levels of pollutants; it's difficult to find a wide variety of organic foods year-round; and modern life affords few the time to regularly prepare wholesome home-cooked meals. Given these realities, taking a good quality multivitamin-multimineral supplement appears necessary. Identifying which, if any, foods you are allergic to is very important and is covered in Chapter Six. If candidal overgrowth in the bowel is suspected, a physician of natural or holistic medicine should be consulted to diagnose the root cause and develop a treatment program, which may require the use of anti-fungal drugs.

The third step is to use extra amounts of specific nutrients and herbs that help rev up the immune system when extra immune power is needed (see Figure 4-4). It is important to understand, however, that these immune aids should only be used for short periods to help stimulate the immune response during an acute infection, to cure a chronic infection, or when trying to reestablish a properly functioning immune system.

Nutritional Support for the Immune System

Without doubt, good nutrition is the mainstay of a well-functioning immune system; yet, even in supposedly healthy adults consuming a nutritionally adequate diet, simply providing a modest level multivitamin-multimineral supplement dramatically decreases the incidence of infection. For example, in a study of 96 healthy adults given either a multivitamin-multimineral supplement or placebo, the supplemented group had an amazing 50% decrease in the number of days of illness due to infection, and 8 of 12 objective measures of immune function improved.[61] Remarkable results for little effort and no danger.

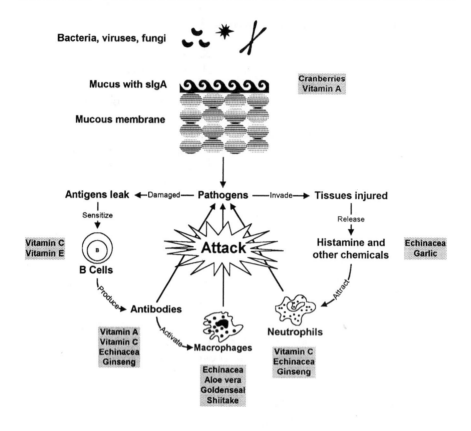

Figure 4-4 *Herbs and Nutrients That Strengthen the Immune System*

Following are my recommendations for special foods and nutritional supplements that can be used to boost the immune system when extra help is needed. Think of them as an extension on a ladder that allows immune defenders to climb to new heights. And, remember, supplements can only optimize immune function when the body's basic needs are met by adequate nutrition, i.e., a whole-foods diet. It's practically impossible to climb a ladder when the lower rungs are missing.

Vitamin A

Vitamin A supplementation has been shown to stimulate and/or enhance numerous immune processes, including inducing the activity of cell-mediated immune defenders that destroy cancerous cells, natural killer cell activity, lymphocyte production, phagocytosis (the ingestion and digestion of bacteria), and antibody production.[62,63] These effects are not due simply to a reversal of vitamin A deficiency, since many of them are further enhanced by the administration of (supposedly) excessive levels of vitamin A. In addition, vitamin A prevents and reverses stress-induced shrinkage of the thymus gland; supplementation with vitamin A can actually promote thymus growth.[64] Retinol, a form of vitamin A present in animal tissue, has also been shown to be very effective in eliminating viral infections.[65]

Considerable research is currently examining the relationship between both vitamin A and carotenes and the incidence of epithelial cancer, i.e., cancer of the lungs, gastrointestinal tract, genitourinary tract, and skin. Tissue enzymes induced by exposure to carcinogens such as excessive sunlight may degrade vitamin A thus leaving the epithelial tissue more susceptible to cancer. High doses of vitamin A may help prevent the depletion caused by these enzymes. High doses of vitamin A, however, should not be consumed over an extended time (no more than a month or two) since it is stored in the body. Long-term supplementation with high doses of vitamin A can lead to toxicity, resulting in symptoms of pressure headaches, nausea, dizziness, dry skin, and joint pain.

- *Typical dosage:* maintenance dose of 20,000 iu per day; 50,000 iu per day during infection (for no more than one month). Pregnant women should first discuss vitamin A supplementation with their doctor because some research suggests even as little as 10,000 iu per day may increase the risk of fetal abnormalities.

Carotenes

Epidemiological studies have demonstrated an inverse relationship between the intake of carotene (the yellow pigment in carrots and other orange fruits and vegetables) and cancer incidence. Besides being converted into vitamin A by the body, carotenes function as antioxidants, with beta-carotene being a very potent quencher of singlet oxygen, a particularly destructive free radical.[66] Since the thymus gland is so susceptible to free radical damage, beta-carotene may be even more helpful in protecting the immune system than vitamin A. Beta-carotene, although the most publicized and possessing the highest vitamin A activity, is only one of more than 500 carotenoids. For example, canthaxanthin is a carotenoid that does not have any vitamin A activity but is a potent antioxidant, especially for the retina of the eye.

Carotenes appear to protect against cancer. Specifically, they have been found to inhibit squamous cell carcinoma (a type of skin cancer) in cell culture. In animal models, beta-carotene supplements have reduced the incidence of mammary tumors. In addition to their antioxidant properties, which help prevent tissue and DNA damage (prerequisites for the initiation of cancer), carotenes also stimulate enzymes that destroy carcinogens, enhance white cell function, and stimulate the body's ability to metabolize toxic substances, transforming them into harmless chemicals.[67]

Supplementation with large amounts of beta-carotene (100,000 to 200,000 iu per day) results in significant increases in helper T cells in healthy adults as well as HIV-infected subjects.[68] Even at this high a dosage, no toxicity was noted.[69] Unlike vitamin A, the only problem that has been observed resulting from an excessively high intake of carotenes is a carrot-color tinge to the skin, similar to that produced by some self-tanning lotions, which quickly fades when carotene intake is reduced.

- *Typical dosage:* 50 mg per day

Vitamin C

Supplementation with extra vitamin C has been shown to help fight infections from virtually all pathogens. Although this is still not accepted by the mainstream medical profession, vitamin C really does help prevent and decrease the duration of the common cold, as concluded by a researcher who reviewed all the published studies on the clinical use of vitamin C for the common cold.[70] It is well-known that blood levels of both white cells and vitamin C drop significantly during the common cold.[71] It is also interesting to note that toxins released by bacteria during infection instantly inhibit white cell uptake of vitamin C, making the white cells more easily damaged during infection.[72]

Although vitamin C has been shown to be directly antiviral[73] and antibacterial,[74] its main beneficial effect is probably via improvement in host resistance. Vitamin C's ability to stimulate the immune system has been demonstrated in many ways, including enhancing the production of lymphocytes; enhancing the movement of lymphocytes to the scene of battle; and increasing interferon levels, antibody responses, antibody production, and the secretion of thymic hormones. Vitamin C is also necessary for the integrity of ground substance (the material that occupies the intercellular spaces in fibrous connective tissue, cartilage, and bone), which mechanically inhibits the spread of infections.[75] Vitamin C also has biochemical effects similar to interferon.[76] Interferon works by binding to cell surfaces and stimulating the synthesis of proteins that prevent viruses from entering the cells.

Even modest levels of vitamin C supplementation in apparently healthy elderly adults on a supposedly adequate diet results in significant immune enhancement. In one representative study, 57 elderly subjects were given a very modest dose of 200 mg of vitamin C per day or a placebo. The supplemented patients fared significantly better than those receiving the placebo. The improvement in immune response was particularly evident in those who were the most severely ill, many of whom had low plasma and white cell concentrations of vitamin C.[77]

- *Typical dosage:* 1,000 mg per day maintenance; 5,000 mg per day during infection

Vitamin E

Possibly vitamin E's most important immune-enhancing role is protecting the immune system from the free radical effects of infection: both those generated by the invading microbe and those resulting from the body's immune reaction, which involves the release of free radicals to kill the invaders. Vitamin E supplementation enhances the non-specific immune response, increases the number of B cells (the immune cells that produce antibodies), and increases the destruction of bacteria by white cells.[18]

Some very important recent studies have shown that vitamin E supplementation may be of special help in reversing the immune depression commonly seen in aging. In one interesting experiment, vitamin E supplementation in aging animals actually caused several indicators of immune function to revert to the same level as found in young animals.[78] Another research study found an inverse correlation between serum vitamin E levels and the incidence of infections in the elderly.[79] In yet another study, 32 healthy adults older than 60 were placed in a double-blind placebo-controlled trial of vitamin E (800 mg per day) for 30 days. Only the vitamin-E supplemented group showed several signs of improved immune function: increased antibody production, increased lymphocyte response, and increased production of interleukin II (a chemical that helps activate the immune system). These data are extremely important as they show that vitamin E enhances immune function, even in healthy elderly individuals consuming the recommended daily allowances of vitamin E in their diets.[80]

Be careful though and don't use too much vitamin E. One research study found that at a dose of 300 mg per day, 18 healthy male volunteers suffered decreased bactericidal activity of neutrophils and decreased responsiveness of lymphocytes in tissue cultures after three weeks. However, the results of this study are questionable since skin testing did not show any depression in immunological response, and synthetic rather than natural vitamin E was used in the research.[81]

In general, the amount of vitamin E needed to support immune function is dependent upon a person's lifestyle. For example, those who are heavy exercisers, whose jobs expose them to chemicals, who work outside in direct sunlight, or who smoke or consume alcoholic beverages frequently will need significantly more vitamin E than someone whose lifestyle results in less free radical generation. Moderate exercisers who neither drink or smoke and who are not exposed to lots of sunshine will have a lower requirement for vitamin E.

- *Typical dosage:* 200 iu per day maintenance

Zinc

Zinc supplementation has been shown to enhance immune function, even in those with normal serum zinc levels. In one experiment, 83 apparently healthy men and women were given 150 mg of zinc a day. After four weeks, they showed a significant increase in T cell function. Because there was no correlation between serum zinc levels and the degree of response, the authors argued that the effect was not due to deficiency.[82] However, serum zinc is a very poor measure of zinc status, so my interpretation is that the effect could have been due to normalizing a zinc deficiency, a state which is very common, but not commonly recognized.

Zinc is especially important in the elderly, who are often deficient in zinc and whose immune systems are already suffering from a shrinking thymus. Zinc supplementation in supposedly healthy elderly subjects resulted in increased numbers of T cells and enhanced cell-mediated immune responses. In mice, even age-related thymic atrophy is reversible by zinc replacement.[83] This suggests that the chronic zinc deficiency of the elderly might account for their thymus degeneration.

As useful as zinc is, once again, it is important not to use too much. Typically, in persons with normal zinc levels (as tested in white cells, a better indicator of zinc status than serum), supplementation with 75 mg of elemental zinc a day will inhibit immune function after a few months; 150 mg twice a day will depress immune response within six weeks.[84]

- *Typical dosage:* 25 mg per day maintenance; 75 mg per day for one week during an infection

Selenium

The damaging effects of a deficiency of selenium on immune function have been well-documented, but relatively little research has been done to determine the effects of selenium supplementation. However, some recent research looks quite promising. One study evaluated selenium supplementation at 200 mcg per day in healthy college students for eight weeks compared to placebo. The researchers found that supplementation resulted in a remarkable 118% increase in lymphocyte killing of tumor cells and an 82.3% increase in natural killer cell activity. Interestingly, supplementation did not significantly alter plasma selenium levels (which is probably a poor measure of selenium status).[85]

- *Typical dosage:* 200 mcg per day maintenance

Breast feeding

While it's too late for those of us who did not have the opportunity as infants, we can certainly ensure that our children have the best possible start in life for their immune system—breast feeding. A large amount of research has conclusively demonstrated that breast-fed infants have fewer infections and fewer problems with allergies. Breast milk is very high in a variety of nutrients needed for the infant's optimal health, particularly his or her still-developing immune cells and antibodies. The most prevalent immunoglobulin in breast milk is secretory IgA. This antibody is especially important because it helps protect the baby's mucous membranes from invading pathogens. Since these antibodies are coming from the mother, who is likely to be exposed to the same pathogens as the infant, they provide precisely the protection needed. Breast milk also provides B and T lymphocytes, macrophages, and neutrophils, all of which help the infant fight infection.

Another beneficial aspect of a mother's antibodies is that they don't harm the normal healthy bacteria of the infant's intestines; indeed, breast milk contains bifidus factor, which stimulates the growth of healthy intestinal bacteria.

As might be expected, when a breast-fed infant is exposed to a pathogen or develops an infection, he or she develops higher levels of antibodies and other measures of immune response than a bottle-fed baby does.[86] In addition, breast feeding greatly decreases the incidence of food allergy, which has such a devastating impact on the immune system.[87]

Herbs That Stimulate the Immune System

Herbs have been used for millennia by all the peoples of the earth to help fight infections and promote health. More and more research is providing compelling documentation of the valuable effects of herbs on improving immune system function. My favorite immune-potentiating herbs are *Echinacea*, goldenseal, and shiitake mushroom.

Echinacea species

Perhaps the most widely used Western herb for enhancement of the immune system is *Echinacea*. Studies have shown that two species, *Echinacea angustifolia* and *Echinacea purpurea*, have profound immune-enhancing effects. *Echinacea* strengthens the immune system, including the thymus gland (the master gland of the immune system), in many ways probably because it contains a diverse range of active constituents.

Root extracts of *Echinacea* have been shown to possess interferon-like activity and direct antiviral activity against influenza, herpes, and vesicular stomatitis viruses.[88]

The most important immune-stimulating components of *Echinacea* are large polysaccharides, such as inulin, that activate the alternative complement pathway (one of the immune system's non-specific defense mechanisms) and increase the production of immune chemicals that activate macrophages. The result is increased activity of many key immune parameters: production of T cells, macrophage phagocytosis, antibody binding, natural killer cell activity, and levels of circulating neutrophils.[89,90,91] *Echinacea* polysaccharides have also been shown to directly destroy tumor cells in tissue culture and inhibit *Candida albicans* infection in rats that were infected intravenously with a lethal dose of *C. albicans*.[92]

Echinacea contains other components, such as fat-soluble alkylamides (which have shown even more potent enhancement of macrophage phagocytosis) and caffeic acid derivatives that are also thought to contribute to the herb's immune empowering effects.[93] The juice of the flower and stem portion of *E. purpurea* has lower concentrations of polysaccharides and higher concentrations of these fat-soluble immune stimulants as compared to the root.

Echinacea strengthens the immune system even in healthy people. For example, oral administration of an *E. purpurea* root extract (a dose of 30 drops three times daily) to healthy males for five days resulted in a remarkable 120% increase in leukocyte phagocytosis.[94] In another study of healthy volunteers aged 25 to 40 years, a 22% alcohol *E. purpurea* extract was found to increase the phagocytosis of *Candida albicans* by 30 to 40%; it also increased the migration of white cells to the scene of battle by 30 to 40%.[95]

Besides immune support, *Echinacea* also helps prevent the spread of bacteria by inhibiting a bacterial enzyme called hyaluronidase. This enzyme is secreted by bacteria in order to break through the body's first line of defense, the protective membranes such as the skin or mucous membranes, so the organism can enter the body.

Currently, over 300 *Echinacea*-containing products are sold worldwide. The chemistry and clinical applications of *Echinacea* have been the subject of almost 400 scientific studies. Clinical research has shown *Echinacea* to be an effective therapeutic agent in many infectious conditions, including influenza, the common cold, upper respiratory infections, and urogenital infections.[96] In general, *Echinacea* appears to offer benefit for nearly all infectious conditions.

An exception to this statement may be AIDS. It is unclear at this time if *Echinacea* should be recommended for AIDS. Although this condition is associated with widespread depression of the immune system, presumably due to the human-immunodeficiency virus (HIV), stimulation of T cell replication by *Echinacea* may stimulate replication of the virus as well. While there are some anecdotal reports of *Echinacea*'s efficacy in HIV-infected individuals, more research is necessary to determine its effects on HIV.

- *Typical dosage:* one-half oz flower extract or 4 (500 mg each) capsules of root every three hours until symptoms resolve

Aloe vera

Acemannan (acetylated mannose), a water-soluble, long-chain polysaccharide extracted from the *Aloe vera* plant, is a potent immunostimulant. It increases the phagocytic activity of macrophages, T cell response to invading pathogens, and the production of interferon and other immune-enhancing chemicals.[97,98]

- *Typical dosage:* 800 mg of acemannan or one quart of juice per day

Astragalus membranaceus

Astragalus is a traditional Chinese medicinal herb used for viral infections. Research in animals has shown that it apparently works by stimulating several factors of the immune system, particularly in those whose immune system has been damaged by chemicals or radiation. In immunodepressed mice, *Astragalus* has been found to reverse the T cell abnormalities caused by cyclophosphamide (a cancer drug), radiation, and aging. It also increases T cell activity in normal mice.[99] Happily, similar results have been shown in cancer patients whose immune systems have been damaged by chemotherapy.[100]

- *Typical dosage:* 3 (500 mg each) capsules three times a day

Hydrastis canadensis (Goldenseal)

Although goldenseal is primarily used for its direct antibacterial properties, it has also shown remarkable immune system-enhancing activity. Foremost is its ability to increase the blood supply to the spleen, thus promoting the spleen's release of immuno-potentiating compounds.[101] Berberine, the primary alkaloid in goldenseal, has also been shown to be a potent activator of macrophages, the cells responsible for engulfing and destroying bacteria, viruses, fungi, and tumor cells.[102]

- *Typical dosage:* 3 (500 mg each) capsules three times a day

Lentinus edodes (Shiitake mushroom)

The shiitake mushroom has been used for centuries in traditional Chinese medicine to increase resistance to infection. Research has found that much of its activity appears to be due to a polysaccharide complex called lentinan. Lentinan is nontoxic and has demonstrated significant immuno-stimulating and antitumor activity.[103] It stimulates macrophages, increases interferon production, increases T cell production, enhances helper T cell activity, and increases the bacteria-killing activity of macrophages.[104,105] It has also been shown to increase natural killer cell activity in patients aged 14 to 77 suffering from "low natural killer syndrome." Interestingly, these patients had not responded to conventional medical fever treatments or antibiotics.[106]

- *Typical dosage:* 3 (500 mg each) capsules three times a day

Allium sativum (Garlic)

Garlic's use for infectious problems predates written history. Sanskrit records reveal garlic remedies used 5,000 years ago, and the Chinese have been using garlic more than 3,000 years. In the West, the use of garlic for numerous ailments can be traced back to Hippocrates, Aristotle, and Pliny.

A large amount of research has shown that garlic has many immuno-potentiating properties, most of which are thought to be due to volatile factors composed of sulfur-containing compounds: allicin, diallyl disulfide, diallyl trisulfide, and others. Fresh garlic, commercial products containing allicin, and aged garlic preparations have all shown these properties. Garlic enhances the pathogen-attacking activity of T cells, neutrophils, and macrophages; increases the secretion of interleukin; and increases natural killer cell activity.[107,108,109,110] The increase in natural killer cell activity was a remarkable 140% in those eating the equivalent of two bulbs a day and 156% in those consuming 1,800 mg of odorless aged garlic. In addition, garlic (but not in the aged forms) has been shown to have broad-spectrum antimicrobial activity against many types of bacteria, viruses, worms, and fungi.[111]

- *Typical dosage:* one-half bulb three times a day or the equivalent in processed garlic products

Panax ginseng (Korean ginseng)

Although best known for its help with stress, ginseng also offers benefits for the immune system, even for those who are apparently healthy. In one study, three groups of 20 healthy volunteers were given either 100 mg of a water extract of ginseng, 100 mg of a lactose placebo, or 100 mg of a standardized ginseng extract (4% ginsenosides) every 12 hours for eight weeks. Within four weeks, the ginseng groups showed increased numbers of lymphocytes in the blood and increased phagocytosis of pathogens. The immune stimulation was even greater after eight weeks. The standardized Panax ginseng extract was the most effective, probably due to its higher content of ginsenosides, ginseng's most important active constituents.[112] Ginseng has also been shown to restore the immune system when damaged by cyclosphamide, a highly toxic drug used in chemotherapy treatment of breast cancer.[113]

In one study of mice, oral administration of large dosages for five to six days resulted in dramatic increases in antibody formation (IgG and IgM increased by 50 and 100%, respectively), natural killer cell activity (44 to 150% increase), and interferon production.[114] The results were dosage dependent. Such dramatic immune system enhancement seems incredible. However, the dosages (equivalent in human adults of 500 to 125,000 mg per day) are far outside those normally used and safely recommended. Ginseng is best used for long-term strengthening of the immune system.

- *Typical dosage:* 3 (500 mg each) capsules three times a day

Eleutherococcus senticosus (Siberian Ginseng)

The other ginseng, known as Siberian ginseng, also improves immune function. In 36 healthy volunteers, 10 ml (one third of an ounce) of a standardized alcohol extract of Eleutherococcus senticosus resulted in a dramatic increase in the number of immune cells in the blood. Particularly elevated were the T lymphocytes (especially the helper/inducer T cells) and cytotoxic and natural killer cells. Not only were there more T lymphocytes, but their activity increased.[115]

- *Typical dosage:* one third ounce of fluid extract or 3 (500 mg each) capsules three times a day

Bromelain

Although bromelain does not enhance immune function per se, it is nonetheless a valuable aid to the immune system when fighting some infectious conditions. Bromelain, the enzyme extracted from the stem of the pineapple plant (Ananas comopsus), has several effects, the most important of which are increasing the absorption of antimicrobial agents and dissolving the mucus that bacteria use to protect themselves from the immune system.[116] Some studies found that bromelain was as effective as antibiotics in treating a variety of infectious processes, e.g., pneumonia, perirectal abscess, cutaneous staphylococcus infection, pyelonephritis, and bronchitis.[117]

- *Typical dosage:* 3 (2,500 mcu each) capsules three times a day between meals

Thymus extracts

As discussed above, the thymus, the master gland of the immune system, degenerates with age and stress. Fortunately, this can be at least partially reversed by taking extracts of calf thymus. As a vegetarian, I don't usually recommend using animal products, but at times they are quite useful. A modest amount of research has now shown that thymus extract supplements can improve immune function, decrease food allergies, and improve resistance to chronic respiratory tract infections.[118]

- *Typical dosage:* 3 (500 mg each) capsules three times a day

Exercise

Regular, moderate exercise augments immune surveillance through heightened cell-mediated immunity.[119] Positive benefits have been demonstrated even in such immunological disasters as HIV infection. However, excessive exercise can depress immune function by decreasing the number of available white cells.[120]

Fighting Bacterial Infections Naturally

How to Tell When You Have a Bacterial Infection

Bacterial infections usually occur in the skin and mucous membranes and are usually accompanied by fever and swollen lymph nodes. Common bacterial infections include impetigo (a highly contagious skin infection in children characterized by weepy honey-colored lesions on the skin) and boils and carbuncles (large boils). More serious are cellulitis (a bacterial infection deep into the tissues characterized by large areas of swelling and redness that are very serious if accompanied by red streaks), pneumonia, and strep throat (any throat infection that continues for a few days or is associated with high fever and swelling of several lymph nodes in the neck requires the immediate attention of a physician).

Antibacterial Herbs

Many botanicals, especially essential oils, have been shown to be very effective antimicrobial agents. My favorite is goldenseal, which can be used both internally and externally.

The Power of Goldenseal

Ed was rarely sick and primarily saw me for health maintenance. So when he called and told me he was so ill he couldn't come to see me in my office, I was quite concerned and went to visit him at his home. As soon as I saw him it was obvious that Ed was quite sick. This normally vital man was lying limply in bed and his glazed eyes, sweating, and red forehead suggested a high fever due to some kind of severe infection. Examining him, I saw a large inflamed abscess on his knee with several red streaks running up his thigh. I immediately recognized this as cellulitis (infection and inflammation in the tissues around the wound) complicated with lymphadenitis (infection and inflammation in the lymph vessels draining the infected area). Such a condition can be very dangerous and if treatment is delayed or ineffective, it can progress to septicemia (infection in the blood), overwhelming infection, and death. It appeared to me that he was close (or perhaps had already progressed) to septicemia. I recommended immediate antibiotics and warned him that if he didn't rapidly improve we would have to hospitalize him for intravenous antibiotics.

Unfortunately, Ed was a fanatic who refused to use synthetic drugs or see a medical doctor. This was normally a good strategy for him because he was quite conscientious and took good care of himself. The problem started when he had badly cut his knee on a coral reef while diving in Hawaii. Such wounds commonly become infected due to the constant wetness and irritating chemicals from the coral. Functioning effectively, his immune system worked hard and after a week had walled off the wound, forming a fairly large abscess. Over the next week the abscess was slowly resolving and Ed thought all was well. Then he fell on his knee during a basketball game and broke open the abscess, spreading the infectious materials throughout the tissues of his knee. This rapidly overwhelmed his immune system. He tried to treat it himself with extra vitamin C and some *Echinacea* tea—but it was too little too late.

Since I was unable to talk him into antibiotics, I immediately instituted a very aggressive natural medicine program: 2,000 mg of vitamin C, one-half ounce of *Echinacea* fluid extract and six (500 mg) capsules of goldenseal root powder every two hours. A goldenseal paste (root powder mixed with tincture) was applied directly to the abscess. I didn't recommend extra vitamin A or zinc since I knew his nutritional status was already very good. Before leaving, I told his wife to immediately call me if he got worse (at which point I would have refused to treat him at home any longer).

When I saw him the next day, I found that the red streak was only half as long, and Ed was already feeling better. Within a few days, he was out of bed and the abscess then quickly resolved. While this is a remarkable example of just how strong herbs can be, don't try to treat cellulitis, septicemia, or lymphadinitis at home by yourself! These are dangerous diseases that require immediate expert medical intervention.

■ *The message*: Goldenseal is a remarkably effective herbal antibiotic but don't be too fanatical—medical intervention really is needed at times to save your life.

Hydrastis canadensis (Goldenseal)

Goldenseal is a remarkably effective and safe antibacterial herb and has been referred to as the "naturopathic antibiotic." Goldenseal was a mainstay of the Native American medicine man from whom the Eclectic physicians of the 18th century and, later, naturopathic physicians learned of its use. Most research has focused on *berberine sulfate*, the most active antibacterial alkaloid in goldenseal. Although not as potent as many prescription antibiotics (which typically are synthesized or come from fungi), berberine exhibits a broad range of antibiotic action. Berberine has shown antimicrobial activity against many bacteria, protozoa, and fungi.[121,122,123,124,125]

Its action against some of these pathogens is actually stronger than that of commonly used antibiotics. Also, unlike many antibiotics, goldenseal leaves the good bacteria (lactobacilli) in our intestines alone. In addition, berberine inhibits candida as well as other pathogenic bacteria that grow as a common side effect of antibiotic use. Table 4-4 lists the *in vitro* (meaning "in a test tube") sensitivity of various organisms to berberine sulfate. Berberine sulfate has been used for centuries as an effective antimicrobial agent in China and India.

Berberine is a more effective antimicrobial agent in an alkaline than an acid solution.[126] At a pH of 8.0 (which is alkaline), its antimicrobial activity *in vitro* is typically two to four times greater than it is at a pH of 7.0 (which is neutral). At an acid pH of 6.0, berberine is only one-fourth as strong as at a neutral pH. This suggests that alkalinization will improve its clinical effectiveness, particularly in the treatment of urinary tract infections. Alkalinity can be increased by consuming less animal products and more plant foods, especially fruits. While this may seem to be a contradiction because most fruits are acidic, digestion of the fruit uses up all their acid components, leaving an alkaline residue.

Also of interest is berberine's ability to block the adherence of bacteria-like *Streptococci* (which causes strep throat) to human cells. This is a very helpful defense, since bacteria need to attach to mucous membranes and skin cells before they can penetrate into our bodies.[127]

■ *Typical antibiotic dosage*: 3 (500 mg each) capsules three times a day; make a paste with tincture and root powder for local application.

Table 4-4 Bacteria Inhibited by Berberine Sulfate

Bacterium	
Bacillus cereus	Pseudomonas mangiferae
B. cereus	P. pyocyanea
B. subtilis	Salmonella paratyphi
Corynebacterium diphtheria	S. typhimurium
Enterobacter aerogenes	Shigella boydii
Escherichia coli	Staphylococcus aureus
Klebsiella sp.	Streptococcus pyogenes
K. pneumoniae	Vibrio cholerae
Mycobacterium tuberculosis	Xanthomonas citri
Proteus sp.	

Allium sativum (Garlic)

As far back as 1944, researchers have found that both garlic and garlic products containing allicin inhibited the growth of Staphylococcus, Streptococcus, Bacillus, Brucella, and Vibrio species, even at low concentrations.[128,129] Table 4-5 shows additional types of bacteria that are killed by garlic. In these studies, the antimicrobial effects of garlic were found to compare favorably to commonly used antibiotics such as penicillin, streptomycin, chloramphenicol, erythromycin, and tetracycline. Besides confirming garlic's well-known antibacterial effects, the studies also demonstrated garlic's effectiveness in inhibiting the growth of some bacteria that had become resistant to one or more of the antibiotics. Garlic has been shown to significantly reduce the number of coliforms and anaerobes in the feces, very important in decreasing toxic bacteria in the intestines.[132]

- *Typical antibiotic dosage:* one-half clove three times a day or the equivalent in capsules; apply the juice locally; insert peeled clove in vagina overnight for vaginal infection.

Aloe vera

Aloe has demonstrated effective activity against many common bacteria in several studies. In the most detailed of these studies, Robson et al. assayed the antimicrobial properties of an Aloe vera extract and reviewed the work of others.[133] Both mean inhibitory and mean lethal concentrations were determined and compared with silver sulfadiazine, a potent antiseptic used in the treatment of

Table 4-5 Bacteria Inhibited by Garlic[130,131]

Alpha- and beta-hemolytic Streptococcus	Mycobacteria
Citrobacter sp.	Proteus vulgaris
Escherichia coli	Salmonella enteritidis
Klebsiella pneumoniae	Staphylococcus aureus

Table 4-6 Bacteria Inhibited by *Aloe vera* Extract Compared to Silver Sulfadiazine (measured as mm of inhibition zone—the bigger the number the better)

Organism	Aloe vera	Silver Sulfadiazine
Bacillus subtilis	19 mm	14 mm
Enterobacter cloacae	14	12
Escherichia coli	16	12
Klebsiella aeruginosa	17	12
Klebsiella pneumoniae	14	6
S. agalactiae	16	12
S. faecalis	6	11
Staphylococcus aureus	18	12
Streptococcus pyogenes	16	12

extensive burns. As evident in Table 4-6, the antimicrobial effects of *Aloe vera* compare quite favorably to silver sulfadiazine. Other studies showed aloe inhibited *Mycobacterium tuberculosis*, *Trichophyton species*, and *Bacillus subtilis*.[134] Against common skin pathogens, the antimicrobial activity of *Aloe vera* gel in a cream base was shown to be slightly better than silver sulfadiazine.

- *Typical antibiotic dosage:* apply undiluted juice locally or use as a douche

Glycyrrhiza glabra (Licorice root)
Although best known for its antiviral activity, alcohol extracts of licorice root have displayed antimicrobial activity *in vitro* (in a test tube) against the bacteria listed in Table 4-7.[135] The majority of the antimicrobial effects are due to licorice's flavonoid components.

- *Typical antibiotic dosage:* 3 (500 mg each) capsules three times a day

Melaleuca alternafolia (Tea tree oil)
The oil extracted from the tea tree has been used for decades in the treatment of infections. As can be seen in Table 4-8, tea tree oil is effective against a wide range of organisms.

- *Typical antibiotic dosage:* apply oil (dilute with olive oil if your skin is sensitive) locally several times a day

Table 4-7 Microorganisms Inhibited by *Glycyrrhiza glabra*

Candida albicans
Mycobacterium smegmatis
Staphylococcus aureus
Streptococcus mutans

Table 4-8 Bacteria Inhibited by *Melaleuca alternafolia*[136]

Bacillus subtili	*Lactobacillus acidophilus*
Bacteroides fragilis	*Mycobacterium smegmatsi*
Branhamell catarrhalis	*Pseudomonas aeruginosa*
Clostridium perfingens	*Serratia marcescens*
Enterococcus faecalis	*Staphylococcus aureus*
Escherichia coli	

Fighting Viral Infections Naturally

How to Tell When You Have a Viral Infection

The most frequent infections we suffer are viral. Common examples include the common cold, influenza, herpes, warts, and gastroenteritis. More serious examples include AIDS, hepatitis, and meningitis. Most viral infections are mild and resolve within a few days, especially if your immune system is working well. However, any infection that continues for more than a few days or is getting progressively worse requires the immediate attention of a physician.

Antiviral Herbs and Nutrients

Although there are few effective antiviral drugs, the world of botanical medicine has many safe and effective antiviral agents. In fact, there really is a cure for the common cold! Licorice root is my favorite and most clinically reliable antiviral herb.

Glycyrrhiza glabra (Licorice root)

Licorice root works both by supporting the immune system and by directly inhibiting various viruses. Glycyrrhizin and glycyrrhetinic acid, two active constituents of licorice root, have been shown to induce interferon.[137] The induction of interferon leads to significant antiviral activity, because interferon binds to cell surfaces where it stimulates synthesis of cellular proteins that inhibit the attachment of viruses to the cell, thereby blocking the production of viral DNA in infected cells. Interferon also increases the activity of macrophages and natural killer cells.

Glycyrrhizin has been shown to directly inhibit the growth of several DNA and RNA viruses in cell cultures (see Table 4-9) and to inactivate the *Herpes simplex* virus irreversibly.[138] Glycyrrhizin also inhibits the thymus-damaging and immunosuppressive action of cortisone.[139] Caution should be exercised in its use, however. Long-term use of large dosages (greater than three grams of root daily for more than six weeks) will increase blood pressure in some people. This hypertensive effect can by avoided if the nutrient glycine is taken along with the licorice root.[140]

Table 4-9 Viruses Inhibited by *Glycyrrhiza glabra*

Hepatitis viruses	Newcastle disease
Herpes simplex types 1 and 2	*Vaccinia virus*
Human immunodeficiency virus (HIV)	*Vesicular stomatitis virus*

- *Typical antiviral dosage:* 3 (500 mg each) capsules three times a day; apply ointment (3% glycyrrhetinic acid) locally until symptoms resolve

Melissa offinalis (Lemon balm)

Lemon balm has a long history of use for feverish conditions, which often occur during viral infections. Reputable double-blind clinical studies have demonstrated that oral consumption of extract of lemon balm is effective in treating several viral infections, those listed in Table 4-10. Polyphenols and tannins have been shown responsible for these antiviral effects. In addition, a cream containing 1% dried lemon balm extract applied five times a day was found to shorten the time needed to heal herpes infections. However, it was only effective if applied early in the infection.[141]

- *Typical antiviral dosage:* 3 (500 mg each) capsules every three hours; cream containing 1% dried lemon balm extract applied locally

Aloe vera

Acemannan, the polysaccharide extracted from the *Aloe vera* plant, is not only an immune stimulant, it is also antiviral. Acemannan has been shown to be active against many viruses, including HIV, influenza virus, and measles virus.[142] Perhaps its most interesting clinical application is with AIDS patients when used in conjunction with AZT. In these patients, it appears to act synergistically, decreasing the amount of drug needed with resultant decreased toxic effects and cost. The clinical results with AIDS patients have, however, been inconsistent, with some studies showing improvements in several measures of the immune system as well as increased longevity of AIDS patients, while other studies showed little effect.[143]

Table 4-10 Viruses Inhibited by *Melissa officinalis*

Newcastle disease
Herpes simplex
Mumps
Vaccina virus

Table 4-11 Viruses Inhibited by *Aloe vera*

Feline leukemia virus
Human immunodeficiency virus (HIV)
Influenza virus
Measles virus

Acemannan in injectable form has been approved for veterinary use in fibrosarcomas and feline leukemia. Its action in feline leukemia is quite impressive. Feline leukemia, like AIDS, is caused by a retrovirus (Feline leukemia virus or FeLV). The virus is so lethal that once cats develop clinical symptoms, they are usually euthanized. Typically, over 70% of cats will die within eight weeks of the onset of clinical signs. In a study of 44 cats with clinically confirmed feline leukemia, acemannan was injected (2 mg/kg) weekly for six weeks, and the cats were re-examined six weeks after termination of treatment.[144] At the end of the 12-week study, 71% of the cats were alive and in good health.

- *Typical antiviral dosage:* 800 mg of acemannan or one quart of *Aloe vera* juice per day

Astragalus membranaceus
Astragalus is a Chinese herb traditionally used to treat infections. Some research supports its antiviral activity. In one study, ten patients suffering from a very serious disease, Coxsackie B viral myocarditis, with depressed natural killer cell activity were treated with *Astragalus*. After three to four months of intramuscular injection, natural killer cell activity improved 12 to 45%, while the untreated patients' natural killer cell activity did not change. In addition, the clinical condition of the *Astragalus*-treated patients improved.[145]

- *Typical antiviral dosage:* 3 (500 mg each) capsules three times per day

Allium sativum (Garlic)
The *in vitro* virucidal effects of various forms and components of garlic have been determined against a variety of viruses. The virucidal effectiveness of garlic's components was found to be:

agoene (most effective) > allicin >
allyl methyl thiosulfinate > methyl allyl thiosulfinate

Agoene is found in oil extracts of garlic, but not in fresh garlic extracts. Fresh garlic extract, however, was still found to be virucidal against all viruses tested. Commercial products vary greatly in their composition. Those with the highest level of allicin and other thiosulfinates had the best virucidal activity.[146] Table 4-12 lists the viruses known to be susceptible to garlic.

- *Typical antiviral dosage:* one-half clove three times a day or the equivalent in capsules

Table 4-12 Viruses Inhibited by Garlic

Herpes simplex type 1	*Parainfluenza virus* type 3
Herpes simplex type 2	*Vaccinia virus*
Human rhinovirus type 2	*Vesicular stomatitis virus*

Echinacea angustifolia

Although *Echinacea*'s primary value is as an immune stimulant, it does have some direct antiviral effects. Table 4-13 list the viruses inhibited by *Echinacea*.

- *Typical antiviral dosage:* one-half ounce of juice of flower or 4 (500 mg each) capsules of root three times per day

Zinc

Zinc inhibits *in vitro* the growth of several viruses, including: rhino (cold), picorna and toga (encephalitis, rubella), *Herpes simplex* (oral and genital herpes) and *Vaccinia virus* (cowpox).[147] A double-blind clinical study demonstrated that zinc gluconate lozenges (containing 23 milligrams of zinc) significantly reduced the average duration of the common cold by seven days.[148] The patients were instructed to dissolve one lozenge in their mouths every two waking hours after an initial double dose. After seven days, 86% of the 37 zinc-treated subjects were asymptomatic, compared to 46% of the 28 placebo-treated subjects. The authors hypothesized that the local zinc concentration was high enough to inhibit the replication of the cold viruses. The topical application of a 0.01 to 0.025% zinc sulfate solution has been shown to be effective in both ameliorating symptoms and inhibiting recurrences of *Herpes simplex* infection.[149]

- *Typical antiviral dosage:* 1 (15 mg each) zinc lozenge every two hours; topical application of ointment containing 0.05% zinc

Fighting Fungal Infections Naturally

How to Tell When You Have a Fungal Infection

Fungi are the most common chronic infections of the skin. Typical examples include ringworm, nail infections, athlete's foot, and jock itch. Fungi can also infect the mucous membranes of the intestines and vagina. Vaginal yeast infections are characterized by an itchy, cheesy odorous discharge.

Table 4-13 Viruses Inhibited by *Echinacea*

Herpes
Influenza
Vesicular stomatitis virus

Antifungal Herbs

The essential oils of virtually every herb are antifungal. However, some are far more effective than others. Tea tree oil is my favorite.

Melaleuca alternafolia (Tea tree oil)

While tea tree oil is a very effective antibacterial agent, its greatest clinical use appears to be in the topical treatment of fungal infections. One of the most reliable antifungal herbs, the oil extracted from the tea tree has been used for decades in the topical treatment of fungal infections such as *Candida albicans*. Clinically, tea tree oil is used for skin infections, vaginal infections, and common nail infections.[150] The oil is applied locally for skin and nail infections and a tampon saturated with a 40% solution is used for vaginal infections.

- *Typical antifungal dosage:* apply oil (dilute with olive oil if your skin is sensitive) locally; tampon soaked in a 40% solution of tea tree oil in water used overnight for vaginal infections

Allium sativum (Garlic)

Garlic has been shown to have a broad spectrum of activity against 17 strains of fungi and was more effective than nystatin (a drug frequently prescribed for fungal infections) against pathogenic yeasts.[151] Highly concentrated extracts of garlic containing 34% allicin, 44% total thiosulfinates, and 20% vinyldithiins were found to be effective against the fungus *Cyrptococcus neoformans*.[152] From a clinical perspective, inhibition of *Candida albicans* has the most significance; both animal and *in vitro* (in a test tube) studies have shown garlic to be more potent than nystatin, gentian violet, and six other reputed antifungal agents.[153,154,155] In one study at a major Chinese hospital, garlic therapy alone was used effectively in the treatment of cryptococcal meningitis, one of the most serious fungal infections known.[156]

- *Typical antifungal dosage:* 1 clove three times a day or the equivalent in capsules

Hydrastis canadensis (Goldenseal)

Although goldenseal is used primarily as an antibacterial agent, it is also quite effective against several fungi. I find it useful when applied as a paste (made

Table 4-14 Fungi Inhibited by Goldenseal

Candida utilis	*Saccharomyces cerevisiae*
C. albicans	*Sporothrix schenkii*
Cryptococcus neoformans	*Trichophyton mentagrophytes*
Microsporum gypseum	

from mixing the tincture and root powder) directly to the infected area and then covered to keep it from being wiped off.

- *Typical antifungal dosage:* 3 (500 mg each) capsules three times per day; paste made of root powder and tincture applied locally

Fighting Parasitic Infections Naturally

How to Tell When You Have a Parasitic Infection

Parasitic infections are far more common than generally realized. The number of infections is increasing due to increased travel abroad and immigration from Third World countries. Unfortunately, most doctors miss these infections because they are not well-covered in medical school, and few laboratories are willing to be rigorous in their testing (it requires working with feces—not very pleasant!).

Parasite infections are often asymptomatic. They are most easily recognized when the worm is seen in the stool or when chronic inexplicable symptoms develop after visiting a Third World country or coming into close contact with someone who has.

Antiparasitic Herbs

Allium sativum (Garlic)
Raw garlic and garlic extracts have been shown to effectively destroy common intestinal parasites, including *Ascaris lumbricoides* (roundworm) and hookworms.[157]

- *Typical antiparasitic dosage:* 1 clove three times a day or the equivalent in capsules

Hydrastis canadensis (Goldenseal)
The plant alkaloid, berberine, which is found in several plants, especially goldenseal, has been found to inhibit the growth of several common parasites that invade the intestine and vagina (see Table 4-15).[158] Goldenseal has demonstrated experimental and clinical efficacy against internal and skin leishmaniasis (a type of parasite) and has been used effectively to treat cholera, giardiasis, and amoebiasis.

Berberine appears to be particularly of value for children because the medical drug of choice, metronidazole (Flagyl) has many significant side effects. In a study in India, children with giardiasis (a common intestinal infection, which causes chronic diarrhea, intestinal pain, and fatigue) were given either berberine sulfate (10 mg/kg/day) or metronidazole. After ten days, 90% of the berberine-treated group no longer had *Giardia* in their stools as compared to 95% in the Flagyl-treated group. Unlike the Flagyl-treated group, those receiving berberine suffered no negative side effects.[159]

- *Typical antiparasitic dosage:* 3 (500 mg each) goldenseal root capsules three times per day

Table 4-15 Parasite Sensitivity to Berberine Sulfate

Entamoeba histolytica	Giardia lamblia
Erwinia carotovora	Trichimonas vaginalis
Leishmania donovani	

Extra Help for Serious Infections

Even for those with very serious infections, herbal medicines can help. In an interesting study, a flavonoid extract, Ginkgolide B, from the leaves of Ginkgo biloba proved to be quite helpful for patients hospitalized with sepsis, a very serious infection of the blood. In this study, 262 patients were treated with antibiotics and then randomly provided either a placebo or the Ginkgo extract. For those patients with gram negative infections, 52% of the placebo patients died, while the mortality rate of those given the Ginkgo extract decreased to 33%—a remarkable improvement.[160]

How to Treat Some Common Infections

The following provide examples of specific therapies of value for some common infectious diseases. Please note: I am assuming that you have already used the above guidelines for strengthening your immune system, i.e., the factors that damage the immune system have been controlled and your nutrition has been optimized.

Sinusitis

Chronic sinusitis is one of our most common health problems, affecting 15 to 20% of the adult population. The most common predisposing factor in acute bacterial sinusitis is viral upper respiratory infection, i.e., the common cold. However, allergic rhinitis (nasal allergy) typically precedes the cold, especially for those with chronic sinus problems. In fact, anything that causes swelling of the mucous membranes may result in obstruction of sinus drainage. The fluids that build up in the sinuses are an excellent growth medium for a wide range of organisms, with Streptococci, Pneumococci, Staphylococci, and Haemophilus influenzae being the most common. A long-term cure requires control of these predisposing factors—simply killing the bacteria provides only short-term relief.

In acute sinusitis, the therapeutic goals are to reestablish normal drainage and clear up the acute infection. Drainage can be increased by local application of heat and steam with volatile oils such as eucalyptus. The infection can be eliminated through the use of immune support and antibacterial botanicals such as goldenseal, used both internally and as a nasal douche. Acute sinusitis also responds well to bromelain (the enzyme extracted from pineapples), probably due to bromelain's ability to help clear the mucus that was blocking drainage. In one study, good-to-excellent results were obtained in 87% of bromelain-treated patients, compared with 68% of the placebo group.[161]

In chronic sinusitis, an allergic condition is almost always present, and in 25%, there is an underlying dental infection. Although antihistamines can provide short-term relief, their chronic use is contraindicated, not only because they eventually stop working but also because there is usually a reflex increase in congestion following discontinuation. Long-term control is dependent on isolation and elimination of the allergenic food or air-borne allergens.

Suggested treatment

To support the immune system, for one week use 50,000 iu per day of vitamin A or beta-carotene (200,000 iu per day), 1,000 mg of vitamin C every two hours during the acute stage, and 25 mg per day of zinc. Swallow one teaspoon of a tincture composed of *Echinacea angustifolia* (three parts) and *Hydrastis canadensis* (two parts) or three (500 mg each) capsules of *Echinacea* and two (500 mg each) capsules of goldenseal every two hours. If the infection is especially bad, douche your nose with a tea made of goldenseal (2 tsp of root powder plus 250 mg of vitamin C per cup). This douching can be accomplished by spraying the tea into your nose with a syringe. Finally, (this therapy might eliminate your social life), chew half a clove of garlic every few hours. If chewing garlic alone is too unpalatable, mix the garlic clove with bread or some other food to moderate the taste.

Urinary Tract Infection (Cystitis)

Urinary tract infections are common in women, affecting 21% of women in the U.S. every year. For an unfortunate 2 to 4%, their urinary tract infections are essentially continuous. Women visit physicians over 5 million times a year for this uncomfortable condition. Obviously, improving the immune system will help considerably. However, urinary infections will still occur at times, and because the antibiotics commonly used for this condition have undesirable side effects, botanicals are a welcome therapeutic alternative. In addition, some botanicals can be of great help to women who suffer from chronic urinary tract infections.

Suggested treatment

One of the natural treatments with the longest history of use is to simply drink cranberry juice, also known as *Vaccinum macrocarpon*. In a reputable study, 153 women (average age 78.5 years) with chronic urinary tract infections were entered in a randomized, double-blind, placebo-controlled trial testing the effect of regular cranberry juice consumption on the level of bacteria and white blood cells in their urine (both measures of infection). They drank 10 ounces of cranberry juice per day or a placebo drink. Both contained vitamin C and were sweetened with saccharin (the latter is important considering the negative impact on the immune system of the amount of sugar in regularly sweetened juice). The results were dramatic, with the women drinking cranberry juice having only 42% the level of bacteria and white cells of the placebo group.[162] Another study showed that as little as 4 to 6 ounces of cranberry juice a day significantly prevented urinary tract infections in the elderly.[163] The cranberry juice apparently works though several mechanisms: inhibiting the adherence of bacteria to the urinary tract mucosa, direct antibacterial effects, and increasing the acidity of the urine.

Inhibiting the adherence of bacteria to the mucosal cells of the bladder is one key mechanism by which cranberry juice works.[164] Interestingly, blueberry juice may be just as effective in blocking adherence. In a study of seven juices (cranberry, blueberry, grapefruit, guava, mango, orange, and pineapple) only cranberry and blueberry blocked the adherence of *Esherichia coli*.[165]

The basic approach is to prevent infection through support of the immune system with optimal nutrition, the regular consumption of large amounts of fluids, and inhibition of bacterial growth by drinking 6 to 10 ounces of cranberry juice a day and ingesting 3 (500 mg each) capsules of *Echinacea* three times a day. If an infection does develop, large dosages of *Hydrastis canadensis* (1 tsp of root powder in a tea every three hours) and garlic (two cloves a day) are very effective.

While many cases of urinary tract infections will respond well and rapidly to this type of treatment, it is always wise to have a physician make sure the infection has cleared up. Even in antibiotic-treated urinary tract infections, some patients progress to kidney infections, with serious consequences.

Influenza and the Common Cold

Although influenza and viral rhinitis (common cold) affect almost everyone one or more times a year, there is no effective medical drug for their treatment. There are, however, several herbs that actually help us to recover more rapidly from these common infections. One of the best is *Echinacea*. While not considered a strong antiviral herb, it's been shown to be effective for both the flu and the common cold.

In an illustrative study, 180 patients with influenza aged 18 to 60 were given either *Echinacea purpurea* extract at a dose of 450 mg, *E. purpurea* at a dose of 900 mg, or placebo. Those taking the 450 mg dosage did no better than the placebo, while those taking the larger dose experienced a significant reduction in symptoms.[166] This provides support for the common wisdom that large dosages of *Echinacea* need to be used for efficacy. In another study, 108 patients with recurrent colds received either an extract of the fresh juice of *Echinacea purpurea* (Echinacin), 4 ml twice a day, or placebo for eight weeks. During this time, 35.2% of the *Echinacea* group remained symptom-free as compared to 25.9% of the placebo group. The length of time between infections in the *Echinacea* group was 40 days, but only 25 days for the placebo. The *Echinacea* patients who got colds had less severe symptoms and recovered more quickly. Those patients with the weakest immune system (i.e., helper T cell to suppresser T cell ratio <1.5) benefited the most.[167]

Herpes

Over 90% of us have had a herpes infection on our lips by age five, and some continue to have recurrent attacks throughout their life. There is no medical treatment to prevent recurrence or shorten the length of an attack. Fortunately, *Echinacea purpurea* can help decrease the frequency of attacks and licorice root can reducing healing time and pain.

Suggested treatment
One ounce of *Echinacea* flower juice or six (500 mg each) capsules of the root powder every three hours used immediately upon experiencing the earliest symptoms of a herpes (neuralgia and pain) can not only abort the outbreak, but, when used consistently, can decrease the frequency of attacks.[168]

Topical application of extracts from licorice root (an ointment made with 3% glycyrrhizinic acid) has also been shown to be quite helpful in reducing the healing time and pain associated with recurrent oral and genital herpes.[169,170] Rub the ointment on the affected area several times a day until symptoms cease. As mentioned above, glycyrrhizin inactivates *Herpes simplex* virus irreversibly and stimulates the synthesis and release of interferon.

Nail Fungal Infections

Fungal infections of the fingernails can be a very frustrating health problem. While improving immune function is, of course, very important, it's often just not enough. Fortunately, some herbs have been found to be especially effective. The herb receiving perhaps the most research in this area is the oil of the tea tree plant.

Suggested treatment
In a double-blind study of 117 patients with distal onychomycosis (the technical name for fungal infections of the fingernails), patients either applied tea tree oil (100% solution) or placebo twice a day for six months. After six months, 50% of the treated group had partial or complete resolution as compared to essentially no improvement in the placebo group.[171] Tea tree oil is strong medicine and can be irritating to sensitive skin. Younger children and those with sensitive skin should use a solution diluted in olive oil.

Chronic Trichomonal or Candidal Vaginitis

Chronic vaginitis from candida or trichomonas is a common problem for women. Improving immune function and using herbs locally can help a lot.

Serious Acute Infection

One evening, I was called to the home of Mary, a 30-year-old who had once seen me for chronic depression, but had not followed through on her program. The previous week, she had had a cold, but although she took extra vitamin C, it was lingering on. She now felt quite sick and did not want to get out of bed. She had a high fever (103.5°F), no energy, felt like she couldn't catch her breath, and was coughing up sputum that looked like it was stained with rust. A quick listen to her lungs confirmed my diagnosis: pneumonia, which later lab studies demonstrated to be bacterial.

While I could have used nutrition and herbal medicine to treat this, her infection was so well-established and she was so debilitated, that we simply didn't have enough time. For this patient, my prescription was penicillin, which worked well, and within three days she felt considerably better. After her health stabilized, we developed a plan to strengthen her immune system and deal with her depression.

- *The message:* High fever, debility, and/or organ dysfunction (e.g., difficulty breathing) indicate a serious infection requiring immediate professional intervention; improve immune function after the acute problem is resolved.

Suggested treatment

Besides scrupulously avoiding sugar and any other immune depressant, inserting a tampon saturated with a 40% solution of tea tree oil in water is very effective, with all women experiencing either a compete cure or dramatic reduction in symptoms after leaving the tampon in overnight.[172]

When to See a Physician

While most acute infections are either self-limiting, i.e., the body will cure itself, or self-treatable with natural medicines, sometimes professional intervention is necessary. In general, see a doctor when a fever is high (above 102°F) for over two days; you are having trouble with an organ system, e.g., difficult breathing (possible pneumonia), severe urine pain associated with back or flank pain (possible kidney infection), an infection in an eye; or the symptoms are just not resolving very quickly.

Summary

A well-functioning immune system is absolutely essential for optimal health. Without an active immune system we suffer from frequent and chronic infections and will likely ultimately succumb to cancer. Fortunately, there is much we can do to strengthen our immune system.

First, use Table 4-2 to identify and correct any aspect of your diet, lifestyle, or environment that is damaging your immune system. Second, ensure you are taking an extra amount of the nutrients key to proper functioning of your immune system. This can be done by taking a good quality multivitamin and mineral supplement, by taking extra vitamins A (50,000 iu) and C (2,000 mg) and zinc (25 mg), or eating extra amounts of foods high in these nutrients.

Finally, until your immune system is running at full speed, regularly take the herbs recommended here to boost your immune system. My preferences are *Echinacea* (4 [500 mg each] capsules or ½ tsp of fluid extract three times a day), shiitake mushroom (2 [500 mg each] capsules three times a day), and ginseng (100 mg of a standardized ginseng extract—4% ginsenosides—three times a day).

If you need to treat an acute or chronic infection, use the herbs recommended in the sections above for bacterial, viral, fungal, and parasitic infections.

Chapter Five

Decreasing Toxicity

Study this chapter if you suffer from any of the following:

- *Symptoms*

  Chronic headaches

  Foul smelling breath or stools

  Chronic fatigue

  Feeling of toxicity (dull headaches, chronic hangover as if from too much alcohol)

  Sensitivity to chemicals

  Caffeine-containing drinks and foods keep you awake

  Chronic allergies

  Unexplained itching

- *Diseases*

  Acne

  Anemia

  Autoimmune disease (e.g., lupus erythematosis, rheumatoid arthritis)

  Cancer

  Eczema

  Gallstones

  Gilbert's syndrome

  Inflammatory bowel disease

  Psoriasis

  Toxemia of pregnancy

  Hives or urticaria (an itchy skin rash usually caused by allergic reaction)

  Liver disease, especially acute or chronic hepatitis

Behaviors that increase risk:

- Using birth control pills or other hormones
- Diet deficient in vitamin C, the B vitamins, magnesium, or zinc
- Using drugs (prescription, over-the-counter, and recreational)
- High levels of exposure to environmental toxins
- Use of broad-spectrum antibiotics, e.g., tetracycline
- Drinking large amounts of grapefruit juice
- Regular consumption of more than one alcoholic drink a day*

*1995 U.S. dietary guidelines define moderate intake as no more than one drink per day for women and two for men; one drink is 12 oz of beer, 5 oz of wine, or 1.5 oz of 80-proof liquor.

Thumbnail: Quick Support for Your Detoxification Systems

- *To directly neutralize toxins, especially free radials:*
  Beta-carotene: 25 mg per day
  Vitamin C: 2,000 mg per day
  Vitamin E: 600 iu per day
  Chlorophyll: 10 mg per day

- *To decrease the toxic load from the intestines:*
  Lactobacilli supplements (500 mg capsule twice a day between meals)
  Eat fructooligosaccharide-rich foods, such as onions, asparagus, and bananas
  Eat fiber-rich foods and take fiber supplements (40 or more gm of fiber each day)
  Avoid all allergenic foods

- *To improve the liver's detoxification abilities:*
  Regularly consume garlic and onions
  Take *Silybum marianum* (120 mg three times a day)
  Eat brassica family foods (cabbage, broccoli, brussels sprouts)
  Take glutathione (100 mg per day)

- *To detoxify systemically:*
  Do a modified fast (see discussion below)
  Take an extended sauna (see discussion below)

You're being poisoned. Bacteria in your intestines, toxins in the environment, food additives, and incomplete metabolic processes—all put poisons in your body that drain your energy and make you more susceptible to disease or even directly cause disease. Virtually every natural healing system, especially Ayurvedic medicine from India and naturopathic medicine in the U.S., recognizes the profound contribution of toxins to disease. Even conventional medicine is finally becoming aware of this problem and has coined the term *xenobiotic* to describe the toxins that come into our bodies from the environment.

While the concept of "toxicity" may sound quaint and unscientific, a surprising amount of research has documented its validity. The presence in the body of various types of toxic chemicals, heavy metals, partially broken down metabolites, bacterial toxins, and bacterial cell wall components has now been correlated with specific diseases and syndromes. These toxins are a serious threat to our health.

Toxicity is typically recognized in the bowel and liver and systemically throughout the body. In the bowel, the most common type of toxicity is called intestinal dysbiosis, which means that the bowel contains excessive levels of toxin-producing bacteria and inadequate amounts of normal health-promoting bacteria. Intestinal dysbiosis is typically caused by the use of broad-spectrum antibiotics, eating contaminated foods, not being breast fed, and/or a low fiber diet. The toxic effects of intestinal dysbiosis are diverse, ranging from chronic fatigue to autoimmune disease.

The other primary organ involved with toxicity is the liver. The liver is responsible for eliminating toxins from the blood or absorbed from a toxic bowel, either by disassembling them or by chemically converting them to less toxic forms more easily excreted by the kidneys. Our modern environment seriously overloads our liver, resulting in increased levels of circulating toxins in the blood, which damage most of our body's systems. A toxic liver sends out alarm signals, which manifest as acne, chronic headaches, inflammatory and autoimmune diseases, and chronic fatigue.

Chemicals can damage the body in an insidious and cumulative way. Once the detoxification system becomes overloaded, toxic metabolites accumulate, and we become progressively more sensitive to other chemicals, some of which are not normally toxic. This accumulation of toxins can wreak havoc on our normal metabolic processes.

The conventional medical approach of using drugs to merely alleviate symptoms not only doesn't deal with the underlying cause of the disease but compounds the problem by adding more toxins into the body. Putting drugs that also need to be detoxified into an already overloaded detoxification system increases systemic toxicity (identified as side effects) and can actually increase the individual's chemical sensitivity.

An effective detoxification system is a necessity for everyone. Even a person eating a natural whole-foods diet requires a healthy detoxification system because even healthful fruits and vegetables contain natural toxins that our bodies have, over the aeons, evolved metabolic processes to neutralize. The vast majority of chemicals consumed by humans are natural. According to some researchers, 99% of the pesticides we eat are naturally present in plants to ward off insects and other predators.[1] Even cooking our foods (especially frying), results in the production of toxic chemicals that our bodies must neutralize. If our detoxification systems are overloaded or aren't working properly because critical nutrients are lacking, toxicity results.

Fortunately, we have excellent defense enzymes, most of which the body will produce more of when we need them. Unfortunately, it takes time for the liver to synthesize these enzymes, so the first exposure to a toxin is the worst.

Real-Life Messages About Toxicity and Detoxification

Ted Got Sick Every Summer

Ted worked his way through college by painting houses every summer. At the end of every summer he was always sick, although no specific disease could be found by the doctors he visited. He would become chronically fatigued, he would have trouble thinking clearly, and he would lose his appetite. Finally, on the recommendation of a friend, he came to see me at the end of one summer. After hearing his story and physically examining him (he was very thin and his liver was tender) I quickly recognized that he was probably suffering from a combination of heavy metal poisoning from the paint he was scraping off houses and solvent toxicity inhaled from the paint as it dried. (Evaporating latex paint also gives off mercury.)

We took a sample of hair from the nape of his head and sent it to a laboratory to analyze it for heavy metals. As I expected, his levels of lead and mercury were greatly elevated. Since such an elevation in head hair lead can sometimes come from direct contamination of the hair from dust in the air rather than through the blood, we repeated the test on his pubic hair since it is protected by clothing. It was also elevated. Unfortunately, at the time, no test was available for measuring solvent damage to the liver.

I put him on a program to chelate the heavy metals out of his body and improve the function of his liver. For the heavy metals, I had him greatly increase his consumption of beans, vitamin-C–rich foods, pectin, and seaweed products. These foods contain compounds that bind to heavy metals, thus helping the body excrete them.

For his liver, I had him drink dandelion tea and supplement his diet with vitamins C and B complex. In addition, he took the herb milk thistle.

After a few months, his symptoms improved, and hair analysis showed that the heavy metals slowly left his body. He continued to paint each summer, and each summer his heavy metal levels would go up. But not as much as they had because he continued the program to help remove these toxins from his body and therefore didn't get as sick.

Ted was so impressed by the results and the better understanding of his body that he developed, that after graduating from the university he enrolled in Bastyr University and eventually graduated as a naturopathic doctor!

An Interesting Case of Pesticide Poisoning

Originally published by detoxification specialist Dr. William Rea, a leading clinician and researcher in environmental medicine, is an interesting case study of a 41-year-old, white, female nurse who developed inexplicable severe spasming of her muscles; spasming of the blood vessels supplying her heart (causing angina) and legs (causing pain and cramping); and low levels of T lymphocytes in her blood. Dr. Rea placed her in an environmental control unit (a special totally clean room with purified air, water, and food) for elimination of all toxins and allergens. This resulted in alleviation of her muscle cramps and artery spasms and her T lymphocytes increased.

She was then experimentally exposed to a pesticide. All her vascular and muscle spasm problems, including angina, returned and her T-lymphocyte count decreased by 19%. Her arterial spasming reaction was so severe, Dr. Rea couldn't even find a pulse in her legs. It took another four days on a pesticide-free diet, pure water, and a clean atmosphere for her symptoms to resolve and her T cells to return to normal.[2]

The Case That Introduced Me to Naturopathic Medicine

When I first came to Seattle, I got a job working as a research associate in the Department of Rheumatology of the University of Washington School of Medicine. I really enjoyed research and couldn't imagine a much better job than working together with M.D.s and Ph.D.s looking for a cure for rheumatoid arthritis.

Then came an event that changed my life forever. The woman who married my college roommate was cured of her juvenile rheumatoid arthritis by someone called a naturopathic doctor. I was stunned! How could this unknown practitioner "cure" my friend of an incurable disease from which she had suffered for over a decade? I "knew" rheumatoid arthritis was incurable since tens of millions of dollars were being spent nationwide looking for a cure for this disease, which afflicted 3% of the population.

I decided to visit this doctor and ask him what he had done. He offhandedly remarked, "Oh, I just detoxified her liver." Weird! But the more we talked, the more I came to appreciate a different way of thinking about patients and disease. I came to understand that the root cause of many chronic conditions is an overburdened, undernourished liver. What did this naturopathic doctor do for my friend's wife? Read on . . .

How the Detoxification System Works

The body eliminates toxins either by directly neutralizing them or by excreting them in the urine or feces (and to a lesser degree from the lungs and skin). Toxins that the body is unable to eliminate build up in the tissues, typically in our fat stores. The intestines, liver, and kidneys are the primary organs of detoxification (see Table 5-1).

Naturally occurring dietary toxins and contaminants, environmental chemicals (such as tobacco products, drugs, pesticides, food coloring, and food additives), and mutagens (derived from cooking, excess hormones in meat, and invading microbes) pose a serious threat to health. Enzymes in healthful intestinal bacteria and the cells lining the intestine transform many of these chemicals, either into immediately harmless metabolites or into even more toxic substances, which are then shunted to the liver where they are disarmed. About 25% of detoxification occurs within the cells lining the intestine; the remainder occurs in the liver.

The Liver

The liver is a complex organ that plays a key role in most metabolic processes, especially detoxification. To a very large extent, our health and vitality are

Table 5-1 Major Detoxification Systems

Organ	Method	Typical Toxin Neutralized
Skin	Excretion through sweat	Fat-soluble toxins such as DDT, heavy metals such as lead
Liver	Filtering of the blood	Bacteria and bacterial products, immune complexes
	Bile secretion	Cholesterol, hemoglobin breakdown products, extra calcium
	Phase I detoxification	Many prescription drugs (e.g., amphetamine, digitalis, pentobarbital), many over-the-counter drugs (acetaminophen, ibuprofen), caffeine, histamine, hormones (both internally produced and externally supplied), benzopyrene (carcinogen from charcoal-broiled meat), aniline (the yellow dyes), carbon tetrachloride, insecticides (e.g., Aldrin, Heptachlor), arachidonic acid (from animal fats)
	Phase II detoxification: Glutathione conjugation	Acetaminophen, nicotine from cigarette smoke, organophosphates (insecticides), epoxides (carcinogens)
	Amino acid conjugation	Benzoate (a common food preservative), aspirin
	Methylation	Dopamine (neurotransmitter), epinephrine (hormone from adrenal gland), histamine, thiouracil (cancer drug)
	Sulfation	Estrogen, aniline dyes, coumarin (blood thinner), acetaminophen, methyl-dopa (used for Parkinson's disease)
	Acetylation	Sulfonamides (antibiotics), mescaline
	Glucuronidation	Acetaminophen, morphine, diazepam (sedative, muscle relaxant), digitalis
	Sulfoxidation	Sulfites, garlic compounds
Intestines	Mucosal detoxification	Toxins from bowel bacteria
	Excretion through feces	Fat-soluble toxins excreted in the bile
Kidneys	Excretion through urine	Many toxins after they are made water-soluble by the liver

determined by the health and vitality of our liver. The liver is constantly bombarded with toxic chemicals, both those produced internally and those coming from the environment. The metabolic processes that make our bodies run normally produce a wide range of toxins for which the liver has evolved efficient neutralizing mechanisms. However, the level and type of internally produced

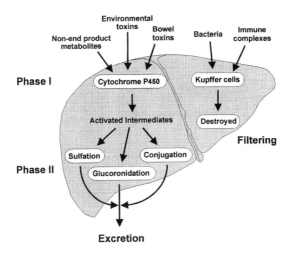

Figure 5-1 *The Liver's Detoxification Pathways*

toxins increases greatly when metabolic processes go awry, typically as a result of nutritional deficiencies.

Many of the toxic chemicals the liver must detoxify come from our environment: the content of our bowel, the food we eat, the water we drink, and the air we breathe. The polycyclic hydrocarbons (e.g., DDT; dioxin; 2,4,5-T; 2,4-D; PCB; and PCP), which are components of various herbicides and pesticides, are one example. Yet, as mentioned above, even those eating unprocessed organic foods need an effective detoxification system because even organically grown foods contain naturally occurring toxic constituents.

The liver plays several roles in detoxification: It filters the blood to remove large toxins, synthesizes and secretes bile full of cholesterol and other fat-soluble toxins, and enzymatically disassembles unwanted chemicals. This enzymatic process usually occurs in two steps referred to as Phase I and Phase II, with Phase I chemically modifying the chemicals to make them an easier target for one or more of the several Phase II enzyme systems. These processes are summarized in Figure 5-1.

Having an effective detoxification system is absolutely necessary for everyday health and prevention of chronic disease. For example, many diseases—including cancer, the autoimmune disorders (e.g., lupus erythematosis and rheumatoid arthritis), neurological disorders (e.g., Alzheimer's disease, Parkinson's disease), and the impairment of the immune system seen with aging—have been shown to be linked to a poorly functioning liver detoxification system.[3]

Proper functioning of the liver's detoxification systems is especially important for the prevention of cancer. Up to 90% of all cancers are thought to be due to the effects of environmental carcinogens, such as those in cigarette smoke, food, water, and air, combined with deficiencies of the nutrients the body needs for proper functioning of the detoxification and immune systems. Our levels of exposure to environmental carcinogens varies widely as does the efficiency of our detoxification enzymes. High levels of exposure to carcinogens coupled with sluggish detoxification enzymes significantly increases our susceptibility to cancer.

The link between our detoxification system's effectiveness and our susceptibility to environmental toxins, such as carcinogens, is exemplified in a study of Turin, Italy chemical plant workers who had an unusually high rate of bladder cancer. When the liver detoxification enzyme activity of all the workers was tested, those with the poorest detoxification system were the ones who developed bladder cancer.[4] In other words, all were exposed to the same level of carcinogens, but those with poor liver function were the ones who developed the cancer.

Fortunately, the detoxification efficiency of the liver can be improved with special nutrients and herbs, as I'll discuss later this chapter. Ultimately, your best protection from cancer is to avoid carcinogens and make sure your detoxification system is working well in order to eliminate those you can't avoid before they can hurt you.

Filtering the Blood

Almost two quarts of blood pass through the liver every minute for detoxification. Filtration of toxins is absolutely critical for the blood from the intestines because it is loaded with bacteria, endotoxins (toxins released when bacteria die and are broken down), antigen-antibody complexes (large molecules produced when the immune system latches on to an invader to neutralize it), and various other toxic substances.

This filtration is accomplished by Kupffer cells along with liver cells called hepatocytes. Together, these special cells, *when working properly*, clear 99% of the bacteria and other toxins from the portal blood before it is allowed to re-enter the general circulation.[5] The Kupffer cells are macrophages just like those found in the blood, except that they stay in the liver. High-speed motion pictures of the Kupffer cells show them engulfing bacteria in the portal vein in less than 0.01 seconds after contact. A very effective system! Immune complexes and large macro-molecular bacterial products are engulfed and destroyed by the Kupffer cells, while smaller molecules are taken up and transported to the bile by the hepatocytes. It appears that the Kupffer cells don't react to foreign proteins (antigens) in the blood by forming antibodies like some other white cells—they engulf and destroy them instead. This helps prevent us from over-reacting to antigens, such as food particles, absorbed from the gut, which could result in developing food allergies.[6]

When the liver is damaged, this filtration system breaks down. For example, patients with liver disease, especially chronic active hepatitis, have significantly increased levels of antibodies to *E. coli*, *Bacteroides*, and dietary proteins.[7] These findings suggest that a diseased liver is unable to adequately eliminate the antigens absorbed from the gut, thus allowing them entry into the systemic circulation, where they then provoke an immune system response. When the immune system's alarms are set off constantly, the result is excessive antibody formation and constant inflammation, which disrupts normal metabolic processes and leads to disease.

If the diet is low in antioxidants, the Kupffer cells can be a source of inflammation themselves since, when they come into contact with toxins from the intestines and other sources, they release inflammatory chemicals and free radicals as a side effect of their detoxification processes. These free radicals are used by the Kupffer cells as weapons but must be neutralized by antioxidants after they destroy the toxins or they can damage the liver.

The Bile

The liver's second detoxification process involves the synthesis and secretion of bile. Each day the liver manufactures approximately one quart of bile, which serves as a carrier in which many toxic substances are effectively eliminated from the body. Sent to the intestines, the bile and its toxic load are absorbed by fiber and excreted. However, a diet low in fiber means these toxins are not bound in the feces very well and are reabsorbed. Even worse, bacteria in the intestine often modify these toxins so that they become even more damaging.

The bile is also the major route for excretion of cholesterol and excess calcium. Besides eliminating unwanted toxins, the bile emulsifies fats and fat-soluble vitamins in the intestine, improving their absorption.

Phase I Detoxification

The liver's third role in detoxification involves a two-step enzymatic process for the neutralization of unwanted chemical compounds. These include not only drugs, pesticides, and toxins from the gut, but also normal body chemicals—such as hormones and inflammatory chemicals (e.g., histamine)—which if allowed to build up would be toxic. Phase I enzymes directly neutralize some chemicals, but many others are converted to intermediate forms that are then processed by Phase II enzymes.[8] Unfortunately, these intermediate forms are often much more chemically active and therefore more toxic, so if the Phase II detoxification systems aren't working adequately, these intermediates hang around and are far more damaging.

Phase I detoxification of most xenobiotics (toxins) involves a group of enzymes called mixed function oxidative enzymes, which, collectively, have been named cytochrome P450. Some 50 to 100 enzymes make up the cytochrome P450 system. Each enzyme works best in detoxifying certain types of chemicals, but with considerable overlap in activity among the enzymes. In other words, they all metabolize the same chemicals, but with differing levels of efficiency. This fail-safe system ensures maximum detoxification.

The activity of the various cytochrome P450 enzymes varies significantly from one individual to another based on genetics, the individual's level of exposure to chemical toxins, and his or her nutritional status. Since the activity of cytochrome P450 varies so much, so does an individual's risk for various diseases. For example, as highlighted in the study of chemical plant workers in Turin, Italy discussed above, those with underactive cytochrome P450 are more susceptible to carcinogens.[9] This variability of cytochrome P450 enzymes is also seen in the variability of people's ability to detoxify the carcinogens found in cigarette smoke and helps to explain why some people can smoke with seemingly impunity, while others develop lung cancer after only a few decades of smoking. Those who develop cancer are typically those who are exposed to a lot of carcinogens and/or those whose cytochrome P450 isn't working very well.

The level of activity of Phase I detoxification varies greatly, even among healthy adults. One way of determining the activity of Phase I is to measure how efficiently a person detoxifies caffeine. Using this test, researchers have found a surprising five-fold difference in the detoxification rates of apparently healthy adults![10]

When cytochrome P450 metabolizes a xenobiotic, it tries to either chemically transform it to a less toxic form, make it water-soluble, or convert it to a more chemically active form. The best result is the first option, i.e., simply neutralizing the toxin. This is what happens to caffeine. Making a toxin water-soluble is also effective because this makes it easier for the kidneys to excrete it in the urine. The final option is to transform the xenobiotic to more chemically reactive forms, which are more easily metabolized by the Phase II enzymes. While ultimately very important for our health, this transformation of xenobiotics into more chemically active toxins can cause several problems.

A significant side effect of all this metabolic activity is the production of free radicals as xenobiotics are transformed. In other words, for each xenobiotic metabolized by Phase I, a free radical is generated. As discussed more fully below, free radicals are extremely damaging. Without adequate free radical defenses, every time the liver neutralizes a toxin, it is damaged by the free radicals produced.

This is how poisonous mushrooms damage the liver: the liver produces so many free radicals while neutralizing the mushroom's poisons that the liver cells are overwhelmed and destroyed in the process. The damage can be so extensive that the majority of the liver is destroyed, which is why people can die from eating poisonous mushrooms. These damaging free radicals are also produced whenever we eat a food to which we are allergic. This powerfully demonstrates the crucial importance of adequate levels of antioxidants to the liver.

The most important antioxidant for neutralizing the free radicals produced as Phase I by-products is the sulfur-containing peptide, glutathione. In the process of neutralizing free radicals, however, glutathione (GSH) is oxidized to

Table 5-2 Nutrients Needed by Phase I Detoxification

Copper	Vitamin C
Magnesium (deficiency substantially increases toxicity of many drugs)[11]	Vitamins B_2, B_3, B_6, B_{12}
	Folic acid
Zinc	Flavanoids

glutathione disulfide (GSSG). Glutathione is required for one of the Phase II detoxification processes, glutathione conjugation. When high levels of toxin exposure produce so many free radicals from Phase I detoxification that all the glutathione is used up, Phase II glutathione conjugation stops working.

Another potential problem occurs because the toxins transformed into "activated intermediates" by Phase I are far more toxic. Some, for example, become carcinogens that can bind to DNA and proteins. Unless quickly removed from the body by Phase II detoxification mechanisms, they can cause widespread problems. Therefore, the rate at which Phase I produces activated intermediates must be balanced by the rate at which Phase II finishes their processing. Unfortunately, some people have a very active Phase I detoxification system but very slow or inactive Phase II enzymes. These people are described as "pathological detoxifiers" because their overactive Phase I results in a build-up of the more harmful intermediate products, which Phase II cannot disarm quickly enough. The end result is that these people suffer severe toxic reactions to environmental poisons.

An imbalance between Phase I and Phase II can also occur when a person is exposed to large amounts of toxins or exposed to lower levels of toxins for a long period of time. In these situations, so many toxins are being neutralized that the critical nutrients needed for Phase II detoxification get used up, which allows the highly toxic activated intermediates to build up.

Recent research shows that cytochrome P450 enzyme systems are found in other parts of the body, especially the brain cells. Inadequate antioxidants and nutrients in the brain result in an increased rate of neuron damage, such as seen in Alzheimer's and Parkinson's disease patients.

As with all enzymes, the cytochrome P450s require several nutrients, listed in Table 5-2, in order to function. A deficiency of any of these means more toxins floating around doing damage.

A considerable amount of research has found that various substances activate cytochrome P450 (see Table 5-3) while other substances inhibit it (see Table 5-4).

Inducers of Phase I detoxification

Cytochrome P450 is induced by some toxins and by some foods and nutrients. Obviously, it is beneficial to improve Phase I detoxification in order to get rid of the toxins as soon as possible. This is best accomplished by providing the

Table 5-3 Substances That Activate Phase I Detoxification

Drugs	Alcohol
	Nicotine in cigarette smoke
	Phenobarbital
	Sulfonamides
	Steroids
Foods	Cabbage, broccoli, and brussels sprouts
	Charcoal-broiled meats (due to their high levels of toxic compounds)
	High-protein diet
	Oranges and tangerines (but *not* grapefruits)
Nutrients	Niacin
	Vitamin B_1 (riboflavin)
	Vitamin C
Herbs	Sassafras (probably due to toxic constituents)
	Caraway and dill seeds
Environmental toxins	Carbon tetrachloride
	Exhaust fumes
	Paint fumes
	Dioxin
	Pesticides

needed nutrients and non-toxic stimulants while avoiding those substances that are toxic. However, stimulation of Phase I is *not* a good idea if your Phase II systems aren't ready to finish the job or if you are a pathological detoxifier.

All of the drugs and environmental toxins listed in Table 5-3 activate P450 to combat their destructive effects, and in so doing, not only use up compounds needed for this detoxification system but contribute significantly to free radical formation and oxidative stress.

Among foods, the brassica family, i.e., cabbage, broccoli, and brussels sprouts, contains chemical constituents that stimulate both Phase I and Phase II detoxification enzymes. One such compound is a combination of vitamin C with a chemical called indole-3-carbinol. It is a very active stimulant of detoxifying enzymes in the gut as well as the liver.[12] The net result is significant protection against several toxins, especially carcinogens. This helps explain the inverse correlation between cancer incidence and brassica vegetable consumption.

Oranges and tangerines (as well as the seeds of caraway and dill) contain limonene, a phytochemical that has been found to prevent and even treat cancer in animal models. Limonene's protective effects are probably due to the fact that it is a strong inducer of both Phase I and Phase II detoxification enzymes that neutralize carcinogens. However, limonene's promotion of regression of breast cancer in rats may also be due to its stimulation of cells to revert to more normal forms by some as yet unknown mechanism.[13]

Table 5-4 Inhibitors of Phase I Detoxification

Drugs	Benzodiazapine antidepressants (e.g., Centrax, Librium, Prozac, Valium, etc.)
	Antihistamines (used for allergies)
	Cimetidine and other stomach-acid secretion blocking drugs (used for stomach ulcers)
	Ketoconazole
	Sulfaphenazole
Foods	Naringenin from grapefruit juice
	Curcumin from the spice turmeric
	Capsaicin from red chili pepper
	Eugenol from clove oil
Other	Aging
	Toxins from inappropriate bacteria in the intestines

Inhibitors of Phase I detoxification

Many substances inhibit cytochrome P450, making toxins more damaging because they remain in the body longer before detoxification. For example, if you are taking drugs or are exposed to elevated levels of toxins, *don't* eat grapefruits or drink grapefruit juice. Grapefruit juice decreases the rate of elimination of drugs, such as cyclosporin (a drug used to suppress the immune system after organ transplants), from the blood.[14] One research study found that after drinking just 8 oz of grapefruit juice a day, six of fourteen healthy adults were found to have a greater than 50% increase in their blood cyclosporin levels compared to when they just drank water! Further research found that a compound in the grapefruit juice, called naringenin, decreased their cytochrome P450 activity by a remarkable 30%. The common inhibitors of Phase I detoxification are listed in Table 5-4.

Curcumin, the compound that gives turmeric its yellow color, is interesting because it inhibits Phase I while stimulating Phase II. This turns out to be useful for preventing cancer. Curcumin has been found to inhibit carcinogens, such as benzopyrene (the carcinogen found in charcoal-broiled meat), from inducing cancer in several animal models. It appears that the curcumin exerts its anticarcinogenic activity by lowering the activation of carcinogens while increasing the detoxification of those that are activated. Curcumin has also been shown to directly inhibit the growth of cancer cells.[15]

Although I've not found any research that has tested this idea clinically, it seems to me that those who smoke should eat lots of curries. This might help because most of the cancer-inducing chemicals in cigarette smoke are only carcinogenic during the period between activation by Phase I and final detoxification by Phase II.

The Phase I detoxification enzymes are less active in old age. (Interestingly, aging has a much smaller effect on Phase II enzymes.) Aging also decreases blood flow though the liver, further aggravating the problem. Lack of the physical activity necessary for good circulation combined with the poor nutrition commonly seen in the elderly add up to a significant impairment of detoxification capacity, which is typically found in aging individuals. This helps to explain why toxic reactions to drugs are seen so commonly in the elderly—they are unable to eliminate them fast enough, so toxic levels build up.

To ensure Phase I is working well: Eat plenty of brassica family foods (cabbage, broccoli, and brussels sprouts), B-vitamin rich foods (nutritional yeast, whole grains), vitamin-C rich foods (peppers, cabbage, and tomatoes) and citrus foods (oranges and tangerines, but not grapefruits).

Phase II Detoxification

Unlike Phase I detoxification, which essentially involves oxidizing the toxin, Phase II typically involves a process called conjugation, in which various enzymes in the liver attach small chemicals to the xenobiotic. This either neutralizes it or makes it more easily excreted through the urine or bile. Phase II enzymes act on some xenobiotics directly, while others must first be activated by the Phase I enzymes. There are essentially six Phase II detoxification pathways: glutathione conjugation, amino acid conjugation, methylation, sulfation, acetylation, and glucuronidation. Table 5-1 provides examples of toxins neutralized by each of these pathways. The astute reader will notice that some toxins are neutralized through several pathways. This is not uncommon, although usually only one pathway will do the majority of the work.

In order to work, these enzyme systems need nutrients both for their activation and to provide the small molecules they add to the toxins. In addition, they need metabolic energy to function and to synthesize some of the small conjugating molecules. If the liver cell's energy producing plants, the mitochondria, are not functioning properly (which can be caused by a magnesium deficiency or lack of exercise), Phase II detoxification slows down, allowing the build-up of toxic intermediates. Table 5-5 lists the key nutrients needed by each of the six Phase II detoxification systems. Table 5-6 lists the inducers and Table 5-7 the inhibitors of Phase II enzymes.

Table 5-5 Nutrients Needed by Phase II Detoxification Enzymes

Phase II System	Required Nutrients
Glutathione conjugation	Glutathione, vitamin B_6
Amino acid conjugation	Glycine
Methylation	S-adenosyl-methionine
Sulfation	Cysteine, methionine, molybdenum
Acetylation	Acetyl-CoA
Glucuronidation	Glucuronic acid

Table 5-6 Inducers of Phase II Detoxification Enzymes[12,16]

Phase II System	Inducer
Glutathione conjugation	Brassica family foods (cabbage, broccoli, and brussels sprouts), limonene-containing foods (citrus peel, dill weed oil, and caraway oil)
Amino acid conjugation	Glycine
Methylation	Lipotropic nutrients (choline, methionine, betaine, folic acid, and vitamin B_{12})
Sulfation	Cysteine, methionine, taurine
Acetylation	None found
Glucuronidation	Fish oils, cigarette smoking, birth control pills, phenobarbital, limonene-containing foods

Glutathione conjugation

A primary detoxification route is the conjugation of glutathione (a tripeptide composed of three amino acids—cysteine, glutamic acid, and glycine). The liver enzyme glutathione S-transferase takes sulfur from glutathione and combines (conjugates) it with the toxic substance, making it water-soluble. This water-soluble form, called a mercaptate, is then excreted in the urine. In order to function, glutathione S-transferase needs plenty of glutathione.

Glutathione is also an important antioxidant in the cellular mitochondria, the energy production factories of the cell. Cellular mitochondrial glutathione is our main defense against free radicals produced as a by-product of cellular respiration, i.e., the production of energy in the cells from oxygen and fuel. In addition, glutathione is an important neutralizer of the free radicals produced when the liver neutralizes toxins through the Phase I pathway. Glutathione appears to be especially important in organs exposed to toxins, such as the liver, kidneys, lungs, and intestines. This combination of detoxification and free radical protection results in glutathione being one of the most important

Table 5-7 Inhibitors of Phase II Detoxification Enzymes

Phase II System	Inhibitor
Glutathione conjugation	Selenium deficiency, vitamin B_2 deficiency, glutathione deficiency, zinc deficiency
Amino acid conjugation	Low protein diet
Methylation	Folic acid or vitamin B_{12} deficiency
Sulfation	Nonsteroidal anti-inflammatory drugs (e.g., aspirin), tartrazine (yellow food dye), molybdenum deficiency
Acetylation	Vitamin B_2, B_5, or C deficiency
Glucuronidation	Aspirin, probenecid (a drug used to treat gout)

anticarcinogens and antioxidants in our cells, which means that a deficiency is devastating.[17]

When we are exposed to high levels of toxins, glutathione is used up faster than it can be produced or absorbed from the diet. We then become much more susceptible to toxin-induced diseases, such as cancer, especially if our Phase I detoxification system is highly active.[18]

For example, throat cancer is very high in women in northern Iran. These women have been found to consume large amounts of alcohol and foods contaminated with fungal toxins, while their consumption of fruits and vegetables is very low. This results in increased levels of exposure to activated carcinogens since the alcohol activates Phase I detoxification (increasing the production of activated carcinogens from fungal toxins) and the lack of vitamin C and other important micronutrients results in lowered activity of Phase II, which delays the final neutralization of the activated carcinogens. Finally, the lack of antioxidants results in additional damage from the increased levels of free radicals produced by the activated Phase I system.[19]

Similar detoxification problems are seen in those who consume large amounts of alcohol and are exposed to pesticides. The alcohol increases the rate of formation of activated intermediates from the pesticides by Phase I, but the depletion of glutathione means these toxins hang around longer and more free radicals are released, causing more damage, this time to the liver, brain, and nervous system.[20]

Disease states due to glutathione deficiency are not uncommon. A deficiency can be induced either by diseases that increase the need for glutathione, deficiencies of the nutrients needed for synthesis, or diseases that inhibit its formation. For example, people with idiopathic pulmonary fibrosis, adult respiratory distress syndrome, HIV infection, hepatic cirrhosis, cataract formation, and advanced AIDS have been found to have a deficiency of glutathione, probably due to their greatly increased need for glutathione, both as an antioxidant and for detoxification.[21] Smoking increases the rate of utilization of glutathione, both in the detoxification of nicotine and in the neutralization of free radicals produced by the toxins in the smoke.

Glutathione is available through two routes: diet and synthesis. Dietary glutathione (found in fresh fruits and vegetables, cooked fish, and meat) is absorbed well by the intestines and does not appear to be affected by the digestive processes. Besides supporting Phase II detoxification, dietary glutathione appears to also detoxify substances in the intestines before they can be absorbed into the bloodstream. Dietary glutathione whether in foods or from supplements, appears to be efficiently absorbed into the blood.[22]

The body also synthesizes glutathione. Some substances, such as N-acetylcysteine (NAC), glycine, and methionine, help increase the synthesis of glutathione. Supplementation with N-acetylcysteine not only raises liver levels of glutathione, but also mitochondrial levels of this important antioxidant. Supplementation with large oral and large intravenous dosages of NAC has been used to successfully treat the liver damage caused by drug overdoses, such as happens when large amounts of acetaminophen are taken along with alcohol. N-acetylcysteine has also been shown to help decrease the toxicity of chemotherapeutic drugs used to treat cancer.[23] People with liver disorders, such as cirrhosis, aren't as able to synthesize glutathione, which probably explains why their levels are 30% below normal.[24] A deficiency of vitamin B_6 also results in decreased production of glutathione.

Fresh fruits and vegetables contain 25 to 750 mg of glutathione per pound. Similar quantities are found in cooked meats and fish. However, commercially prepared foods, dairy products (milk has none), most cereals, legumes, and nuts have little glutathione. Among processed foods, frozen foods generally retain their glutathione content. While beer contains moderate amounts of glutathione, it is used up when the body detoxifies the alcohol also in beer. Meat contains a considerable amount of methionine, which the body can convert to glutathione.[25] Longevity has been increased in animals fed cysteine, which increases glutathione synthesis. This is an important observation because studies show that large segments of the elderly have low glutathione levels.[26]

When you are exposed to high levels of xenobiotics, carcinogens, or oxidants, eating glutathione-rich foods and supplementation is especially helpful. Oral supplementation of glutathione for maintenance and antioxidant protection ranges from 100 to 500 mg per day for antioxidant support.[27] Detoxification protocols call for somewhat higher intakes.[28]

To ensure that glutathione conjugation is working well: Eat plenty of glutathione-rich foods (i.e., asparagus, avocado, and walnuts), brassica family foods (cabbage, broccoli, brussels sprouts) and limonene-rich foods (orange peel oil, dill and caraway seeds), which stimulate glutathione conjugation.

Amino acid conjugation

Several amino acids (glycine, taurine, glutamine, arginine, and ornithine) are used to combine with and neutralize xenobiotics. Of these, glycine is the most commonly utilized in Phase II amino acid detoxification. People suffering from hepatitis, alcoholic liver disorders, carcinomas, chronic arthritis, hypothyroidism, toxemia of pregnancy, and excessive chemical exposure are commonly found to have a poorly functioning amino acid conjugation system. For example, using the benzoate clearance test (a measure of the rate at which the body detoxifies benzoate by conjugating it with glycine to form hippuric acid, which is excreted by the kidneys), the rate of clearance is half in those with liver ease compared to healthy adults. This means that in those with liver di all the toxins requiring this pathway stay in the body doing damage twice as long.[29]

Even in apparently normal adults, a wide variation exists in th the glycine conjugation pathway. This is due not only to genetic also to the availability of glycine in the liver. Glycine and acids used for conjugation become deficient on a low-protein diet and when chronic exposure to toxins results in depletion.

To ensure that amino acid conjugation is working well: Eat adequate amounts of protein-rich foods.

Methylation

Methylation involves conjugating methyl groups to xenobiotics. Most of the methyl groups used for detoxification come from S-adenosylmethionine (SAM). SAM is synthesized from the amino acid methionine. This synthesis requires the nutrients choline, vitamin B_{12}, and folic acid.

SAM is able to inactivate estrogens (through methylation), supporting the use of methionine in conditions of presumed estrogen excess, such as PMS. Its effects in preventing estrogen-induced cholestasis (stagnation of bile in the gall bladder) have been demonstrated in pregnant women and those on oral contraceptives.[30] In addition to its role in promoting estrogen excretion, methionine has been shown to increase the membrane fluidity that is typically decreased by estrogens, thereby restoring several factors that promote bile flow. Methionine also promotes the flow of lipids to and from the liver in humans. Methionine is a major source of numerous sulfur-containing compounds, including the amino acids, cysteine, and taurine.

To ensure that methylation is working adequately: Eat foods rich in choline (lecithin, eggs), folic acid (green leafy vegetables), and vitamin B_{12} (animal products or supplements). (Methionine deficiency is not likely to be a problem because it is widely available in the diet.)

Sulfation

Sulfation is the conjugation of xenobiotics that have been bioactivated by the Phase I system with sulfur-containing compounds. The sulfation system is important for detoxifying several drugs, food additives, and, especially, toxins from intestinal bacteria and the environment.

The enzyme that catalyzes sulfation is called sulfotransferase. Sulfation, like the other Phase II detoxification systems, results in decreased toxicity and water solubility of toxins, making it easier for them to be excreted in the bile. Sulfation is also used to detoxify some normal body eliminate steroid hormones (such as estrogen) n't build up to damaging levels. Since sulfaelimination of neurotransmitters, dysfunction development of some neurological disorders. comes from the amino acid cysteine, through ch is called sulfoxidation. Sulfoxidation (dismineral molybdenum to function properly. et and can be synthesized from the amino acid

Many factors influence the activity of sulfate conjugation. For example, the diet needs adequate amounts of methionine and cysteine. A diet low in these amino acids has been shown to reduce the sulfation of acetaminophen—one of the pathways by which the body eliminates this commonly used over-the-counter drug.[31] Sulfation is also reduced by excessive levels of molybdenum (too little molybdenum inhibits sulfoxidation while too much inhibits sulfation) and excessive amounts of vitamin B$_6$ (over about 100 mg per day).[32] In some cases, sulfation can be increased by supplemental sulfate, extra amounts of sulfur-containing foods in the diet, and the amino acids taurine and glutathione.

To ensure that sulfation is working adequately: Consume adequate amounts of sulfur-containing foods, i.e., egg yolks, red peppers, garlic, onions, broccoli, and brussels sprouts.

Acetylation

Conjugation of xenobiotics with acetyl CoA is the method by which the body eliminates sulfa drugs (commonly used antibiotics for urinary tract infections). This system appears to be especially sensitive to genetic variation, with those having a poor acetylation system being far more susceptible to toxic reactions from such drugs as isoniazid (used to treat tuberculosis), p-aminosalicylic acid (used to treat tuberculosis), and the hallucinogenic mescaline. These slow acetylators suffer neurological damage when they take anti-tuberculosis drugs. While not much is known about how to directly improve activity of this system, it is known that acetylation is dependent on riboflavin (vitamin B$_2$), pantothenic acid (B$_5$), and vitamin C.[33]

To ensure that acetylation is working adequately: Eat foods rich in B vitamins (yeast, whole grains) and vitamin C (peppers, cabbage, citrus fruits).

Glucuronidation

Glucuronidation, the combining of glucuronic acid with xenobiotics, requires the enzyme UDP-glucuronyl transferase (UDPGT). Many of the commonly prescribed drugs are detoxified through this important pathway. It also helps to detoxify aspirin, menthol, vanillin (synthetic vanilla), food additives such as benzoates, and some hormones. Glucuronidation appears to work well in most of us and doesn't seem to require special attention, except for those with Gilbert's disease.

A surprising 5 to 7% of us have a genetically weak UDPGT resulting in Gilbert's disease. Those with this genetic weakness are far more susceptible to toxic effects from drugs, environmental toxins, and some normal metabolic products. The main way this condition is recognized is by a slight yellowish tinge to the skin and white of the eye due to inadequate metabolism of bilirubin, a breakdown product of hemoglobin. Gilbert's Syndrome is discussed under How to Treat Common Toxicity Diseases, page 156.

The activity of UDPGT is increased by foods rich in a monoterpene called limonene (citrus peel, dill weed seeds, and caraway seeds). Eating these foods not only improves glucuronidation but has also been shown to protect us from chemical carcinogens. Several studies in animals have shown that limonene not only prevents experimental cancer but even reverses it. One study in rats found a remarkable complete regression of tumors in 90% of the animals after just one to six weeks![34]

To ensure that glucuronidation is working adequately: See Gilbert's Syndrome, page 156.

Sulfoxidation

Sulfoxidation is the process by which the sulfur-containing molecules in drugs (such as chlorpromazine, a tranquilizer) and foods (such as garlic) are metabolized. It is also the process by which the body eliminates sulfite food additives used to preserve foods and drugs. Various sulfites are widely used in potato salad (as a preservative), salad bars (to keep the vegetable looking fresh), dried fruits (sulfites keep dried apricots orange), and in some drugs (such as those used in asthma). Normally, the enzyme sulfite oxidase metabolizes sulfites to safer sulfates, which are then excreted in the urine. Those with a poorly functioning sulfoxidation system, however, have an increased ratio of sulfite to sulfate in their urine.

When the sulfoxidation detoxification pathway isn't working very well, people become sensitive to sulfur-containing drugs and foods containing sulfur or sulfite additives. This is especially important for asthmatics, who can react to these additives with life-threatening attacks. Interestingly, until recently, the inhalers used by asthmatics during attacks actually had sulfite preservatives mixed with the anti-spasmotic drugs!

Dr. Jonathan Wright, one of the leading holistic medical doctors in the country, discovered several years ago that providing molybdenum to asthmatics with an elevated ratio of sulfites to sulfates in their urine resulted in a significant improvement in their condition. Molybdenum helps because sulfite oxidase is dependent upon this trace mineral. Although most nutrition textbooks believe it to be an uncommon deficiency, an Austrian study of 1,750 patients found that 41.5% were molybdenum deficient.[35]

To ensure that sulfoxidation is working adequately: Eat foods rich in molybdenum (dairy products, beans, whole grains).

Example of How a Common Chemical Is Detoxified

Many people freely use acetaminophen for the relief of pain and inflammation. It is clinically effective and, in most circumstances, relatively non-toxic when the liver's detoxification processes are working properly. It is an interesting example of how the liver detoxifies drugs, since it can be metabolized through several pathways as shown in Figure 5-2. Normally, most acetaminophen is first bioactivated by the Phase I detoxification system. This is followed primarily by Phase II conjugation with glutathione, resulting in a water-soluble mercaptate that is easily excreted via the urine. A small amount of the activated acetaminophen is neutralized directly by Phase II conjugation with either sulfate or glucuronic acid, again for excretion from the kidneys. For most of us, these overlapping detoxification pathways work just fine.

However, if the Phase II glucuronidation pathway isn't working adequately, an activated intermediate builds up and again cycles through at Phase I where it is further bioactivated to a compound called N-acetyl-*p*-benzo-quinoneimine (NAPQI). NAPQI is extremely toxic to the liver. The production of NAPQI occurs when liver glutathione reserves are depleted, so Phase II neutralization of the activated intermediates either doesn't occur, or occurs too slowly. As discussed above, liver glutathione reserves are decreased by exposure to high levels of xenobiotics, alcohol, fasting, and poor nutritional status. Glutathione depletion may also be caused by taking large amounts of acetaminophen over long periods of time.[36]

This highlights a crucial concept: Multiple pathways can be used for the detoxification of most xenobiotics. However, for most substances, there is an optimal detoxification process, which eliminates each toxin as rapidly and safely as possible. When the optimal pathway is not working properly, a less effective pathway is used instead. This can result in a toxin staying in the body longer, incomplete detoxification, or production of even more toxic forms. The end result is increased damage and chronic draining of our health and vitality.

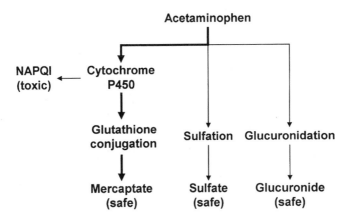

Figure 5-2 *The Detoxification of Acetaminophen*

How to Recognize Dysfunctional Liver Detoxification Systems

The term "sluggish liver" is an old naturopathic concept indicating an impairment of liver detoxification function. Because of the liver's important role in detoxification, however, even minor impairment of liver function can have profound effects. Liver function can be impaired by excessive exposure to toxins (discussed in the next section), by poor production and excretion of bile, and by inadequate functioning of detoxification enzymes due either to nutritional deficiencies or genetic weakness.

Poor Bile Flow

Once the liver has modified a toxin, it needs to be eliminated from the body as soon as possible. However, when the excretion of bile is inhibited (a condition called cholestasis), toxins stay in the liver longer. Cholestasis has several causes, including obstruction of the bile ducts and impairment of bile flow within the liver. The most common cause of obstruction of the bile ducts is the presence of gallstones. Currently, it is conservatively estimated that 20 million people in the U.S. have gallstones. Nearly 20% of the female and 8% of the male population over the age of 40 are found to have gallstones on biopsy and approximately 500,000 gallbladders are removed because of stones each year in the U.S. The prevalence of gallstones in this country has been linked to the high-fat, low-fiber diet consumed by the majority of Americans.[37]

Impairment of bile flow within the liver can be caused by a variety of agents and conditions, as listed in Table 5-8. These conditions are often associated with alterations of liver function in laboratory tests (serum bilirubin, alkaline phosphatase, SGOT, LDH, GGTP, etc.) signifying cellular damage. However, relying on these tests alone to evaluate liver function is not adequate, since, in the initial or subclinical stages of many problems with liver function, laboratory values remain normal. Among the symptoms people with enzymatic damage may complain of are fatigue, general malaise, digestive disturbances, allergies and chemical sensitivities, premenstrual syndrome, and constipation.

Perhaps the most common cause of cholestasis and impaired liver function is alcohol ingestion. In some especially sensitive individuals, as little as 1 oz of alcohol can produce damage to the liver, which results in fat being deposited within the liver. All active alcoholics demonstrate fatty infiltration of the liver.

Methionine administered as SAM has been shown to be quite beneficial in treating two common causes of stagnation of bile in the liver—estrogen excess (due to either oral contraceptive use or pregnancy) and Gilbert's syndrome.[38]

Poor Enzyme Function

While sophisticated blood tests are necessary to prove a dysfunction of a specific liver detoxification system, several signs and symptoms can give us a good

Table 5-8 Causes of Cholestasis

Presence of gallstones
Alcohol
Endotoxins
Hereditary disorders such as Gilbert's syndrome
Hyperthyroidism or thyroxine supplementation
Viral hepatitis
Pregnancy
Certain chemicals or drugs:
   Natural and synthetic steroidal hormones:
   Anabolic steroids
   Estrogens
   Oral contraceptives
Aminosalicylic acid
Chlorothiazide
Erythromycin estolate
Mepazine
Phenylbutazone
Sulphadiazine
Thiouracil

idea of when our liver's detoxification systems are not functioning well or are overloaded. In general, anytime you have a bad reaction to a drug or environmental toxin you can be pretty sure there is a detoxification problem. Table 5-9 lists symptoms that are directly tied to a particular dysfunction.

The strong odor in the urine after eating asparagus (listed in Table 5-9) is an interesting phenomenon because while it is unheard of in China, 100% of the French have been estimated to experience such an odor (about 50% of adults in the U.S. notice this effect). This is an excellent example of genetic variability in liver detoxification function.

Toxins

Toxins bombard us from all directions: the water we drink, the food we eat, and the air we breathe, especially indoors. Even the normal metabolic processes of our bodies regularly produce toxins. As long as the levels of exposure aren't too high, and our detoxification processes are working the way they should, our health continues. Avoidance of toxins is one of the most effective ways to maintain and improve our health. This is true even when our detoxification systems are working well since we waste a lot of needed metabolic energy getting rid of these noxious substances, and their detoxification still causes some damage.

Table 5-9 Recognizing Dysfunctional Liver Detoxification Systems

Symptoms and Diseases	System Most Likely Dysfunctional
Adverse reactions to sulfite food additives (such as in commercial potato salad or salad bars)	Sulfoxidation
Alzheimer's disease	Sulfoxidation
Asthma reactions after eating at a restaurant	Sulfoxidation
Caffeine intolerance (even small amounts keep you awake at night)	Phase I
Chronic exposure to toxins	Phase II glutathione conjugation
Eating asparagus results in a strong urine odor	Sulfoxidation
Fasting	Phase II glutathione conjugation
Garlic makes you sick	Sulfoxidation
Gilbert's disease	Phase II glucuronidation
Intestinal toxicity	Phase II sulfation and amino acid conjugation
Liver disease	Phase II amino acid conjugation
Parkinson's disease	Phase I
Premenstrual syndrome	Phase II sulfation
Prostate cancer	Phase II sulfation
Rheumatoid arthritis	Sulfoxidation
Sulfites, such as in commercial potato salad or salad bars, make you feel ill	Sulfoxidation
Toxemia of pregnancy	Phase II amino acid conjugation
Yellow discoloration of eyes and skin, not due to hepatitis	Phase II glucuronidation
Rapid metabolism of caffeine (you can drink two cups of coffee and still sleep well at night)	Overactive Phase I

Table 5-10 lists key external and internal sources of toxins. For most of us, the most consistent source of toxins is an unhealthy intestine, which, technically, is outside of the body. The intestinal mucosa functions just like our skin, keeping the unwanted contents of the intestines out of our blood and tissues.

Intestinal Toxins

Our intestines have paradoxical functions: they are a digestive/absorptive organ as well as a barrier to toxic compounds and undigested food. The intestinal mucosal membranes accomplish their barrier function through a combination of mechanical exclusion and a specialized intestinal immune defense system. Elaborate immunological and mechanical mechanisms exclude potentially toxic constituents of the diet as well as allergenic food proteins, bacterial products, and infectious microbial organisms.[39,40]

Problems with the intestines basically occur in two ways: Excessive amounts of toxins in the intestines produce what is called a "toxic bowel," and

Table 5-10 Primary Causes of Toxicity

Source	Adverse Effects
Intestinal dysbiosis, i.e., excessive levels of toxin-producing bacteria combined with inadequate amounts of normal bacteria in the intestines; typically caused by the use of broad-spectrum antibiotics or the ingestion of contaminated foods	Bacterial metabolites form toxins; bacterial cell wall components cross-react with normal tissue proteins, disrupting their normal functioning and suppressing the immune system
Environmental pollutants	Poison enzyme systems, directly damage cells and tissues, displace needed nutrients
Free radicals	Destroy enzyme systems, punch holes in cell membranes, transform DNA to abnormal forms
Liver toxicity	Decreased metabolic control resulting in increased levels of circulating immune complexes

damage to the intestinal barrier allows both normal and toxic bowel constituents to leak into the body, a condition referred to as a "leaky gut."

The intestines contain numerous dietary and bacterial products, many of which are quite toxic if they enter the body. In the past, the gastrointestinal system was thought to be impermeable to bowel contents except for nutrients. We now know this is inaccurate.[41] Toxic bowel constituents can pass into the body, causing a wide range of damaging effects. In fact, many diseases are now known to be associated with, and possibly caused by, excessive gastrointestinal permeability (which is discussed more fully below).

The Toxic Bowel

Toxins from the bowel cause problems in many ways. First, many of them directly damage enzymes and tissues, including the brain and nervous system.[42] Second, when some of these xenobiotic substances are detoxified, they trigger the release of chemicals that cause inflammation. Third, the more toxins the body has to detoxify, the more the detoxification enzymes in the liver are activated, which results in increased free radical production. Finally, endotoxins from the gut bacteria activate the liver's Kupffer cells, causing a release of interleukin 2.

Interleukin 2 decreases the activity of the Phase I detoxification enzymes and depletes Phase II amino acid conjugation in the glutamine pathway. That is, a toxic bowel disrupts both Phase I and Phase II detoxification pathways. In other words, toxic bacteria in the intestines make us more susceptible to environmental and bowel toxins.

The gastrointestinal tract contains a large amount and variety of con-stituents of varying degrees of toxicity. The toxic constituents come from essen-tially three sources: food, food additives, and toxic bacteria. Even the average American diet contains significant amounts of toxins from normal constituents of foods and food additives. For example, meat (especially when fried or barbe-cued) contains heterocyclic compounds, which can be converted to carcinogens by normal gut microflora.[43] Pathogenic bacteria in the intestines directly pro-duce toxins (called endotoxins), convert normal food constituents to toxic forms and, when they die, release their constituents into the bowel, which also can be damaging.

Intestinal Dysbiosis (Toxic Bacteria)

The gut microflora is large and varied. About 400 species have been isolated, with the number of microorganisms in the colon being estimated at 10^{10} to 10^{11} per gram of fecal material, suggesting that we have more microbial than human cells.[44] The metabolic processes of these bacteria produce many chemi-cals, some of which are harmful to the body.

Dysbiosis is defined as a disordered microbial ecology that causes disease. This state may exist in the oral cavity, gastrointestinal tract, or vaginal cavity. In dysbiosis, organisms that do not normally cause infection, including bacte-ria, yeasts, and protozoa, induce disease by producing toxins or altering the nutrition or immune responses of their host. Some of the toxic chemicals they produce are carcinogens while others provoke an allergic response.[45,46] Some of these pathogenic organisms even change dietary constituents and liver excre-tion products into carcinogens.[47] Unfortunately, many of the microbial meta-bolic by-products and toxins can pass easily from the intestines into the blood.

Overuse of antibiotics, development of antibiotic-resistant microorganisms, alterations in gut microflora, and the increased incidence of parasites, all con-tribute to the development of abnormal bacteria in the gut. The overuse of broad-spectrum antibiotics has resulted in increased gastrointestinal yeast, fungus, and anaerobic organisms, some of which have become resistant to antibiotics.

Of particular significance is the research which has shown that these unhealthful intestinal microorganisms produce toxic metabolites that poison our body's enzyme systems. Some of these chemicals are very similar to normal Krebs cycle metabolites. The Krebs cycle is the series of chemical processes in the mitochondria that produce energy for the cells to function. Poisoning these enzymes is devastating to the body because, without adequate energy, cellular processes go awry.

Some of these chemicals also mimic the neurotransmitters that make our brain and nervous system work. The leakage of abnormal forms or inappropriate levels of neurotransmitters into the body can cause significant brain dysfunction and alterations in behavior. Some of these chemicals can even be hallucinogenic. Interestingly, many of these abnormal chemicals have been found in the urine of

Table 5-11 Diseases in Which Intestinal Dysbiosis Is Implicated

Autoimmune joint disease	Inflammatory bowel disease
Chronic fatigue syndrome	Irritable bowel syndrome
Colon and breast cancer	Psoriasis
Cystic acne	Steatorrhea
Eczema	Vitamin B_{12} deficiency

autistic patients. Table 5-11 lists common diseases that have been shown to be associated with, and possibly caused by, intestinal dysbiosis.

For example, patients with psoriasis who have been found to have high levels of circulating endotoxins from bacteria[48] rapidly improve when they take the drug cholestyramine, a strong binder of endotoxin in the gut.[49] In a controlled study of 92 patients, an endotoxin-binding saponin (sarsasaponin) from *Similas officinalis* (sarsaparilla) markedly improved 62% of the patients and resulted in complete clearance in 18%.[50]

The research on intestinal dysbiosis has progressed to the point that correlations are now being seen between specific types of bacteria in the intestines and certain diseases (see Table 5-12). For example, there is a correlation between intestinal infection with *Shigella*, *Salmonella*, *Yersinia*, or *Campylobacter* and Reiter's syndrome, an inflammatory condition of the joints and eye.[51] This suggests that the body reacts to these bacterial proteins by forming antibodies, which then also react with the tissues of the joints.[52] Studies have demonstrated that patients with ankylosing spondylitis, rheumatoid arthritis, and vasculitis have increased intestinal permeability, which may be an important factor in the development of these disorders.[53,54]

The Leaky Gut

The problem with bowel toxins becomes even worse when the intestinal mucosal barrier becomes damaged. Not only does this allow more toxins to enter, but it also allows the entry of viable bacteria, pieces of dead bacteria and yeasts, and dietary proteins.[61] This results in a huge overload for the liver. It also results in food allergies. The term "leaky gut" has been coined to describe this condition.

In the past few years, the association between intestinal inflammation and intestinal leakage and many chronic diseases, including autoimmune diseases, has become well-established. As can be seen from Table 5-13, a leaky gut has been found in diseases as diverse as infection, food allergy, Crohn's disease, eczema, and autoimmune diseases, such as rheumatoid arthritis and ankylosing spondylitis. In some diseases, such as AIDS, the disease appears to cause the increased permeability, while in others such as eczema, increased permeability appears to be a major cause.

Table 5-12 Intestinal Microorganisms Associated with Chronic Diseases[55,56,57,58,59,60]

Microorganism	Toxic Reaction	Disease
Bacteroides	Separate B_{12} from intrinsic factor	Pernicious anemia
Campylobacter	Cross-reacts with collagen	Reiter's syndrome
Candida albicans	Increase prostaglandin synthesis	Irritable bowel syndrome
Escherichia coli	Cross-reacts with insulin receptors	Diabetes mellitus
	Cross-reacts with nerve acetyl-choline receptors	Myasthenia gravis
Klebsiella pneumoniae	Cross-reacts with nerve acetyl-choline receptors	Myasthenia gravis
	Cross-reacts with joint tissues	Rheumatoid arthritis
Nisseria meningitidis	Cross-reacts with nerve cell membranes	Meningitis
Proteus vulgaris	Cross-reacts with nerve acetyl-choline receptors	Myasthenia gravis
Salmonella	Cross-reacts with collagen	Reiter's syndrome
Shigella	Cross-reacts with collagen	Reiter's syndrome
Yersinia enterocolitica	Cross-reacts with thyroid plasma membrane and collagen	Arthritis, enterocolitis, erythema nodosum, Graves' disease, Hashimoto's disease, Reiter's syndrome, iritis

When the intestines are damaged, from infection, inflammation, or food allergy, leakage into the body of substances that are normally excluded increases dramatically. This is especially a problem in chronic intestinal inflammatory diseases such as Crohn's disease, where the absorption of toxins increases as much as six-fold.[69,70]

The permeability of the gastrointestinal tract can be measured by a procedure called the lactulose/mannitol absorption test.[71] In this test, intestinal leakage is measured by the rate of absorption of lactulose, a molecule so large that it normally does not enter the body in any appreciable amount.

Studies of a wide range of illnesses have demonstrated that increases in intestinal absorption of lactulose correlate well with clinical and pathological conditions, often returning to normal values as the condition improves and worsening as the condition worsens. For example, when Crohn's disease patients are placed on a totally synthetic diet, their previously elevated lactulose/mannitol ratios fall significantly, coinciding with marked clinical improvement.[72] Researchers have consistently reported a correlation between intestinal permeability and bowel inflammation.[73]

In diseases of the small intestine such as gluten-sensitive enteropathy (a severe allergy to wheat, also known as coeliac disease), permeability to large

Table 5-13 Clinical Conditions Associated with Altered Intestinal
Permeability[62,63,64,65,66,67,68]

Aging	Inflammatory joint disease
Alcoholism	Intestinal infections
Ankylosing spondylitis	Irritable bowel disease
Asthma	Malabsorption
Chemotherapy	Malnutrition
Coeliac disease	NSAID-induced intestinal damage
Crohn's disease	Psoriasis
Eczema	Reiter's disease
Endotoxemia	Rheumatoid arthritis
Food allergy	Schizophrenia
Giardiasis	Thermal injury (severe burns)
Hives	Trauma
HIV positive	Ulcerative colitis
Infantile colic	Urticaria (hives)
Inflammatory bowel disease	

molecules increases and, paradoxically, permeability to small molecules decreases. This latter effect is due to the destruction of the microvilli, the minuscule folds in the intestines that greatly increase the absorptive surface area of the intestines. While the surface area of a person with a normal intestine is a remarkable 2,000 square feet (about the size of a tennis court), the patient with untreated coeliac disease has an 80% smaller surface area, one that is not very good at discriminating what passes through it.

After exposure to a single oral dose of gluten (the protein in wheat that makes it gluey), the intestinal permeability of people with coeliac disease becomes significantly abnormal. Remarkably, when all gluten is scrupulously avoided, their intestines heal incredibly rapidly and permeability returns almost to normal within one week.

How the Gut Can Be Damaged

Many factors damage the gut: food allergy, drugs (e.g., alcohol), aging, intestinal infections, nonsteroidal anti-inflammatory drugs (e.g., aspirin), chemical toxins ingested with foods, and maldigestion.[74,75] (Maldigestion is covered extensively in Chapter Seven.)

Food Allergy

A very common condition causing, and caused by, a leaky gut, is food allergy. Whether or not a person will develop a food allergy depends on many factors, including heredity, gut permeability, an overly sensitive immune response, poor digestive function, and excessive exposure to a limited number of foods. While

Grains and the Immature Digestive Tract

A case I saw in the teaching clinic when I was a young medical student at the National College of Naturopathic Medicine had a huge impact on my clinical thinking. Charlotte brought her four-year-old son Michael into the clinic and laid him on my examining table. While his older brothers bounced around the examining room, Michael lay listlessly on the table— very uncharacteristic of a young child! Michael had suffered from diarrhea and debility for three years. His mother had taken him to countless doctors, specialists, and hospitals and spent thousands of dollars, yet his diarrhea and debility continued. I saw a passive child with dark circles under his eyes, a sallow complexion, a protruding belly, bowed legs, and what looked like a ricketic rosary (lumps at the ends of his ribs).

I, and this child, had the great fortune of having Dr. John Bastyr supervising in clinic that shift. (Dr. Bastyr, who died recently at the age of 83, was a wonderful healer and physician who inspired several generations of naturopathic doctors-to-be. He had such a powerful impact on us that when we decided to start a new naturopathic school in 1978, we named it in his honor to provide a guiding spirit for the institution.)

After examining Michael and asking his mother about his diet, Dr. Bastyr quickly recognized the cause of his problems: food allergies. Michael's mother had introduced grains into his diet before his digestive system had matured enough to digest them properly. He told Charlotte to stop feeding her son grains, not just wheat, but also rye, barley, oats, corn, and rice. In addition, he told her to feed her son only equal amounts of carrot juice and raw goat's milk (one of Dr. Bastyr's famous concoctions) for one week and then to bring him back for re-evaluation.

One week later, Michael had dramatically improved. His diarrhea had stopped, and he was bouncing off the walls, just like his brothers. Unfortunately, over the next year, Charlotte would, despite my admonitions to the contrary, try feeding him grains, and each time he would again develop diarrhea.

- *The message:* Food allergies can cause serious chronic damage to the body, yet don't turn up on conventional medical evaluation.

conventional medical texts assert that only about 1% of the population has food allergies, nutritionally oriented physicians will tell you that half of all patients they test are allergic to at least one food, some many more. Chronic inflammatory skin diseases, such as eczema, also appear to be associated with food allergy and a leaky gut. Patients with atopic dermatitis and/or urticaria demonstrate increased permeability when given an oral challenge of the food(s) that provoke their symptoms.[76]

Most people are unaware that they are sensitive to foods because most only think of allergies as an immediate reaction, like hives or asthma attacks. Far more common are what are called "masked" or "delayed" reactions, which occur hours, or even days, after the food is ingested. This delay makes it very difficult to connect the eating of a specific food with the reaction. Immediate reactions are mediated by IgE type antibodies while IgG and IgM antibodies mediate the delayed reactions. Unfortunately, most conventional allergists believe food allergies are only mediated by IgE and ignore delayed food reactions. Patients who have had their chronic, "incurable" diseases cured by avoiding the foods that they are allergic to know otherwise.

There are two basic ways of detecting food allergies: laboratory methods, which attempt to measure antibodies in the blood to various foods, and experiential clinical tests, where a person eats a suspected food according to a special protocol and watches for reactions.

Laboratory procedures for diagnosing food allergy

Table 5-14 summarizes the strengths and weaknesses of the currently available laboratory procedures. These procedures require the assistance of a physician.

Experiential tests for food allergy

Many physicians, including myself, believe that the oral food challenge is the best method (the "gold standard") for diagnosing food intolerance. I use the term "intolerance" rather than allergy because some people have a reaction to a food that is not mediated by antibodies and, technically, a reaction is not an allergy unless there are antibodies involved. The food challenge is an accurate and useful procedure when used appropriately. As might be expected, there are a wide variety of protocols among the physicians using this method.

There are two broad categories of food provocation challenge testing: (1) elimination diet (meaning only a few, relatively low allergenic foods are eaten) followed by food reintroduction and (2) pure water fast followed by food challenge. Food challenge may be performed in an open, single-blind, or double-blind manner.

Please note: Food challenge testing should *not* be used by those with symptoms that are potentially life-threatening (such as the airway constriction found in asthma or severe anaphylaxis).

The typical procedure is pretty straightforward:

1. For four days either eat no food of any kind (except liberal amounts of water) or only a few foods or a synthetic hypoallergenic formula (such as UltraClear).
2. On the fifth day, begin eating one new food each day, alternating between the suspected foods and foods that are usually safe. My recommended order is wheat, carrots, corn, cabbage, milk, pears, cheese, avocado, peanuts, apples, soy, grapes, tomatoes, cucumbers, and beef.

Table 5-14 Laboratory Food Allergy Tests

Procedure	Advantages	Disadvantages
RAST	Convenient Good for inhalants Office kits available	Low sensitivity Expensive Detects IgE only
RASP	Convenient Good sensitivity	Expensive Not widely available Detects IgE and only some IgG
FICA	Patient convenience Good sensitivity Detects IgG	Expensive Not widely available Little research
Cytotoxic	Convenient Moderate cost Many foods easily tested	Poor reproducibility Limited availability
ELISA/ACT	Patient convenience Good sensitivity Detects both immediate and delayed reactions	Expensive Not widely available Little research
Skin prick	Widely available Good for inhalants	Poor sensitivity for food allergens Inconvenient
Provocation	Good for chemicals Office procedure Facilitates therapy	Expensive Time-consuming
EAV Acupuncture	Inexpensive Easily applied	No scientific basis Little research
Kinesiologic	Inexpensive Easily applied	No scientific basis Little research

3. Very carefully keep track of symptoms, not only on the day the food is introduced but also the next morning. Fortunately, most people react within an hour, but some people react as much as two or three days later, making detection more complicated.
4. Continue until all foods in the diet have been tested.

The first four days are considered the cleansing period, with the gastrointestinal tract being cleared of previously ingested foods, thus decreasing food sensitivity reactions. On the fifth or sixth day, symptoms due to food allergy usually start to disappear (if the allergic food was eliminated) and the person generally feels better.[77]

During the first two to three weeks after stopping a food, a person will actually become even more sensitive, or hyper-reactive, to the offending foods. This explains why the reintroduction of foods may produce more severe or more easily recognizable symptoms. Foods are usually reintroduced in the order of probability, with a person's favorite food, especially a food they crave, being the most likely suspect. While it is beyond the scope of this book to fully explain why this happens, the short answer is that due to physiological adaptation the person usually becomes addicted to the foods causing the most trouble. When I bring up the idea of food allergy to a patient, very often he or she will say "Well I know it can't be 'x' as I always feel better when I eat it." Virtually always, 'x' is their worst food allergen!

In order for this procedure to work, great care must be exercised in keeping track of symptoms and ensuring that only pure foods are eaten. Many of the foods we eat contain food additives that are at times the real culprits and sometimes other foods are hidden in the food being tested. For example, various corn, wheat, and dairy products are often added to other foods, without their presence being listed on labels. Keeping a careful daily-symptom diary, noting when various foods were introduced, is absolutely necessary for the recognition of reactions.

Challenge testing is great for those wanting to take more control of their health, those with limited financial resources, and those with less severe health problems. Another advantage is the dramatic increase in symptoms you feel after eating the food to which you are allergic. It makes it much easier to avoid the offending foods when you have such a direct experience with how damaging they can be to your health. A disadvantage is that it is time-consuming and requires considerable discipline. The fewer the allergenic foods, the greater the ease of establishing a diagnosis with an elimination diet.

In general, better results can be achieved by eliminating all foods and just drinking water for four days. However, you are much more likely to experience "withdrawal" symptoms and a feeling of toxicity, which will usually subside by the fourth or fifth day. This method is only advisable for those who are physically and mentally capable of the more rigorous water fast.

Alcohol

Drinking more than moderate amounts of alcohol damages the mucous membranes of the intestinal tract—the more you drink, the worse the damage. Alcoholics' intestinal permeability is elevated and this dysfunction persists for up to two weeks after they stop drinking.[78] Their increased permeability may account for some of widespread damage commonly found in alcoholics. The leaky gut also exposes the liver to more toxins from the bowel, which aggravates alcohol-induced liver disease.

Aging

In rats and other laboratory animals, aging results in a diminished capacity to prevent larger molecules from penetrating the intestinal mucosa, possibly allowing antigenic or mutagenic compounds to reach the systemic circulation.[79]

Intestinal Infections

Many intestinal infections cause increased permeability.[80] Studies show that the body's responses to these infections result in increased passage of micro-organisms and endotoxins into the systemic circulation.[81] Several researchers believe that this breach of the mucosal barrier is an important aspect in both the acute and chronic systemic effects of intestinal infection.

Severe Burns

Researchers have found that intestinal permeability increases in human beings after a major burn.[82] This occurs even in the absence of infection of the burned areas. In addition, increasing evidence shows that the gut barrier's failure to function may play a role in initiating the multiple-organ-failure syndrome that occurs after major trauma. Loss of blood supply to the intestines due to the trauma probably explains the mucosal changes.

Non-Steroidal Anti-Inflammatory Drugs

Numerous studies have shown that non-steroidal anti-inflammatory drugs (NSAIDs) disrupt the intestinal barrier function and cause increased perme-ability.[83] This is of particular importance in arthritic patients treated with NSAIDs because the increased permeability probably contributes to the pro-gression of their disease; a sad example of relieving the symptoms at the cost of aggravating the underlying disease. The most common NSAIDs are listed in Table 5-15.

Constipation

Constipation significantly increases the toxicity of the body because the longer toxins stay in the bowel, the more time they have to damage the intestinal mucosa and leak into the body. Constipation has several causes, the most important being a low-fiber diet and food allergies.

Transit time, the time taken for passage of material from the mouth to the anus, is greatly reduced on a high-fiber diet. Cultures consuming a high-fiber diet (100 to 170 gm per day) usually have a transit time of 30 hours and a fecal

Table 5-15 Common Non-Steroidal Anti-Inflammatory Drugs

Acetaminophen (e.g., Tylenol)	Meclofenamate (e.g., Baprosyn)
Aspirin	Phenylbutazone
Fenoprofen (e.g., Nalfon)	Piroxicam (e.g., Feldene)
Ibuprofen (e.g., Advil, Motrin, Nuprin)	Sulindac (e.g., Clinoril)
Indomethacin (e.g., Indocin, Indometh)	Tolmetin (e.g., Tolectin)

weight of 500 gm (a little over a pound). In contrast, Europeans and Americans, who typically eat a low-fiber diet (20 gm per day) have a transit time of greater than 48 hours and a fecal weight of only 100 gm.[84]

The dietary fiber supplements I recommend most frequently are psyllium seed and oat bran.

Besides a low-fiber diet, allergy to cow's milk may be a significant cause of chronic constipation. A group of researchers in Italy studied 27 children under three years of age who suffered from chronic constipation. No changes were made in their diet, other than substituting soy milk for cow's milk. The results were quite impressive, with 21 showing a significant improvement, i.e., an increased number of stools per day, softer stools, and elimination or decrease in intestinal discomfort and anal and perianal fissures. The children improved within three days but their symptoms returned rapidly when cow's milk was reintroduced.[85]

Other Sources of Toxins

Free Radicals

Our life depends on the easy availability of oxygen, which is required for many critical metabolic processes. For example, our mitochondria, the cells' energy-producing factories, use oxygen to convert fuel (from food) to energy, and white blood cells use oxygen to destroy invading microbes. However, oxygen is such a powerful reactant that it creates free radicals, which do considerable damage when not properly controlled. This results in damage to our enzyme systems, cell membranes, and DNA. Free radical attack and cumulative oxidative damage are associated with more than 100 degenerative conditions, the most common of which are summarized in Table 5-16.

Ischemia (loss of blood supply), reperfusion (re-establishment of blood supply after ischemia), burns, trauma, cold, exercising to excess, toxins, inflammation, radiation, and infection—all release free radicals. But being implicated does not necessarily mean that they are the initiating factor. Sometimes the free radicals are just a consequence of tissue injury. However, if not immediately quenched, they keep the damage going. Once an initial event generates free radicals, a cascade ensues, producing ever more free radicals, which continue to snowball unless held in check by antioxidant defenses.[86]

In addition to free radicals, the body generates other powerful oxidizing agents, including hydrogen peroxide (H_2O_2), lipid peroxide (ROOH), hypochlorite (OCl^-—the same powerful oxidizer found in commercial bleach), chloramines (RNHCl), and several other highly reactive oxidizing chemicals. All of these various oxidizing molecules are referred to here by the term *free radicals*.

Targets of free radicals include polyunsaturated fatty acids in membranes, serum lipoproteins, proteins, and even DNA. The products may be lipid peroxides

Table 5-16 Conditions Mediated by Free Radical Damage[87,88,89,90,91,92,93,94]

Alcohol-induced damage	Liver cirrhosis
Atherosclerosis	Myocardial infarction
Autoimmune diseases (rheumatoid arthritis and others)	Nephrotoxicity
	Nutrient deficiencies
Cancer	Obstructive lung disease
Contact dermatitis	Parkinson's disease
Diabetic cataracts	Premature aging
Drug toxicity	Premature retinopathy
Emphysema	Senile dementia and neurologic degeneration
Hypertensive cerebrovascular injury	Stroke
Immune deficiency of aging	Thermal injury
Inflammatory bowel disease	Viral infections, including AIDS
Iron overload disease	

(oxidized fats implicated in cardiovascular disease), protein carbonyls (oxidized proteins that are carcinogenic), or altered purines (DNA components). The consequences are often subtle, such as damage to cell membrane receptor proteins, which alters cellular regulatory mechanisms so that enzymes required for ATP production are inactivated, leading to low energy.

Production of Free Radicals
As listed in Table 5-17, free radicals are produced by external sources, such as radiation and environmental pollution, as well as normal internal metabolic and defense processes. These add up to a surprisingly heavy load of free radicals.

Inflammation represents a major source of oxidants, especially during a chronic disease process. Infection, immune complexes, bacterial toxins, toxic exposure, ischemia (low blood supply), trauma—all activate phagocytes, the immune cells that surround and destroy undesirable cells and substances. This triggers the local production and release of highly reactive free radicals to destroy damaged tissues, viruses, bacteria, and toxic chemicals. While many toxins can be neutralized this way, unfortunately, some are converted to even more reactive forms.[97] As discussed in more detail in Chapter Six, inflammation also activates the arachidonic acid cascade, which produces the inflammatory prostaglandins and leukotrienes, which contribute to the free radical load. The continuous production of free radicals by activated phagocytes during chronic (even undetected low level) inflammation will eventually deplete antioxidant defenses, thus allowing free radicals to damage cells.

The term "oxidative stress" refers to an increase in the ratio of pro-oxidants to antioxidants. The oxidative overload is due to excessive free radical production or inadequate antioxidant defenses. Increased oxidative stress results in chronic tissue injury and progressive damage to metabolic processes. The body's ability to protect itself from oxidative stress is affected by the degree of exposure

Table 5-17 The Production of Free Radicals[95,96]

Source	Mechanism
Air pollution	Ozone and nitrogen oxides are strong oxidants.
Radiation	Cosmic rays and radiation produce free radicals when they impact body tissues.
Energy production	Up to 2% of oxygen molecules passing through mitochondria end up as superoxides instead of energy. This generates about 10 gm of superoxide per day.
Fatty acid oxidation	Cells contain little organs that oxidize fatty acids as part of metabolizing fat with the side effect of producing hydrogen peroxide. Drugs such as clofibrate increase the activity of these organelles.
Metabolism of DNA, RNA, and ATP	The metabolism of DNA, RNA, and ATP relies on the enzyme xanthine oxidase, which produces superoxide.
Metabolite and xenobiotic detoxification	Phase I detoxification generates free radicals. Metabolism of drugs, such as penicillamine and phenylbutazone, and environmental poisons, such as paraquat and alloxan, produce free radicals. These oxidative products account for the liver damage caused by many pesticides and drugs.
Inflammatory response	Iron and copper are released from storage sites during inflammation and injury. These ions catalyze the spontaneous production of free radicals.
Immune response	White cells produce free radicals as part of their defensive mechanism.

to pollutants, the level of dietary consumption of antioxidants, one's age and genetic factors. When free radical production exceeds the ability of the neutralizing systems, progressive cellular damage occurs. When this damage is severe or long lasting, a downward spiral from health to chronic disease results.

Americans consume relatively low amounts of the antioxidant nutrients: vitamins C and E, beta-carotene, zinc, selenium, copper, and manganese. This is probably because fewer than 10% eat the recommended five daily servings of fruits and vegetables.[98,99]

Food Additives

Irregularities in the detoxification system may make individuals especially sensitive to natural compounds in foods and to synthetic food additives. Symptoms include chronic urticaria (hives), angioedema, asthma, rhinitis, nasal polyps, headaches, upper abdominal pain, and mood changes. Offending additives include benzoates, tartrazine and other synthetic colors, and acetylacetic acid.[100]

Drugs

Virtually all drugs need to be detoxified by the liver. Adverse side effects are experienced by 15 to 30% of those taking medications (both over-the-counter and prescription), and drug reactions account for 20 to 30% of hospital admissions. Often the side effects people experience are from the damage these foreign chemicals cause to the liver. This damage can be caused directly by the drugs, or indirectly as a result of the liver's detoxification of the drug or the effect of the drug on the metabolism of other drugs. This is one reason why the mixing of prescription drugs can cause so many problems and is widely discouraged.

Benzodiazepines

Benzodiazepines (e.g., Centrax, Librium, Prozac, Valium, etc.) are drugs widely prescribed to relieve the symptoms of anxiety and insomnia. While modestly clinically effective, they cause significant problems for the elderly, where their use is associated with the development of neurological damage in the brain. This may in part be due to benzodiazepines' suppression of Phase I detoxification enzymes, both in the liver and in the brain. This results in slower metabolism of some neurotransmitters that the body needs to regularly eliminate lest they reach toxic levels.

The combination of bacterial toxins from the intestine, poor liver detoxification processes, and the addition of drugs such as benzodiazepines that further aggravate the toxicity problem appears to result in greatly increased risk of brain and nervous system dysfunction, called by some "brain toxicity."

Acetaminophen

Although normally relatively safe, combining acetaminophen with either alcohol or fasting can damage your liver. The danger appears to start at about three drinks per day.[101] This toxicity reaction can also happen in those with very poor nutrition and by taking large amounts over long periods of time.

Heavy Metals

All metals in our environment are toxic at some level of exposure. Even metals that are required nutrients, such as iron, are toxic at high levels, while some, such as lead, are toxic at any level of exposure.

Aluminum

More and more research is showing that aluminum poses a serious health problem for humans. We now know that aluminum catalyzes free radical damage to the nervous tissue in the brain. This is especially a problem for those with Alzheimer's disease, because their ability to transport and detoxify aluminum appears to be impaired.[102] However, a high exposure to aluminum is probably a problem for everyone. For example, miners given aluminum powder as prophylaxis against silicotic lung disease between 1944 and 1979 were found during a later study to perform less well on cognitive state examinations as compared to non-exposed miners, with their level of impairment directly related to the duration of the aluminum exposure.[103]

As might be expected, those who work with aluminum experience problems also. When 25 workers from an aluminum smelting plant were evaluated for neurologic symptomatology, 88% reported frequent loss of balance, 84% reported memory loss, 84% had signs of coordination loss, 75% showed mild or greater impairment on memory tests, and 89% were depressed according to the Minnesota Multiphasic Personality Inventory. The researchers also found a correlation with the degree of exposure and coordination loss.[104]

Those on dialysis for kidney failure are commonly poisoned by aluminum. A side effect of the chemicals used for the procedure is the leakage of aluminum salts into the body tissues. When the aluminum builds to a toxic level, these people develop a condition known as dialysis encephalopathy. This manifests as dementia, speech disorders, jerking muscles, seizures, and psychotic episodes. Before symptoms occur, their EEGs (a measure of electrical activity in the brain) become abnormal as the aluminum starts to disrupt brain neurochemistry.[105]

Mercury

Mercury is highly toxic, especially to the nerves. The saying "mad as a hatter" came from stories of hatters in England in the nineteenth century. The hatters used a mercury compound to help stiffen the cloth used to make hats. Unfortunately, they absorbed some of the mercury and developed such mental dysfunction they became psychotic.

The tendency of mercury to concentrate in the nervous tissue is well-documented and the role of mercury-containing tooth fillings as a chronic source is cause for serious concern. Autopsy samples of the central nervous system (especially the olfactory [smelling] region and the pituitary gland) and kidney cortex have revealed a high concentration of mercury in those having amalgam fillings when compared to amalgam-free cadavers.[106] The association between amalgam load and the accumulation of mercury in tissues is thought to be caused by swallowing and inhalation of mercury vapor released from amalgam fillings. Because the vaporization rate is low, blood and urine mercury levels (the indicators used by the dental and amalgam representatives to claim that amalgams are safe) remain low and are a poor diagnostic indicator of body burden.[107] Although the exposure is low, it is constant and cumulative and our nervous system is especially sensitive.

Even in those without overt disease, research suggests that the mere presence of mercury amalgams in the teeth has an impact on mental symptoms. In one study, 50 university students with amalgam fillings were compared to 51 with no dental fillings. The amalgam group was found to have 201% higher mercury levels in the urine and 26% higher in the hair. Health questionnaires showed an increase in the number of subjective physical and mental complaints. Removal of their fillings resulted in a significant improvement in their symptoms.[108] Many dentists are now aware of this problem and are replacing amalgam fillings with safer plastic and ceramic alternatives.

Lead

Lead, the oldest known environmental pollutant, continues to be a serious problem for our society. While changing gasoline from leaded to unleaded certainly has helped, lead continues to contaminate our environment: the typical person has 100 to 1,000 times as much lead in his or her body as our prehistoric ancestors. No level of lead exposure has been shown to be safe.

Research over the past decade has substantially increased our understanding of lead toxicity, and we now recognize that levels previously considered safe are not. Subclinical toxicity can cause inhibition of enzymes, kidney damage, hypertension, sperm malformation, slowing of nerve conduction, and central nervous system dysfunction. All these effects have occurred in apparently healthy workers at levels of exposure to airborne lead below OSHA's (Occupational Safety and Health Administration) supposedly safe exposure levels.[109]

Common sources of lead in the environment include leaded paint, water, copper-leaded pipes, leaded gasoline, batteries, and lead smelters. Another very significant source is cigarettes, with smokers having twice the body load of nonsmokers.[110] Two of the many toxic effects of lead of particular importance are the blockage of hemoglobin formation (hence the anemia and chronic tiredness) and the inhibition of glutathione regeneration resulting in increased susceptibility to environmental chemical toxins. Children and those on a calcium-deficient diet are the most susceptible to lead.

Fortunately, treatment with chelating agents can be used to reduce blood and tissues levels of toxic heavy metals. In a recent animal study, the combined use of prescription drugs EDTA and meso 2,3-dimercaptosuccinic acid was more beneficial in reducing blood and liver lead compared to treatment with these drugs alone.[111] However, as these drugs cause lead to be excreted through the kidneys, care must be exercised that the rate isn't too fast which could damage the kidneys.

Recognizing heavy metal overload

While acute poisoning or high levels of heavy metal toxicity are easy to recognize, chronic low level exposure can be difficult to recognize since the symptoms can be subtle and pervasive. Table 5-18 lists the common signs and symptoms of heavy metal toxicity. As can be seen, many of the common discomforts of life can be caused by heavy metals, making diagnosis from symptoms alone difficult and unreliable.

A simple and inexpensive test, hair analysis, can easily warn us of exposure. Unfortunately, hair analysis has developed a controversial reputation because some misguided practitioners have inappropriately used this procedure to evaluate nutritional status. The research is clear: With a few exceptions

Table 5-18 Signs and Symptoms of Heavy Metal Toxicity[112]

Toxic Metal	Symptoms
Aluminum	Colic, dementia, esophagitis, gastroenteritis, liver dysfunction, loss of appetite, loss of balance, kidney damage, muscle pain, psychosis, shortness of breath, weakness
Cadmium	Anemia, dry and scaly skin, emphysema, fatigue, hair loss, hypertension, joint soreness, kidney stones, liver dysfunction, loss of appetite, osteoporosis, pain in back and legs, yellow teeth
Lead	Abdominal pain, anemia, anxiety, bone pain, confusion, depression, difficult concentration, dizziness, drowsiness, fatigue, headaches, hypertension, incoordination, indigestion, irritability, loss of appetite, memory impairment, muscle pain, restlessness, tremors
Mercury	Anemia, colitis, depression, dermatitis, dizziness, drowsiness, emotional instability, fatigue, headaches, hearing loss, hypertension, incoordination, insomnia, irritability, loss of appetite, loss of balance, kidney dysfunction, memory impairment, metallic taste, numbness, psychosis, inflamed gums, strange sensations in hands, tremors, vision impairment, weakness
Nickel	Apathy, blue color of lips, diarrhea, fever, headaches, insomnia, nausea and vomiting, shortness of breath, very rapid heart rate

(chromium, manganese, and selenium), hair analysis is not a reliable tool for measuring mineral status and is absolutely worthless for measuring vitamin status.[113] It is, however, very useful and reliable for detecting heavy metal exposure and is sensitive enough to detect exposure before it is bad enough to cause significant clinical symptoms. Hair analysis is useful for recognizing exposure to mercury, lead, iron, and arsenic.[114,115]

Helicobacter Pylori

Helicobacter pylori infection is associated with stomach cancer and other health problems (see Table 5-19). It is estimated that 50% of the population over the age of 60 in the U.S. is infected with *H. pylori*.[116] For most of those infected, their mucosal resistance factors are working just fine and they are asymptomatic. For others though, it contributes to both peptic ulcer disease and the risk of gastric adenocarcinoma.

Some research is helping us understand why some people develop stomach ulcers and stomach cancer while others effectively resist *H. pylori*. One research group found that while users and non-users of nonsteroidal anti-inflammatory agents (NSAIDs) had the same incidence of *H. pylori*, those taking NSAIDs had a four-fold increased risk of ulcers. In other words, aspirin and other NSAIDs inhibited the stomach's ability to protect itself from *H. pylori*.[118] Coffee consumption also appears to help the *H. pylori* cause trouble.[119]

Table 5-19 Effects of *Helicobacter Pylori* Infection[117]

Change Induced by H. pylori	Effect
Hyperproliferation of gastric mucosa	Greater opportunity for mutagen integration and fixation Greater susceptibility to carcinogen formation and activity
Altered pH	Impairs digestion
Genetic changes in host mucosal tissue	Impairs normal repair process
Denaturation or oxidation of mucosal cell ascorbic acid, setting the stage for vitamin C deficiency	Enhanced formation of nitrosamines which are carcinogenic
Enhanced mutagenic/carcinogenic insult	Increased risk of cancer
Atrophic gastritis, with loss of parietal cells and hypochlorhydria	Hyperproliferation of nitrosamine-forming bacteria in small bowel and release of toxic substances Alteration of GI flora, affecting steroid deconjugation and, therefore, the metabolism and activity of estrogenic hormones

H. pylori infection also causes destruction of vitamin C. In a study of 19 patients with H. pylori, their gastric juice ascorbic acid concentrations were 75% lower than uninfected controls. These patients also had a significant increase in inflammation in the stomach and intestines. Eradicating the H. pylori resulted in an increase in gastric juice ascorbic acid concentration. In other words, the infection uses up vitamin C. This is especially important because vitamin C neutralizes nitrosamines, carcinogens thought to be the primary cause of stomach cancer.[120]

Also of interest is the research that shows that a 5 to 10% per volume solution of manuka honey completely inhibits H. pylori in vitro after 72 hours of incubation.[121] Human studies are now needed to determine if this will be clinically useful.

Silicone Implants

Silicone (polydimethylsiloxane) is used for body implants for the breast, penis, and muscle enhancement and in replacement joints. Unfortunately, a growing body of evidence shows that silicone molecules leach from the implants and are picked up by macrophages. This results in their transport throughout the body where they combine with normal proteins to form abnormal proteins that activate an autoimmune reaction. These then initiate an inflammatory response, which continues unabated due to continued stimulation. The silicone particles also suppress natural killer cell activity, which returns to normal after removal of the implant.[122] Unfortunately, the body has no detoxification system for these man-made molecules.

Pesticides and Herbicides

Farmers have an increased incidence of certain types of cancers, particularly those of the stomach, connective tissue, skin, brain, prostate, and lymphatic and blood-forming system. Herbicide exposure may be the cause. A large study of over 69,000 Saskatchewan farmers, ages 35 or older, found a strong correlation between the use of herbicides and the incidence of non-Hodgkin's lymphoma. Mortality from non-Hodgkin's lymphoma rose in proportion to the number of acres sprayed with herbicides. The association was specific in that the incidence of non-Hodgkin's lymphoma was not correlated to education, income, ethnicity, fuel expenditure, use of fertilizers, or insecticides.[123]

Another disconcerting study looked at the association between various childhood cancers and the home and yard use of pesticides. They found significant association between the use of pest strips and leukemias, brain tumors, and lymphomas. Yard pesticides were associated with soft tissue sarcomas while house insect extermination was associated with lymphoma.[124]

How to Recognize When Your Detoxification Systems Are Overloaded or Aren't Working Adequately

Many of the daily discomforts we suffer, as well as several diseases, are the result of unrecognized toxicity, either due to excessive exposure or inadequate detoxification. Table 5-20 shows a list of common symptoms that indicate the build up of toxins.

Supporting the Detoxification Systems

No mater how good our food or how pure an environment we live in, we will always be exposed to toxins. They naturally occur in foods, are produced as a normal by-product of metabolism, and are even secreted by health-promoting bacteria in the intestines as unwanted chemicals. The bottom line is that we need our detoxification systems to work well.

Enhancing the Liver's Detoxification Functions

The liver has remarkable regenerative and detoxification properties, if given the chance. Optimizing liver function focuses on protecting the liver from toxins, increasing the excretion of toxins from the liver, normalizing the liver's detoxification systems, and protecting the liver from the build-up of fat. Liver-protecting substances include many nutritional and herbal compounds that

Table 5-20 Signs and Symptoms of Toxicity

Acne, especially cystic acne	Foul-smelling stools
Autoimmune disease	Generalized pruritis (itching)
Bad breath	Intolerance of garlic
Chronic degenerative disease with	Irritable bowel syndrome
unknown cause	Liver disease
Chronic fatigue	Nausea and vomiting during pregnancy
Chronic fatigue syndrome	Premature development of "age spots"
Chronic headaches	Psoriasis
Colon and breast cancer	Sensitivity to chemicals
Eczema	Toxic headache

prevent the damage to the liver associated with detoxifying harmful chemicals. Lipotropic factors are, by definition, substances that hasten the removal or decrease the deposit of fat in the liver. Choleretics are agents that stimulate bile secretion by the liver, while cholagogues are agents that stimulate gallbladder contraction in order to improve the excretion of bile into the intestines.

Protecting the Liver from Virus- and Toxin-Induced Damage

As noted above, whenever the liver metabolizes toxins, free radicals are produced. In order to prevent damage to the liver, these must be neutralized as soon as possible. Following is a discussion of a few of the free radical quenchers that are especially important for the liver. A more complete discussion of free radical quenching nutrients, enzyme systems, and herbs are discussed later this chapter.

Nutrients

The nutritional antioxidants—i.e., vitamins C and E, bioflavonoids, carotenoids, glutathione, and selenium—are essential for protecting the liver from the free radicals produced during the neutralization of toxins. The protective effects of these antioxidant nutrients can be substantially augmented by increasing the diversity and magnitude of other antioxidants such as coenzyme Q and catechin.[125] Also of particular value are several flavonoids from herbs, which have the surprising property of being concentrated in the liver, just where they are most needed and most effective.

Phospholipids (a kind of fat found in cell membranes) are of special value because they protect the liver from chronic exposure to organic solvents. This appears to be due to the incorporation of phospholipids into cellular membranes, resulting in improved membrane fluidity, activation of membrane-dependent enzyme processes, and regeneration of damaged liver cells.[126] The phospholipids that protect the liver include phosphatidylcholine, phosphatidylethanolamine, and phosphatidylserine. These important nutrients are found in egg yolks and lecithin and can be obtained from dietary supplements.

Silybum marianum (Milk thistle)

Silybum is possibly the most potent liver protective agent known. It is so effective in protecting the liver that in experiments with mice, if silybum is given within a few minutes of ingestion of the deadly *Amanita phalloides* mushroom, death is not only prevented, but little liver damage is found! It works by preventing free radical damage (several time stronger than vitamin E) and by stimulating protein synthesis and production of new liver cells. The constituents that provide this protection are a mixture of three flavanolignins collectively referred to as silymarin.[127] The concentration of silymarin is highest in the fruit, but it is also found in the seeds and leaves.

The clinical efficacy of silybum has been well-documented in large clinical studies. For example, in one multicenter trial, 2,637 patients with various liver disorders (56.1% fatty infiltration of the liver, 19.3% hepatitis and cirrhosis, and 22.6% no clear diagnosis) were given an average of four tables (140 mg of silymarin per tablet) of standardized milk thistle extract daily. After eight weeks, 63% of the patients reported a complete disappearance of their symptoms (nausea, pruritis, abdominal distention, lack of appetite, and fatigue). Laboratory evaluation confirmed the subjective results with the level of liver enzymes in the blood (a measure of liver damage) decreasing by an average of 40%. Those with liver enlargement also had their liver decrease in size. Only 0.8% complained of side effects (stomach upset, nausea, and light diarrhea) and stopped their herbal medication.[128]

Other clinical trials have shown that silymarin is effective in treating cirrhosis, chronic hepatitis, fatty infiltration of the liver (chemical and alcohol induced), and inflammation of the bile duct.[129] The therapeutic effect of silymarin in all of these disorders has been confirmed by histological (biopsy), clinical, and laboratory data.

Silymarin protects the liver from such diverse toxic chemicals as alcohol, carbon tetrachloride, amanita mushroom toxin, galactosamine, and praseodymium nitrate.[130,131] Silybum is also particularly helpful for those having to take drugs for various reasons. For example, many of the psychotropic drugs used for patients with psychiatric disorders cause significant damage to the liver. In one study of 60 patients receiving long-term drug treatment with phenothiazines and butyrophenones, 90 days of treatment with 800 mg per day of silymarin resulted in significantly reduced levels of liver damage. The silymarin did not interfere with the clinical efficacy of the psychotrophic drugs.[132]

■ *Dosage:* 120 mg silymarin three times a day

Catechin

Catechin is a flavonoid extracted from the herbs *Acacia catechu* (black catechu) and *Uncaria gambier* (pale catechu, gambier). It is widely used in Europe for treatment of liver disease. In the laboratory, catechin has been shown to directly inactivate endotoxins and quench free radicals produced by bacterial endotoxins.[133] Supplementation has been shown to be effective in treating a variety of liver diseases, including chemical damage (such as from carbon tetrachloride poisoning), alcoholism, bacterial toxin damage (such as those secreted by gram-negative bacteria in the intestines), autoimmune hepatitis, viral hepatitis, and cirrhosis.[134] However, clinical trials have shown inconsistent results in chronic hepatitis with it appearing to be effective in treating hepatitis B and C, but not acute hepatitis A. It has also been shown to protect against some chemical carcinogens in experimental mice models.[135]

Catechin, however, is one nutrient that must be used with caution because some people will develop hemolytic anemia after high dosages or long periods of use.[136] The major dietary source of catechin is green tea.

- *Dosage:* 250 mg catechin twice a day or 2 cups of green tea a day

Protecting the Liver from Fat Buildup

The first step in protecting the liver from fat infiltration is dietary: Decrease the consumption of saturated fats (which increase the risk of developing fatty infiltration and the build-up of bile in the liver and gallbladder) and increase dietary fiber, particularly the water-soluble fibers (which promote increased bile secretion). Alcohol consumption must also be limited because excessive consumption stimulates the build-up of fat in the liver.

The next step is to ensure adequate consumption of lipotropic factors, because these nutrients are required by the liver to metabolize toxins, other metabolites, and fatty acids. Lipotropic factors appear to be especially indicated in women taking oral contraceptive agents, women who are pregnant, and anyone exposed to toxic compounds, especially organic solvents and polycyclic hydrocarbons, such as pesticides and herbicides, since these put an additional load on the lipotropic-dependent metabolic processes of the liver.

Compounds commonly employed as lipotropic agents include choline, methionine, betaine, folic acid, carnitine, and vitamin B_{12}. One of the best supplements for protecting the liver from toxins, especially alcohol, is carnitine.

Carnitine is a vitamin-like compound that we get from our diet (mainly from meat) or synthesize from the amino acids lysine and methionine, with the help of vitamin C, iron, niacin, and vitamin B_6. Since carnitine normally facilitates the conversion of fatty acids to energy, a high level of carnitine in the liver is needed to handle the increased fatty acid load produced by alcohol consumption, a high-fat diet, and/or chemical exposure. Carnitine supplementation is one of the few therapies that significantly inhibits alcohol-induced fatty liver disease. Chronic ethanol consumption, chemical exposure, and heavy exercise result in a deficiency of carnitine.[137] By supplementing L-carnitine, this functional deficiency state is reversed, leading to normalization of fatty acid transport and alleviation of fatty acid infiltration within the liver.

A Very Sick Boat Builder

Seattle claims to have one of the highest per capita rates of boat ownership in the world. As might be expected, there are many boat builders in the area. Jack was a wooden boat builder in Port Townsend, Washington. Although a young man, he was becoming progressively debilitated, a problem that he noted was far worse in the winter. He had become so weak, he was having problems getting out of bed in the morning to do his work. At the urging of friends, he took the two-hour trip to Seattle to seek my advice. As usual, he had seen several medical doctors, and none could provide an effective therapy for his ailments because they could find no recognizable disease. By the time he came to see me, he was very weak, felt like he had the flu all the time, and was desperate because he had a wife and young children to support. A bit of detective work quickly pinpointed the cause of his problems.

Wooden boat builders are exposed to several very toxic chemicals, especially solvents in varnishes and heavy metals in special paints used to keep barnacles from growing on the bottom of the boat. While this was not much of a problem for him in the summer, in the winter he would close all the doors and windows in his workshop to keep the heat in. As might be expected, this also kept the toxins in, despite the vents. Since his workshop had been approved by OSHA, he assumed the chemicals he worked with weren't a problem. Not only was he not using a mask, he wasn't even wearing gloves most of the time, and his living space was right next-door and smelled of solvents!

On examination, I found that he had an enlarged and very sensitive liver. His hands were discolored as was his complexion, which appeared waxen. I immediately put him on an intensive detoxification program. First, we eliminated all toxin exposure: He stopped working for one week, moved his family several blocks away from his workshop, added a heater, opened all doors and windows in the workshop, and began using both gloves and a chemical mask.

Next, we stimulated his detoxification processes. For one week Jack went on a modified fast, consuming only raw and cooked fruits and vegetables. To this he added large dosages of vitamin C and B-complex. Finally, he took two herbs for detoxification, *Chionanthus virginicus* (fringe tree) and *Chelidonium majus* (tetterwort). These herbs have been traditionally used by naturopathic doctors for detoxification of the liver. They are both powerful cholagogues, meaning that they help eliminate bile from the liver while stimulating its detoxification actions. (Since I've not been able to find any modern research supporting the clinical use of these herbs, I now use others, such as *Silybum marianum*, which have more documentation.)

Jack had a good constitution and responded rapidly to the therapy. Within a few weeks he was back to his normal energetic self. By improving the ventilation in his workshop and having him rigorously limit contact exposure, he was able to continue building his beautiful wooden boats.

■ *The message:* The chemical solvents in our home and work environments progressively damage our health in direct proportion to exposure.

One toxin that is particularly damaging to carnitine metabolism is valproate, one of the primary anti-epileptic drugs given to children. Supplementation with carnitine reverses most of the toxicity commonly seen with this drug.[138] Another problem is the common food additive sodium benzoate, which is added to many foods and drinks as a preservative (look at the label). It also causes trouble by interfering with the synthesis of carnitine.[139]

- *Dosage:* 250 mg carnitine, 500 mg choline, B-complex (with an average of 25 mg of each of the B vitamins)—all twice a day

Increasing the Flow of Bile

One of the best ways to detoxify and protect the liver is to get toxins out of it as soon as possible. This is done by increasing the excretion of bile from the liver, because that's where the liver puts the toxins. Several herbs do this quite effectively. However, they are most effective for those on a high-fiber diet since there isn't much point in excreting bile into the intestine unless there is fiber there for it to bind to for elimination from the body.

Taraxacum officinale (Dandelion root)
While many consider the common dandelion to be an unwanted weed, herbalists all over the world have revered this valuable liver remedy for centuries.[140] Dandelion is regarded as one of the finest liver remedies, both as food and medicine. Studies in humans and laboratory animals have shown that dandelion enhances the flow of bile, improving such conditions as liver congestion, bile duct inflammation, hepatitis, gallstones, and jaundice.[141] Dandelion's action on increasing bile flow is two-fold. It causes an increase in bile production and flow to the gallbladder (choleretic effect) and stimulates the gallbladder to contract and release the stored bile (cholagogue effect) into the intestine. Dandelion's beneficial effect on a wide variety of conditions is probably closely related to its ability to increase the elimination of toxins from the liver.

- *Dosage:* 4 gm of dried root or 4 to 8 ml fluid extract of *Taraxicum officinale* three times a day

Cynara scolymus (Artichoke leaves)
Artichoke leaf extracts increase the excretion of bile from the liver. Clinical research comparing artichoke to placebo has demonstrated significantly more bile excretion for two to three hours after administration of a standardized extract containing 0.06% cynarin (a constituent of artichoke leaves).[142] This effect is so potent, that artichoke extracts are now used as cholesterol lowering agents, since cholesterol is eliminated from the body through the bile. In one study of 30 patients, 500 mg per day of cynarin lowered blood cholesterol by 20% and triglycerides by 15%.[143]

- *Dosage:* 500 mg *Cynara scolymus* extract (15% cynarin) per day

Curcuma longa (Turmeric)

The common spice turmeric contains the yellow pigment curcumin, which has demonstrated protective effects similar to those of silymarin and cynarin, i.e., it increases the flow of bile from the liver and decreases blood cholesterol levels.[144] It is especially effective in lowering cholesterol levels as demonstrated in experiments with rats fed large amounts of cholesterol, where it decreased blood levels a remarkable 50%.[145]

- *Dosage:* Use turmeric liberally as a spice; 300 mg curcumin three times a day

Promoting Liver Regeneration

The oral administration of liquid liver extracts has been used in the treatment of many chronic liver diseases since 1896. Numerous scientific investigations into the therapeutic efficacy of liver extracts have demonstrated that they possess a lipotropic effect, promote liver cell regeneration, and prevent scarring (fibrosis).[146] Clinical studies have demonstrated efficacy in the treatment of chronic liver disease, including chronic active hepatitis.[147] However, as valuable as this extract is, those with gout should probably avoid liver extracts since their high concentration of DNA and RDA may raise blood uric acid levels. This is not a problem for the average person.

- *Dosage:* 500 mg liver extract three times a day

While milk thistle (*Silybum marianum*, discussed above) is best known for its liver protective effects, possibly of even greater value is its use in stimulating regeneration of the liver. Its flavonoid complex silymarin stimulates liver protein synthesis. The result is an increase in the production of new liver cells to replace the damaged old ones.[148]

- *Dosage:* 120 mg silymarin three times a day

Increasing Phase II Detoxification

Sulfur compounds

Supplementing with the amino acid L-cysteine, inorganic sulfate, or taurine helps increase liver sulfation.[149] Since the sulfation system backs up the glutathione system for some toxins, if a person is exposed to such high levels of xenobiotics that all the glutathione is used up, their sulfate stores can also be used up. Garlic and onions are good dietary sources of sulfur compounds.

Glycine

Glycine has been used as an aid for many toxic conditions. As long ago as the 1960s, pioneer nutrition researcher Roger Williams, Ph.D., recommended it for alcoholics and others exposed to high levels of chemical toxins. It works through several mechanisms to support Phase II detoxification.

It is used in direct conjugation of xenobiotics and for the synthesis of glutathione, and indirectly aids in the production of glucuronic acid, which is used in glucuronidation.

Brassica family foods

Brassica family foods (cabbage, cauliflower, and especially brussels sprouts) contain several compounds that greatly improve the functioning of liver detoxification.[150,151] The flavonoids and carbinols contained in these foods increase the activity of the Phase II glutathione-S-transferase detoxification system. These foods are especially valuable in the prevention of cancer.[152]

Vitamin C

Vitamin C is a cofactor in both Phase I and Phase II detoxification processes.[153] Exposure to xenobiotics causes up-regulation of the specific enzymes that detoxify these substances. Because humans lack the ability to produce their own vitamin C, exposure to toxins increases the need for vitamin C. Unfortunately, both smoking and exposure to cigarette smoke deplete the body's vitamin C stores.[154]

Glutathione

Glutathione, utilized in the liver in Phase II conjugation, is available in the diet and synthesized from the amino acids glycine, cysteine, and glutamic acid. Glutathione intercepts toxic compounds by combining with them to form a water-soluble conjugate, which is discharged harmlessly in body wastes. Glutathione is also a component of glutathione S-transferase, a liver enzyme important in alcohol detoxification.[155] *Silybum marianum* not only prevents the depletion of glutathione caused by alcohol and other liver toxins, but has been found to even increase the levels of glutathione in the liver by 35% over controls. This is extremely useful when exposure to toxic substances is high.

Controlling Toxins

We need to decrease our exposure to toxins, and when present, eliminate them from our body as rapidly and safely as possible. This entails a bit of detective work to determine what we are being exposed to. However, this can be difficult, so I recommend concentrating on those that most commonly affect the most people. In general, we need to control four major sources of toxins: bowel toxins, free radicals, heavy metals, and environmental poisons.

Since the intestines are a major consistent source of toxins for most of us, improving the health of the intestines is one of the most effective actions we can take to improve our health. Even though we may be exposed to other sources of toxins, decreasing the load on the liver from the intestines allows the liver to more effectively eliminate the other toxins, whether from the environment or faulty metabolic processes. This entails both decreasing the amount of toxins in the intestines and healing the damaged intestines so they are a better barrier to the toxins they contain.

The other highly effective action we can take is to optimize our free radical defenses, since so many of the damaging effects of toxins are mediated through free-radical damage.

Supporting Intestinal Health

Reestablishing a healthy intestine is critical for health because a leaky gut full of poisonous bacteria and toxic metabolites contributes to many chronic diseases. In addition, an unhealthy intestine can result in malabsorption and malnutrition, leading to a wide range of metabolic dysfunctions. Healing the intestines can rapidly relieve symptoms and gradually improve health and vitality.

Healing the damaged intestinal mucosa requires a comprehensive approach that includes eliminating all factors that injure the intestine (such as toxic bacteria), reestablishing the normal bowel flora, removing toxins from the intestines, improving digestion (see Chapter Seven), decreasing inflammation, and promoting the metabolism and repair of the intestinal-lining cells.

Eliminating Toxic Bacteria and Yeasts

Toxic bacteria in the bowel both directly damage the intestinal lining cells and release toxins that can be absorbed into the body. Most bowel pathogens can be eliminated by the use of two herbs: goldenseal and garlic.

Hydrastis canadensis (Goldenseal)

Goldenseal is a useful herb for all kinds of infections, including those of the intestines. It is especially of value when toxic bacteria are overgrowing the gut. The alkaloid berberine that is found in Hydrastis canadensis, works in two ways: First, it kills abnormal bacteria and second, it inhibits the activity of the bacterial enzymes that damage the intestinal cells. By inhibiting these damaging microbial enzymes (called decarboxylase enzymes) it blocks the production of vasoactive amines such as histamine, tyramine, putrescine, and cadaverine, all of which contribute to increased intestinal permeability.[156] Unlike antibiotics which decimate healthy as well as toxic bacteria, Hydrastis has the remarkable property of leaving the lactobacilli we need for intestinal health alone.

- *Dosage:* 2 gm of goldenseal root three times per day for two weeks

Allium sativum (Garlic)

Garlic is very useful for eliminating toxic microorganisms, especially yeasts, from the intestine. It directly inhibits several toxic intestinal microorganisms, such as *Staphylococcus, Streptococcus, Bacillus, Brucella, Salmonella enteritidis, Candida albicans, Mycobacteria, Cryptococcus neoformans* and *Vibrio* species, even at low concentrations.[157,158,159,160] The most effective extracts of garlic for antimicrobial activity are those that are high in allicin—the aged extracts, while effective for lowering cholesterol, are not effective for killing off pathogens. One caveat: Those with a poorly functioning sulfoxidation enzyme system (see discussion above) need to limit their garlic consumption since they have trouble metabolizing its sulfur-containing compounds.

- *Dosage:* Eat freely as part of a regular healthful diet and take ½ a clove (or equivalent in garlic extract) three times a day

Reseeding the Intestines with Health-Promoting Bacteria

Fundamental to correction of gastrointestinal dysfunction is re-establishment of the appropriate microbial flora of the intestine. The health-inducing bacteria are especially important because they suppress the growth of toxic bacteria. Reseeding the intestines is done through the use of probiotics and prebiotics. Probiotics are the intestinal bacteria found in the healthy intestines. Prebiotics are indigestible substances that help the healthful bacteria grow. Prebiotics also help by increasing the production of secretory IgA in the intestines, which also helps protect against bacteria and food allergens.[161]

Probiotics

The primary beneficial organisms used to reseed the intestines are *Lactobacilli* and *Bifidobacteria*. They play many important roles, a crucial one of which is inhibiting the growth of toxic bacteria, viruses, fungi, yeasts, and parasites.[162] These health-promoting intestinal bacteria also aid in digestion, synthesize vitamins (folic acid and other B vitamins), reduce blood ammonia levels, lower cholesterol levels, neutralize carcinogens, and stimulate the immune system.[163]

As important as these bacteria are to reestablishing the health of the bowel, finding effective products is difficult. One problem is that most of the traditional sources, i.e., fermented products such as yogurt, miso, and some cheeses, no longer contain *lactobacilli* because commercial production has switched to other bacteria that work better for mass production. Unfortunately, the bacterial strains they use have little value for human health. The other problem is that most of the *lactobacilli* products on the market are either the wrong strain or contain so few live bacteria that they have little effect. Two forms I've found to be clinically effective are Eugalin Forte (available in health food stores) and HMF (available from InterPlexus in Kent, Washington 1-800-875-0511).

- *Dosage: Lactobacilli*-containing dairy products and 2 (250 mg each) capsules of *Lactobacilli + Bifidobacteria* twice a day between meals

Prebiotics

An important part of reseeding the intestines is to ensure that the food the health-promoting bacteria need to live on is easily available. One of the best ways to do this is with oligosaccharides, especially fructooligosaccharides.

Fructooligosaccharides are short-chain carbohydrates composed of three to ten molecules of sugars, at least two of which are fructose. This molecule is essentially indigestible by humans. However, the good intestinal bacteria, *Bifidobacteria* and *Lactobacilli*, preferentially utilize fructooligosaccharides to grow and multiply. In contrast, toxic bacteria are unable to use these short-chain carbohydrates.[164] Fructooligosaccharides also help by inhibiting the attachment of toxic and parasitic bacteria to the gastrointestinal mucosa.[165] Foods rich in fructo-oligosaccharides include onions, asparagus, bananas, and maple syrup.

In addition to containing fructooligosaccharides, bananas help heal the damaged intestinal mucosa because they contain water-soluble polysaccharides, pectin, and valuable phospholipids.

- *Dosage:* 1 gm of fructooligosaccharides or two bananas per day

Removing Toxins from the Intestines

Not only do we need to remove toxins from the intestines to help promote health, but we should also try to keep them from accumulating in the first place. A high-fiber diet is one of the most effective ways to keep toxins from accumulating. Fiber consumption is most easily increased by eating a whole-foods diet. However, fiber supplementation also works. Increasing fiber intake (via whole, unprocessed grains, vegetables, and fruits) aids digestion, decreases the amount of time toxins stay in the intestine, and decreases toxin absorption from the gut. Fiber increases the excretion of bacterial breakdown products as well as the protein putrefaction metabolites found in the gut.[166]

Dietary fiber also helps to maintain healthful colonic bacterial flora. A low-fiber intake is associated with an overgrowth of endotoxin-producing bacteria and a lower percentage of *Lactobacilli* and other healthful bacteria.[167] A high-fiber diet provides short-chain fatty acids, which are metabolized by healthful bacteria to provide some of the fuel used by the intestinal mucosal cells.

Pectin (a fiber found in fruit and also available as a supplement) increases the secretion of digestive enzymes (trypsin, chymotrypsin, lipase, and amylase), prevents absorption of toxic molecules in the bowel, and decreases transit time, thus decreasing the opportunity for absorption of toxins.[168]

Protecting the Intestines and Stimulating Repair

The most common non-bacterial causes of intestinal damage are non-steroidal anti-inflammatory drugs (NSAIDs); ingestion of allergenic foods; consumption of alcohol, chemicals, and drugs; trauma; and endotoxemia. The first step in protecting our intestines is to control what we put in our mouth!

Glutathione   Just like in the liver, glutathione is useful in the intestine for helping stimulate cell regeneration and protecting against further damage since it works both as a free radical quencher and as a direct neutralizer of some toxins. When the antioxidant properties of glutathione are being used, extra selenium is needed to help convert it back to its healthy form.[169]

- *Dosage:* 100 mg glutathione twice a day

Quercetin   Cromolyn sodium is a prescription drug that inhibits the release of inflammatory chemicals from sensitized mast cells. It has been used in many clinical trials to reduce the intestinal damage caused by ingestion of food allergens.[170] Quercetin is a natural bioflavonoid with similar metabolic and clinical effects. Quercetin and other bioflavonoids have been shown to inhibit the release of inflammatory chemicals from mast cells, scavenge free radicals, and inhibit irritability of the muscles of the intestines.[171] Naturopathic doctors use quercetin to help control food allergies and heal the damaged intestinal mucosa in chronic inflammatory bowel disease. It's also useful in the treatment of such conditions as acute and chronic diarrhea and stomach ulcers.

- *Dosage:* 500 mg of quercetin 15 to 20 minutes before meals

Anti-Oxidants   A significant portion of the intestinal mucosal damage is due to free radicals produced by the inflammatory reaction to food allergens and intestinal toxins. The problem with free radicals is further aggregated when the blood supply to the intestines is inadequate.[172] Administration of free radical scavengers helps neutralize these toxic chemicals. Some common natural antioxidants are: vitamin E, beta-carotene, ascorbic acid, zinc, selenium, and superoxide dismutase.

Avoiding allergenic foods

Researchers have observed that intestinal permeability increases even after ingestion of an amount of an allergenic food that is not large enough to cause a clinical reaction.[173] In other words, eating any amount of a food allergen appears to damage the intestines, but overt clinical symptoms don't appear until the leakage gets bad enough. Apparently people with food allergies have intestines that are especially sensitive to food allergens. For example, a number of studies have shown that people with food allergies have increased permeability even while fasting and that the permeability further increased after ingestion of an offending allergen. Fortunately, the intestines heal quickly (within a few days) when the offending food is removed.

Digestive aids

A poor digestive function causes many problems: malnutrition, food allergies, and an increased risk of intestinal infections. Most people with food allergies have an inadequate digestive system. Poor digestion (as discussed in Chapter Seven) means large molecules are in the intestine where they don't belong. Digestive aids—such as fungal enzymes, HCl, pepsin, and pancreatin—help to lessen the allergic damage done to the intestines when allergenic foods are eaten by ensuring that the food molecules are broken down the way they should be. As might be expected, patients with low stomach acid have increased gastrointestinal permeability and an increased delivery of bacterial toxins to the liver. Interestingly, maldigestion does not cause as much trouble with fat and carbohydrate absorption as it does with protein and trace mineral absorption.[174] This means people can absorb enough calories to be fat, but not enough nutrients to be healthy and energetic.

When our digestion is functioning properly, the enzymes released by the pancreas digest food constituents (specifically the short-chain fatty acid carboxylic acid) into acetate, propionate and butyrate, all essential nutrients for the intestinal mucosal cells. However, when the digestion is not working properly, bacterial fermentation occurs instead. This results in the production of isobutyrate, valarate, and isovalarate, which are not utilizable by the intestinal mucosa.[175] Butyric acid is manufactured in the lower intestines as a by-product of bacterial fermentation of fiber. It is the main energy source for lower intestinal epithelial cells and is important for the repair and regeneration of damaged cells.[176]

Glutamine

Glutamine (the most abundant amino acid in the blood) is one of the principle fuels used by the intestinal lining cells, accounting for 35% of their energy production. While readily available in the diet and synthesized in the body, supplementation improves the energy metabolism of the gastrointestinal mucosa, thus stimulating regeneration.[177] Glutamine prevents intestinal mucosal damage and has been shown to decrease bacterial leakage across the intestines after they are damaged, presumably by stimulating repair.[178]

Glutamine supplementation is of particular value for healing the serious, even life-threatening, intestinal damage caused by abdominal irradiation.[179] Glutamine is also important any time there are intense demands for cellular repair, such as after major surgery and severe burns. During these times, glutamine levels drop precipitously and blood flow to the intestines is reduced. This adds up to a significant problem for the intestinal cells and is why intestinal degeneration is seen in those with severe trauma, such as burns over large areas of their body. Glutamine supplementation is also of value for enhancing repair of the damage seen in chronic intestinal diseases such as Crohn's disease and colitis.[180]

- *Dosage:* 500 mg glutamine three times a day

Fasting   The intestinal mucosa appears to heal during fasting as indicated by the decrease in intestinal permeability seen in patients who fast. Fasting patients with rheumatoid arthritis decrease their intestinal leakage after only four days. After seven to ten days their joint tenderness, pain and stiffness is reduced as is their sedimentation rate and level of acute phase reacting plasma proteins (both measures of inflammation in the body). However, returning to the same diet results in a return of symptoms and intestinal leakage after only one week.[181] Predictably, the researchers interpreted this to mean fasts were of no long-term value for arthritis. A better interpretation is that they started eating their food allergens again and reestablished the pathology in their intestines and subsequently their joints. Although described as a fast, they were actually on diluted fruit and vegetable juice (2–3 liters per day). Very long fasts, such as over three weeks can result in damage to the intestines and digestive processes and should never be attempted without the guidance of a practitioner highly experienced in supervising fasts. Interestingly, one of the reasons long-term fasting can be a problem is that it causes depletion of glutamine.

Neutralizing Free Radicals

Considering the serious and widespread damage that free radicals cause, it is not surprising that the body utilizes many mechanisms to neutralize them. Most of these processes use antioxidants, i.e., substances that neutralize free radicals. Antioxidants can be either nutrients or enzyme systems, which either directly attack oxidants or regenerate antioxidant nutrients. Table 5-21 lists the antioxidant defenses that protect against free radicals.

Nutrient Antioxidants

A healthful diet provides a wide range of substances, primarily of plant origin, that act as antioxidants. Some have been classified as required vitamins while others appear to be important but have not (yet) been recognized as required.

Table 5-21 Antioxidant Defenses

Nutrient Antioxidants	Vitamin E
	Vitamin C
	Carotenoids
	Xanthophylls
	Flavonoids
Antioxidant Enzymes	Superoxide dismutases (require copper, zinc, manganese)
	Catalases (require iron)
	Glutathione peroxidases (require selenium)
Antioxidants Made by the Body	Glutathione
	Coenzyme Q_{10}
	Melatonin
Herbal Antioxidants	*Silybum marianum* (Milk thistle)
	Picnogenols
	Livotrit

This is probably due to the current bias of the RDAs toward only classifying substances as vitamins if a deficiency results in a specific disease. Unfortunately, this ignores the role of those nutrients whose primary role is to promote health and prevent or ameliorate disease. As might be expected. a diet of whole, unrefined foods, especially those of vegetable origin, contains the highest levels of these important nutrients.

Vitamin E

One of the most important and well-known antioxidants is vitamin E (tocopherol). It actually includes eight fat-soluble compounds, of which alpha-tocopherol is the best known. Vitamin E is a very important antioxidant for the heart, blood lipids, and cell membranes. Vitamin E also inhibits the formation of nitrosamines (highly carcinogenic and inflammatory substances), and decreases inappropriate blood clot formation.[182,183] These protective actions help to ensure proper functioning of the many biological processes needed for health.

The current RDA for vitamin E is 15 iu (10 mg alpha tocopherol equivalents, or TE) for men and 12 iu (8 mg TE) for women, which isn't sufficient. This amount is designed to prevent myopathy and neuropathy, but is far too low to maintain optimal health. Several studies have shown that supposedly healthy people eating diets supplying the RDA of vitamin E have less oxidative damage when supplemented with vitamin E at a modest 150 iu per day.[184] The real daily requirement varies according to the amount of oxidative stress a person experiences. Living in a polluted city, consuming large amounts of polyunsaturated fatty acids (such as fish oils), and heavy exercise—all increase the need for vitamin E and other antioxidants. And even though too low, the RDA still isn't met by the typical U.S. diet.

Because the best sources of vitamin E—unrefined vegetable oils, wheat germ, liver, and eggs—are high-fat foods, it is difficult to provide high levels of vitamin E in the diet without supplementation. Synthetic vitamin E contains a mixture of d and l isomers (meaning they are mirror images of each other). Only the d form is active in the body. Combining vitamin E with acetate, succinate, or palmitate makes it more chemically stable. Whether this makes it more clinically useful has yet to be determined.

Vitamin E itself becomes a free radical after its neutralizes a more toxic free radical. Fortunately, the vitamin E radical does not readily attack lipids and proteins and will decompose. It can also be converted back to the normal antioxidant vitamin E by vitamin C, glutathione, and coenzyme Q_{10}.[185,186]

Topical applications of vitamin E are also very effective. For example, rubbing vitamin E on your skin will greatly decrease the redness, inflammation and skin sensitivity from sunburn, a very visible demonstration of its anti-inflammatory properties.[187]

- *Dosage:* 600 iu mixed tocopherols a day

Vitamin C

Vitamin C is a prominent, water-soluble antioxidant present in body fluids and the cells. It is a very efficient antioxidant and can neutralize a wide range of free radicals including superoxide, singlet oxygen, hypochlorite, and sulfur radicals.[188] Vitamin C protects lipids and cell membranes from oxidative damage by neutralizing peroxyl and hydroxyl radicals. This helps to reduce the risk of cataracts and retinal damage, increase immune function, and decrease heavy metal toxicity.[189,190,191]

Supplementing with vitamin C reduces the gastrointestinal production of fecal mutagens—potent cancer-causing chemicals.[192] This, along with vitamin C's immune potentiation, probably explains why increased vitamin C intake is correlated with a reduced risk of cancer of the cervix, stomach, colon, and lung.[193] Vitamin C supplementation also reduces oxidation of fats in the blood, important for protection from atherosclerosis.[55]

Several research studies have demonstrated that vitamin C supplementation protects cells from radiation-induced transformation to cancerous forms. Vitamin C apparently accomplishes this by quenching the free radicals produced by the irradiation before they can interact with the cell's DNA and other important components. This protective effect has been demonstrated in cells in the laboratory as well as in cells in irradiated animals.[194,195] If you are planning to get a diagnostic x-ray, take your vitamin C first!

Vitamin C works with glutathione and lipoic acid to regenerate vitamin E. Like vitamin E, vitamin C is also converted to a free radical when it neutralizes oxidants. Fortunately, also like the vitamin E radical, the vitamin C radical (dehydroascorbate) is relatively stable, has little tendency to attack cells, and can be converted back to vitamin C.

- *Dosage:* 500 mg vitamin C twice a day

Carotenoids

Carotenoids represent over 500 different plant pigments and are divided into carotenes and xanthophylls (oxygenated carotenes). Beta-carotene is the most abundant carotenoid in nature and is the major carotenoid in the liver, adrenal gland, kidney, ovary, and fat tissues. However, it represents only 25 to 33% of the carotenoids in plasma, possibly because xanthophylls make up 90% of the carotenoids in green leafy vegetables, a major source of dietary carotenoids for humans. Lycopene, a red pigment from tomatoes, is prevalent in the testes, prostate, and human plasma.[196]

In general, carotenoids are versatile antioxidants and lycopene, lutein, and zeaxanthin are all effective quenchers of free radicals, although they do not form vitamin A, as does beta-carotene.[197] Beta-carotene is especially effective at low oxygen levels such as that found in tissues.[198]

The antioxidant effects of carotenoids result in significant health benefits as listed in Table 5-22. The correlation of carotenoid consumption with cancer

Table 5-22 Health Effects of Carotenoids[201,202,203]

Decreased blood lipid oxidation
Protection against coronary artery disease
Decreased risk of age-related macular degeneration, the most common cause of old age blindness
Decreased incidence of some forms of cancer

prevention has received considerable research interest, with 29 of 31 studies showing significant protection.[199] However, a highly publicized study of Finnish men with a long history of heavy cigarette smoking and alcohol use failed to find a reduced risk with beta-carotene supplementation.[200] This unexpected result has several possible explanations: the researchers were using synthetic beta-carotene, which is different from the natural; these people's diet and lifestyle were so bad that the antioxidants might have little effect; and, while high levels of beta-carotene in the blood are certainly associated with a lower incidence of cancer, it may only be a marker for another as yet unrecognized nutrient.

- *Dosage:* 25 mg mixed natural carotenoids a day

Flavonoids

One of the largest classes of dietary antioxidants is the flavonoids. They are found mainly in fruits, vegetables, legumes, and tea. About 5,000 flavonoids have been reported, with quercetin and kaempferol being among the most abundant. Flavonoids directly neutralize free radicals, potentiate the effects of vitamin C (as vitamin C potentiates the action of flavonoids), and protect other easily oxidizable substances.[204] Flavonoids are especially effective antioxidants, several times as powerful as vitamins E and C. Unfortunately, the typical U.S. diet contains only about 23 mg a day.

- *Dosage:* 500 mg mixed flavonoids a day

Table 5-23 Antioxidant Effects of Various Flavonoids[205,206,207,208,209]

Flavonoid	Effect
Rutin, myricetin, and quercetin	Scavenge superoxide and block LDL oxidation
Anthocyanidins (from blueberries and grapes)	Protect collagen from superoxides
Many flavonoids	Bind metals, limiting their ability to catalyze free radical formation
Most flavonoids	Decrease risk of some forms of cancer and cardiovascular disease

Antioxidant Enzymes

Oxidant detoxification enzyme systems occur throughout our cells, tissues, and fluids. Three types detoxify free radicals: superoxide dismutase, catalase, and glutathione peroxidase. These enzymes work together to neutralize oxidants through several steps.

Superoxide dismutase

Superoxide dismutase (SOD) very rapidly converts free radicals into hydrogen peroxide (H_2O_2) before they can damage tissues. Because hydrogen peroxide itself is highly reactive, SOD operates in conjunction with catalase and glutathione peroxidase, which break it down further to water. Several different types of superoxide dismutase exist. The form in the mitochondria requires the trace mineral manganese, while the form in the cell requires copper and zinc. That's why these trace mineral nutrients are often classified as antioxidants, although it is actually the enzyme that they activate that does the antioxidant work. During acute inflammation, the manganese form of SOD increases as part of the body's process to ensure the inflammatory processes do not get out of control.[210]

SOD is a useful therapeutic agent. However, as a supplement it is not very well-absorbed (about 10%) into the body because it is damaged by the digestive processes.[211] Special forms of SOD have now been synthesized to improve its absorption and utilization by the body. In one of these, it is bound up in a liposome (a little ball of fat). Liposomal SOD has been successfully used to treat patients with Crohn's disease.[212] Administering SOD bound to polyethylene glycol together with catalase has been shown to reduce the damage from experimental trauma in animals.[213]

- *Dosage:* 10 mg of manganese, 5 mg of copper, 25 mg zinc per day

Catalase

Catalase is an iron-dependent enzyme that occurs widely in cells. Its primary function is to neutralize hydrogen peroxide. Animal studies with catalase, usually in conjunction with SOD, suggest it provides protection against ischemic (low blood supply) injury to the retina, free radical damage to the intestine, and the free radicals produced by radiation.[214,215,216]

A zinc-dependent version of catalase appears to be especially important for protecting the macula (the part of the eye responsible for acute vision). When compared to matched controls, catalase activity in eyes with signs of macular degeneration is reduced by 32%. Supplementation of zinc in patients with macular degeneration has shown reduced vision loss.[217]

- *Dosage:* 10 mg of iron and 10 mg of zinc per day

Glutathione Peroxidase

This family of enzymes disposes of peroxides, such as hydrogen peroxide. Glutathione peroxidase requires the trace mineral selenium for activation, which is why selenium is sometimes referred to as an antioxidant nutrient. Gluta-thione peroxidase exists in several forms, and more is synthesized when needed. For example, in animal models, exhaustive exercise causes oxidative stress leading to increased levels of SOD, glutathione peroxidase, and gluta-thione transferase. On the other hand, prior supplementation with vitamin E and selenium reduced free radical production and lesser amounts of detoxifica-tion enzymes were produced.[218]

- *Dosage:* 150 μg selenium per day

Antioxidants Made by the Body

The body makes several special compounds that provide antioxidant support, especially in the mitochondria and the cells.

Glutathione (GSH)

Glutathione occurs in high concentrations in most cells, where it is used by the antioxidant enzyme glutathione peroxidase. It also works together with vitamin C to regenerate vitamin E. In addition, glutathione directly neutralizes several free radicals (singlet oxygen, hydroxyl radicals, and superoxide radi-cals). This neutralization results in the oxidation of glutathione (GSSG), which is converted back to the normal form by reductase enzymes.[219] In a healthy person, the ratio of normal to oxidized glutathione (GSH/GSSG) is greater than 100 to 1. However, when a person is exposed to high levels of free radicals (oxidative stress), this ratio is decreased. AIDS patients have substan-tially depressed levels of glutathione in their cells, apparently due to the chronic inflammation they suffer.

- *Dosage:* 100 mg glutathione twice a day

Coenzyme Q_{10} (Ubiquinone)

Ubiquinone are fat-soluble antioxidants. The most common form in humans is ubiquinone-10 or coenzyme Q_{10} (CoQ_{10}). CoQ_{10} protects lipids, especially the very delicate membranes within the cells, against oxidation.[220] It is espe-cially effective in protecting the heart cells from toxic chemicals.[221] In addi-tion, CoQ_{10} can regenerate vitamin E.[222] CoQ_{10} synthesis in the body requires vitamins B_2, B_6, B_{12} and folate, and synthesis is limited in people with low intake of these nutrients. CoQ_{10} deficiencies commonly occur in older persons, being 65% lower in 80 year olds compared to 20 year olds.[223] Because CoQ_{10} is not well-absorbed, increasing plasma CoQ_{10} levels through diet (liver, heart, and germs of grains are rich sources) or supplementation can be difficult.

- *Dosage:* 10 mg of coenzyme Q_{10} per day (people with AIDS have even more trouble absorbing coenzyme Q_{10}, so we recommend 100 mg in our teaching clinic)

Melatonin

Melatonin is best known for its role in setting the circadian rhythms and in helping initiate the sleep process. However, equally important, it is a potent and efficient free-radical scavenger. The central nervous system consumes 20% of the oxygen used daily and generates free radicals at a high rate. Normally present in high concentrations in the nervous system, melatonin appears to play a pivotal part in preventing oxidative damage to the nerves and brain.[224] Aged animals and humans are melatonin-deficient and more sensitive to oxidative stress. Melatonin supplementation and treatments aimed at preserving the endogenous rhythm of melatonin formation appear to retard the rate of aging and the time of onset of age-related diseases.[225]

■ *Dosage:* Start with 1 mg half an hour before going to bed. Increase the dose until effective, but no more than 5 mg.

Herbal Antioxidants

Herbs have been used since antiquity by natural medicine practitioners around the world. Interestingly, modern research suggests that many of their medicinal properties are due to the antioxidants they contain, especially their flavonoid constituents. In fact, some of the most potent antioxidants currently known, such as the flavonoid silymarin from milk thistle, are found in traditional herbal medicines. Another example is the antioxidant activity of procyanidolic oligomers from grape seed skins which is a remarkable 50 times that of vitamin C and vitamin E. Another valuable aspect of these botanical medicines is their tendency to concentrate their antioxidants in specific organs. For example, silymarin from *Silybum marianum* concentrates in the liver, which may explain why it is such an effective protective agent for the liver. This tendency of herbal constituents to concentrate in specific organs has led to the concept of organ specificity of herbs. Table 5-24 lists the antioxidant activity and tissue predilection of several herbs as well as the conditions they help alleviate. All dosages are for the standardized extracts.

How to Decide Which Antioxidant to Use

The extreme diversity of free radicals and the mechanisms and sites for oxidant damage means that no single antioxidant could possibly provide all the protection we need. Also, in general, antioxidants and antioxidant enzyme systems appear to work best synergistically. As might be expected, animal studies indicate that a diversity of antioxidants provides more antioxidant protection than a single nutrient.[226]

Table 5-25 provides my recommended intake of antioxidants for maximum protection from free radicals (based on a comprehensive chapter written by Dr. Robert Ronzio for A *Textbook of Natural Medicine*). Adequate amounts of a broad spectrum of antioxidants are essential to promote optimal health and to minimize the effects of aging, degenerative disease, and toxin exposure.

Table 5-24 Antioxidant Herbs

Herb	Antioxidant Constituents	Target Tissue	Conditions	Daily Dosage
Crataegus oxyacantha (hawthorn berry)	Anthocyanidins and proanthocyanidins (also known as procyanidins)	Heart	Congestive heart failure, athero-sclerosis, hyper-tension	100–250 mg
Ginkgo biloba	Ginkgoflavono-glycosides	Brain	Dementia, Alzheimer's disease, cerebral ischemia	120 mg
Vaccinum myrtillus (blueberry)	Anthocyanidins	Retina of eye	Macular degenera-tion, myopia, glaucoma, cataracts	150 mg
Vitex vinifera (grape seed skins) and pine bark	Procyanidolic oligomers (also known as pycnogenols)	Blood vessels	Varicose veins, diabetic retinopathy, atherosclerosis	50 mg

Removing Heavy Metals

Acute poisoning or the accumulation of high levels of heavy metals requires the immediate expert care of a physician skilled in environmental medicine. Such situations are extremely dangerous and typically require intravenous administration of chelating drugs. Fortunately, such situations are rare. Lower levels of exposure can be effectively treated with nutrition (See Table 5-26), when the heavy metal toxin has been identified and the source of contamination controlled.

Detoxification

Detoxification, simply defined as the removal of toxins from the body, is accomplished by stimulating the body tissues to release toxins and then neutralizing or excreting them as rapidly as possible. Eating a wholesome diet, adopting a healthful lifestyle, and following the advice above for improving the detoxification function of the liver and healing and detoxifying the intestines will result in progressive elimination of toxins over time. However, some may want to accelerate the process. The fastest way is through fasting.

However, before fasting, the routes of elimination from the body must be open and fully functional. There is no point in stirring up toxins if there is no way to eliminate them or if they are released faster than the body can cope with them. This is why the best detoxification results are found when the liver's detoxification enzyme systems are working at their best and the bowel is healthy enough to ensure that toxins excreted into it are quickly removed from

Table 5-25 Recommended Daily Dosages of Antioxidants

Nutrient	Daily Dosage	Potential Toxicity
Mixed tocopherols	600 iu	No significant toxicity for natural tocopherols has been reported. Mild, reversible side effects have been noted at intakes greater than 1,000 mg per day.
Mixed carotenoids	25 mg	Generally, no adverse side effects have been noted other than hypercarotenemia (skin turning yellow) at levels above 30 mg per day.
Vitamin C	2,000 mg	There are generally no adverse effects with long-term consumption of up to several grams of vitamin C daily.
Vitamin A	5,000 iu	Toxicity with chronic consumption of 25,000 retinol equivalents per day can occur rarely. Levels above 100,000 iu per day commonly causes problems.
Copper	5 mg	High copper content in drinking water has been associated with a significantly elevated incidence of atherosclerosis.
Manganese	10 mg	Large amounts may raise blood pressure and chronic overdose may cause neurologic disorders.
Selenium	150 µg	Excessive selenium can be toxic.
Zinc	25 mg	High levels (>75 mg per day) block copper assimilation and are immunosuppressive.
Ginkgo biloba	120 mg	None known
Vaccinum myrtillus	50 mg	None known

the body. Also, great caution should be exercised by those who have high levels of toxins. For example, when patients suffering from significant contamination with fat-soluble toxins, such as DDT, fast, so much DDT is released into circulation that it can reach blood levels toxic to the nervous system.[235]

Fasting

Fasting is a potent and very rapid method for eliminating toxins from our bodies. However, I'm of two minds on fasting and no longer support fasts of over two weeks. For centuries, fasting has been used around the world as an effective therapeutic tool. However, recent research tells us that the toxins released by fasting quickly use up the nutrients in the liver needed for Phase II detoxification. This results in increased toxicity *while* toxins are being released. This problem can be alleviated by using products that support the liver while engaging in a more modest fast.

Although our culture fears fasting and assumes death is imminent after only a few days, as long as water is available, the average adult can actually go

Table 5-26 Nutrients to Chelate Heavy Metals Out of the Body[227,228,229,230,231,232,233,234]

Heavy Metal	Nutrient Chelate	Dosage
Arsenic	N-acetylcysteine (NAC)	1 gm per day
Cadmium	Garlic	1 clove (or equivalent) three times a day
	Selenium	250 µg per day
	Zinc	50 mg per day
Gold	Garlic	1 clove (or equivalent) three times a day
Lead	Garlic	1 clove (or equivalent) three times a day
	Onion	3 oz three times a day
	Pectin	3 gm per day
	Methionine	100 mg per day
	Selenium	250 µg per day
	Thiamin (B$_1$)	100 mg per day
	Zinc	200 mg per day(this dosage should only be used under the supervision of a physician)
Mercury	Garlic	1 clove (or equivalent) three times a day
	Selenium	250 µg per day
	Vitamin E	1,000 iu per day
Silver	Selenium	250 µg per day

without any food for quite a long period of time. As can be seen in Table 5-27, the body has several sources of energy reserve, with protein and fat providing the most. Under extreme circumstances, the average adult can actually survive without food for over two months. This is obviously not recommended! I have supervised water fasts as long as 30 days, although I no longer believe such a long time is healthful. The longest water fast I have done myself was ten days.

What happens during a fast

During fasting, the body's metabolic processes change in several ways, according to the length of the fast. The physiology of fasting is a highly ordered series of events that conserve body energy reserves while maintaining the basic metabolic rate (which decreases by about 1% per day during fasting, until it stabilizes at about 75% of normal).[236] It has been suggested that humans, like other species, have evolved as a survival mechanism special biochemical pathways to subsist for long periods of time without food.[237] Some believe this has also evolved as an important part of the self-healing process.

The body's response to the lack of energy input can be divided into three stages: early fasting, fasting, and starvation. Maintaining adequate energy resources for metabolism during fasting involves several adaptations, which change as the body moves from one stage to the next.

Normally, glucose, fatty acids, and amino acids are the major energy fuels of the body. The initial physiological response to the lack of food is the breakdown of glycogen by the liver to produce glucose for release into the bloodstream.

Table 5-27 Energy Reserve Utilization

Energy Source	Reserve (These estimates are based on 100% utilization of each fuel)
Glucose	1 hour
Food in the digestive tract	4 to 8 hours
Glycogen	12 hours
Amino acids	48 hours
Protein	3 weeks (if protein were the only fuel used for gluconeogenesis) 24 weeks (obligatory loss only)
Triglycerides	8 weeks

Glucose is especially needed by the red blood cells and the brain, which consumes about 65% of the total circulating glucose.[238] Together they consume 100 to 180 gm of glucose per day. Early in fasting, the liver is the sole source of glucose for the bloodstream. However, liver glycogen stores can only supply enough glucose for a few hours. (Although muscle actually contains more glycogen than the liver, it lacks the needed enzymes to convert glycogen to glucose for release into the bloodstream.[239]) The liver then begins converting amino acids to glucose, a process called gluconeogenesis. Interestingly, later in fasting, the glycogen reserves are restored.

Since liver's amino acid stores are also limited, amino acids from other tissues, primarily the muscles, are accessed. As the fast proceeds, the kidneys become progressively more important in the maintenance of blood glucose levels, and eventually the renal cortex synthesizes more glucose from amino acids than does the liver. If the body continued to require its normal 100 to 180 gm of glucose a day for the brain, gluconeogenesis during fasting would quickly use up much body protein, and death would ensue within three to four weeks. During the early stages of fasting, the body converts 60 to 84 gm of protein to glucose per day.

After two to three days, the body converts to using the fat stores as the primary source of energy.[240] At this stage, the liver produces energy from the fatty acids released by the breakdown of triglycerides (the storage form of fat) in the fat cells. The brain also changes its metabolic processes and begins to use fatty acids for energy (technically described as oxidation of beta-hydroxybutyrate) instead of sugar. However, there is still a need for approximately 80 gm of glucose a day for the brain, red cells, muscles, and other tissues. This requirement increases significantly during exercise. Some of the needed glucose is synthesized from glycerol, which is released when the fat cells give up fatty acids. The rest of the glucose requirement is met by the catabolism of 18 to 24 gm of protein a day. These metabolic changes result in the elevation of ketones in the blood, which appear in the urine by the third day.

An average 154-pound male has the fat stores to maintain basic caloric requirements for two to three months of fasting. Starvation occurs when the body's fat reserves are depleted and significant protein catabolism again becomes necessary for energy production. The body's protein stores are adequate for only a few weeks, after which essential proteins are utilized and death occurs.

Why fasting can be beneficial

Unfortunately, most of the fasting research has been focused on understanding how the body maintains energy levels and determining whether it was effective in treating various diseases. However, some tantalizing research suggests the mechanisms by which fasting helps to promote health. Obviously, it is very effective in removing toxins from the fat (and other) stores, because fat-soluble toxins are rapidly released during fasting. However, probably its most useful effects for detoxification are immune system enhancement, removal of immune complexes from the blood, and removal of food allergens from the intestines.

Changes in the immune system during fasting include: increased macrophage activity, increased cell-mediated immunity (T lymphocytes and lymphokines), decreased complement factors, decreased antigen-antibody complexes, increased immunoglobulin levels, increased neutrophil bactericidal activity, depressed lymphocyte blastogenesis, heightened monocyte killing and bactericidal function, and enhanced natural killer cell activity.[241,242] The net effect appears to be an increase in the toxin scavenging activity of the white cells combined with elimination of immune complexes, which can cause widespread inflammatory damage in the body.

The leaky gut syndrome may help to explain why fasting leads to improvement of chronic inflammatory diseases such as rheumatoid arthritis. Fasting reduces gut permeability by allowing the damaged intestines to heal when the offending foods are removed.[243]

Chronic food restriction has been well-documented as increasing longevity and decreasing cancer in animals. This is probably partially due to an increased rate of detoxification. For example, in rat research, it was found that food restriction increased the detoxification of the polycyclic aromatic hydrocarbons (benzopyrene), which are carcinogenic. This detoxification process may be important in the protective action of reduced food intake.[244] Table 5-28 lists diseases that have been alleviated by fasting. Note, however, that some of this research is very old and has not been verified by more recent rigorous standards.

Table 5-28 Diseases Alleviated by Fasting

Arthritis[245,246]	Leaky gut[252]
Autoimmune disease[247]	Obesity[253,254]
Atherosclerosis[248]	Pancreatitis[255]
Diabetes[249,250]	PCB and DDT contamination[256]
Epilepsy[251]	(extreme caution must be exercised)

Classic (water) fasting

Fasting is classically defined as abstinence from all food and drink, except water, for a specific period of time, usually for a therapeutic or religious purpose. Fasting is differentiated from starvation because, when properly implemented, it spares essential tissue and utilizes non-essential tissues (i.e., fat) for fuel. In contrast, starvation is a process in which the body uses essential tissue for fuel. Fasting carried on too long becomes starvation, which in time leads to death. In general, water fasts of up to one week are safe, except in those who are emaciated, children, and pregnant or lactating women. Those with any serious disease—e.g., diabetes, heart disease, cancer, or Gilbert's syndrome—should only engage in a fast under the supervision of a physician experienced with therapeutic fasts.

There are many protocols for water fasting. The protocol I recommend is based on my experience (I have personally fasted for a week or more several times and have supervised a large number of patients on extended fasts) and the advice of Dr. Trevor K. Salloum and Dr. Alec Burton found in the chapter "Therapeutic Fasting" in A *Textbook of Natural Medicine*.

In general, therapeutic fasting of more than five-days duration is probably best conducted under supervision at an in-patient facility. Several facilities now exist in the U.S., Canada, England, and Australia, and these centers follow the standards of care and principles of ethics established by the International Association of Professional Natural Hygienists. The basic procedure I recommend:

1. Days one to two: raw fruits and vegetables
2. Days three to seven: pure water only
3. Day eight: a small amount of fruit several times during the day
4. Day nine: Modest amounts of raw fruit and lightly cooked vegetables
5. Day ten: Back to a healthful diet

Large amounts of pure water (distilled, spring, or reverse osmosis) should be drunk during the fast. While some fasting experts recommend drinking diluted fruit and vegetable juices, such a protocol is considered to be a restricted diet or modified food fast, not a classic fast. Also, the continued consumption of carbohydrates inhibits the body's conversion to ketotic metabolism. Another advantage of drinking only water is that hunger almost totally disappears, conversion to fatty acid utilization occurs more quickly and efficiently, weight loss is more dramatic and is from fat rather than protein stores, healing time is shorter, and you don't feel as debilitated.[257]

The optimal quantity of water to ingest during fasting is best determined by thirst, but should be at least four glasses a day.[258] Large amounts of water are critical since the increased levels of toxins released in the circulation need to be excreted in the urine. If the urine is too concentrated, there is a greater risk of damaging the kidneys. Although it may sound reasonable to use enemas to help eliminate toxins, most fasting authorities discourage their use.

Another very important aspect of fasting is getting adequate rest. Energy conservation is necessary to allow maximum healing and to avoid unnecessary breakdown of protein to supply glucose. Short walks and light stretching can improve one's sense of well-being, but intense exercise will inhibit repair and elimination.

Side effects, other than discomfort, from fasting are rarely serious, but fasting may uncover hidden pathology. Discomfort during fasting may be due to withdrawal from stimulants, withdrawal from food allergens, hypoglycemia, acidosis, and high levels of toxins released into the circulation. Some fasters experience headaches, insomnia, skin irritations, dizziness, nausea, coated tongue, body odor, aching limbs, palpitations, mucus discharge, and visual and hearing disturbances.

In some people, complications occur that necessitate breaking the fast early. Examples of such conditions include a sudden drop in blood pressure, mental confusion, lowered body temperature, extreme weakness, shortness of breath, vomiting, diarrhea, gastrointestinal bleeding, liver dysfunction, kidney insufficiency, gout, a rapid or slow or irregular heart beat, and serious emotional distress.

Modified Fasts

Several products are now on the market that aid the detoxification process. A good example is a product called "UltraClear Plus," produced by HealthComm and designed by Jeff Bland, Ph.D. (Please note, the author derives no commercial benefit from these or other products or supplements mentioned in this book.) When used properly as part of a fast, these products initiate the same detoxification processes, albeit at a lower rate, while ensuring the availability of the critical nutrients needed to maintain energy and the liver's detoxification processes. I strongly advise those interested in fasting to use this methodology first. It is far less uncomfortable, will produce healthful results and appears to place less strain on the liver.

The intensity of a fast can be adjusted according to your needs. At one extreme, the only thing consumed is water and the meal replacement powder. This will produce a detoxification process almost as intense as classic water fasting. At the other extreme, a diet of raw and steamed fruits and vegetables is consumed along with the meal replacement powder. This will also result in detoxification, but at a lowered rate.

Saunas

Saunas are an age-old detoxification therapy. They are based on the concept that as the body sweats, toxins are released through the skin. Prolonged saunas (over an hour at a lower temperature) are thought to increase the excretion of fatty acids through the skin and thus fat-soluble toxins. There is some research that documents this method of detoxification. One group of researchers studied 14 firefighters who had been exposed to highly toxic polychlorinated biphenyls in a transformer fire and who subsequently developed neuropsychological problems six months after the fire. They underwent two to three weeks of experimental detoxification, which was a medically supervised diet, exercise, and sauna program. These men were compared with firefighters from the same department who did not participate in the detoxification program. Those who followed the detoxification program showed significant improvement in scores in three memory tests as compared to those who didn't. Self appraisal for depression, anger, and fatigue, however, did not improve.[259] However, this was a very short period of time for eliminating such toxins and the results do suggest potential benefits.

As valuable as saunas are, they must be used with care because greatly elevating body temperature can cause problems in some situations. Specifically, saunas are contraindicated in pregnant women, young children, adults with heart disease or seizure disorders, immediately after intense exercise, and after drinking alcohol or ingesting cocaine.[260]

How to Treat Common Toxicity Diseases

Toxicity can contribute to virtually every disease. Some diseases appear to be triggered by environmental toxins, some are aggravated by toxins, some are caused by the damage induced by toxins, and some are the direct result of derangement of the detoxification processes.

Gilbert's Syndrome

Gilbert's syndrome is one of the few diseases known to be specifically due to an abnormality in the liver's detoxification system.[261] Specifically, the Phase II glucuronidation pathway doesn't work very well in affected people.[262] This results in a chronically elevated serum bilirubin level and a slight yellowing of the white of the eye in the absence of hepatitis. Previously considered rare, this disorder is now known to affect 5 to 7% of the general population. Although most usually do not have symptoms, some suffer from anorexia (loss of appetite), malaise (weakness), and fatigue—all typical symptoms of impaired liver function. Of particular significance is that those with this syndrome are more susceptible to toxic reactions to xenobiotics and drugs, such as the widely used analgesic acetaminophen, especially if used above the recommended dosages.

This toxicity results because if acetaminophen is not processed rapidly enough by Phase II systems (it can also go through the glutathione conjugation and sulfation pathways, but they are even slower) some of it is processed by Phase I enzymes, which form a far more active and toxic form. This bioactivated form binds to molecules within the cells causing damage and even cell death. The typical person with Gilbert's syndrome has a 31% slower rate of glucuronidation of acetaminophen. Other common drugs that are poorly metabolized by those with Gilbert's syndrome include menthol, clofibrate, and tolbutamide. Those with this syndrome are probably not good candidates for fasting because fasting uses up available glutathione very rapidly. When these people fast for very long, they develop significant jaundice.[263]

Much can be done to help reverse this enzyme dysfunction. The first step is to protect the weakened enzyme from further damage. This can be done by avoiding fluoridated water and other sources of fluoride. Being an enzyme inhibitor, fluoride reduces the activity of glucuronyl even further. One report found that when some patients with Gilbert's syndrome stopped drinking fluoride, their mild jaundice cleared. Drinking fluoridated water caused the jaundice to return.[264]

Methionine, administered as S-adenosylmethionine (SAM), is particularly helpful in treating Gilbert's syndrome because it activates several Phase II pathways. Supplementation (1 gm twice a day) results in a significant decreases in serum bilirubin in patients with Gilbert's syndrome.[265]

A far more serious condition is Crigler-Najjar syndrome, where the glucuronidation enzyme is virtually nonfunctional. Those with no enzyme activity seldom survive into adulthood.

- *Dosage:* 500 mg of S-adenosylmethionine twice a day

Chronic Fatigue Syndrome

Many people are chronically tired, but few actually have chronic fatigue syndrome (CFS). In a random survey of 4,000 members of a health maintenance organization in the Northwest, a surprising 19% of the 77% who responded reported chronic fatigue. Of these 66% had a medical or psychiatric condition that could account for the fatigue. Of the remaining 74, only 3 met the strict Centers for Disease Control criteria for chronic fatigue syndrome (CFS).[266] But those with CFS suffer from a tough disease.

Chronic fatigue syndrome is still not fully understood. Our best understanding is that it is the end result of a viral infection that has damaged the energy-producing mitochondria, brain, and endocrine system. While no cure is known, several natural medicine therapies help substantially.

Improving the function of the liver, gastrointestinal system, and mitochondria is especially important for those with mild-to-moderate chronic fatigue syndrome. Functional tests have demonstrated significant impairment of Phase I and Phase II detoxification and leaky intestines.

Dr. Jeffrey Bland, a leading researcher in the field of preventive and nutritional medicine, recently published an extremely important paper on a successful comprehensive treatment program for 106 patients suffering chronic fatigue, fibromyalgia, and irritable bowel syndrome. His research group of several cooperating clinics across the country found that these patients had both abnormal liver detoxification pathways and abnormal gut permeability. The intervention program they used included avoidance of food allergens, stimulation of repair of the intestinal lining cells, strengthening of the liver detoxification pathways through the use of key nutrients, and a high quality nonallergenic oligoantigenic rice protein formula. Not only did the patient's symptoms improve dramatically (52% reduction after 10 weeks), but so did their laboratory test results.[267]

This is a very difficult condition to treat and virtually always requires the guidance of a physician skilled in nutrition and environmental medicine. The basic protocol is to stop the damage, heal the damaged intestines and liver, reestablish proper mitochondrial metabolism, and regenerate the adrenal glands. The first step is to detect and scrupulously avoid all toxins and food allergens and reestablish healthy flora in the intestines. This can be accomplished by using a meal-replacement product such as UltraClear SUSTAIN, which was used in the Bland research. Based on rice protein, it is very low in allergens. It is also high in the nutrients needed to stimulate liver detoxification (e.g., NAC and glutathione), healing of the damaged intestines (e.g., fructooligosaccharides, insulin and glutamine), and restoration of mitochondrial function (B vitamins and magnesium). These beneficial effects on the liver and intestines can be augmented by eating brassica family foods at least twice a day and using the herb *Silybum marianum* (120 mg of standardized extract three times a day). The final step is to help regenerate the adrenal glands, which are commonly dysfunctional in chronic fatigue syndrome patients. Once again, the UltraClear product has useful nutrients (e.g., pantothenic acid and vitamin C). To this can be added Siberian ginseng (10 ml fluid extract three times a day of standardized *Eleutherococcus senticosus* extract).

The strong correlation between chronic fatigue syndrome, fibromyalgia, and multiple chemical sensitivities suggests that all may respond to hepatic detoxification, food allergy control, and a gut restoration diet.[268]

Multiple Chemical Sensitivities

This condition goes by many names: multiple chemical sensitivities, total allergy syndrome, 20th century disease, cerebral allergy, and chemically induced immune dysregulation. It has been recognized for the past 40 years by physicians who practice clinical ecology. Those with this condition become sick because of toxic effects of chemicals in the environment. These patients are chronically ill and have problems in many systems, often without any objective evidence of standard diseases. However, some suffer from such diseases as allergies, autoimmune diseases, migraine headaches, dysmenorrhea, and cancer. The typical patient is unable to tolerate a large number of foods, drugs, and environmental chemicals. Usually little is found on physical examination of these patients and conventional physicians often suggest, or diagnose, a psychiatric illness.[269]

However, this is a real phenomenon, an unfortunate side effect of modern life. Over 100 research studies published in medical literature support the validity of chemical sensitivity as a significant health problem.[270] The chemically sensitive individual typically has one or more defects or deficiencies in xenobiotic detoxification systems, resulting in their being reactive to chemicals that may not affect others at similar levels of exposure.[271]

One of the reasons this condition is not readily accepted or understood by conventional physicians is that the symptoms these people develop cross specialty boundaries. For physicians to understand the pathophysiology of this disorder, they need to step out of the current medical paradigm, which pigeonholes disease. Chronic exposure to toxins—such as happened in the early 1970's when urea foam formaldehyde insulation was installed in many homes across the country—can produce, in susceptible individuals, almost any symptom. Common symptoms include chronic flu-like symptoms, joint pain, and brain dysfunction, which manifests with such symptoms as confusion, inability to concentrate, fatigue, mood swings, poor memory, depression, spaciness, or dizziness (remember, the brain is the most metabolically active organ in the body so it is not surprising that it is so easily affected).

There are many reasons for the varying susceptibility of people to xenobiotics: genetic variations in detoxification enzymes, deficiencies of key nutrients needed for the detoxification systems, multiple sites of exposure (e.g., a home with urea insulation and a tight building at work), and length of exposure to toxins (which could use up the available Phase II detoxification substances). For example, a person with poor detoxification enzymes living in a toxic home environment may eventually become depleted in the conjugating substances that may help protect him or her. Once depleted, the person becomes progressively more sensitive to chemicals as more and more chemicals and toxic metabolites build up in their system. These people typically respond very poorly to the current drug-treatment paradigm, because no matter how good or appropriate a drug may be, it is seen by the body as yet another addition to its toxic burden. Rather, these people need to decrease their toxic burden while providing key nutrients to support their detoxification pathways.

The basic approach with these patients is to decrease exposure and provide support for all of the liver's detoxification pathways, i.e., vitamins B-complex (25 mg three times a day) and C (500 mg three times a day), selenium (250 µg a day), glutathione (100 mg three times a day), brassica family foods (two or three servings a day, and *Silybum marianum* (120 mg three times a day).

Of particular importance is establishing a safe home and work environment. This can be quite a challenge. Fortunately, several groups around the country have developed expertise in providing guidance for the chemically sensitive (for referral contact the American Environmental Foundation 1-214-361-9515 in Dallas, Texas). Removing chemicals from the home or work environment typically requires replacing soft surface with hard surface building materials. For example, carpets are a common source of continuing pollution as their plastic threads constantly give out gas chemicals (this is what makes them flexible), provide a breeding ground for mites and, in high humidity environments, allow the growth of molds—all common environmental problems for the chemically sensitive. The recommended procedure is to replace these surfaces with tile, which is chemically inert.

Sick Building Syndrome

Sick building syndrome is a special category of illness where people in a specific building suffer from ill defined, but reproducible, illness. It sometimes is confused with multiple chemical sensitivities. In contrast to multiple chemical sensitivity, patients with sick building syndrome become ill quickly whenever they enter the problem building and improve after leaving the building. They do not have intolerance to environmental exposures elsewhere.[272] Typical chemicals found in such buildings include toluene, xylene, benzene, trichloroethene, styrene, phthalates, and pesticides. For example, toluene, which affects the central nervous system and slows metabolism of benzene, a known carcinogen, is released as a gas from paints, carpets, and furniture. Enhanced energy efficiency standards have increased the sick building syndrome problem: the rate of air turnover is far slower, allowing much higher levels of building chemicals to build up.

The approach for treatment is basically the same as for multiple chemical sensitivities: avoid the source of the toxins (this may involve finding a new job) and provide support for your liver's detoxification functions, as discussed earlier this chapter.

Migraine Headaches

Headaches are one of the ten most common complaints that bring people to a doctor. Migraine headaches affect about 17% of women and 5% of men sometime in their life. The disease usually begins in childhood, but during this early period it often does not manifest as headaches. Instead, such nonspecific symptoms as colic, periodic abdominal pains and vomiting, vertigo, or unusually severe motion sickness are the most common complaints. The peak incidence is between 20 and 35 years of age, then gradually declining with age. More than half of the patients have a family history of the illness.

The typical medical approach is to relieve the symptoms through the use of drugs, such as sumatriptan and ergotamine. Sumatriptan works well, improving symptoms in 70% of cases with most side effects being mild except in the 5% who suffer chest pain.[273] However, it has no impact on the frequency of attacks and is extremely expensive. A far better approach is to deal with the underlying cause: food allergies.

Several studies have documented the efficacy of food allergy control in the treatment of migraine headaches, both for children and adults. In a double-blind, controlled trial of 88 children with severe, frequent migraines, 93% showed significant recovery when their diet was modified to eliminate allergenic foods.[274] Associated symptoms—such as abdominal pain, behavioral disorders, fits, asthma, and eczema—also improved in the treated children. In other words, the side effects were better health! In a study of adult patients with migraines, 66% had complete relief within two weeks when the offending foods (an average of six different foods in each person) were eliminated.[275] The six most common allergenic foods were cow's milk, wheat, chocolate, eggs, oranges, and the common food additive benzoic acid.

Summary

No mater how good our food or how pure an environment we live in, we will always be exposed to toxins. Whether from the environment, our intestines, or dysfunctional metabolic processes, toxins are devastating to our health if our detoxification systems aren't working well enough. Total wellness requires decreasing our exposure to toxins, optimizing nutritional status to ensure that our detoxification systems are working, supplementing with the key nutrients and herbs that strengthen detoxification, and removing toxins from our liver, bowels, and whole system.

Chapter Six

Normalizing Inflammatory Function

You need to study this chapter if you suffer from any of the following:
- *Symptoms*
  Allergies
  Chronically impacted ear wax
  Chronically runny nose
  Dry skin, especially behind the ears and around the nose and eyebrows
  Fluid retention
  Pain and stiffness in the morning
  Red eyes
  Swollen ankles

- *Diseases*
  Asthma
  Hay fever
  Hives
  Inflammatory bowel disease (Crohn's disease, ulcerative colitis)
  Lupus erythematosis
  Multiple sclerosis
  Rheumatoid arthritis
  Seborrheic dermatitis

Behaviors that increase risk:
- A high-meat diet
- A diet rich in hydrogenated fats, e.g., margarine and shortening
- Bottle-fed infants
- Eating foods containing additives
- Excessive alcohol consumption
- Inadequate amounts of fruits and vegetables in the diet
- Inadequate amounts of raw nuts and seeds in the diet

Thumbnail: Quick Help for Inflammation

- *To normalize the inflammatory response:*
  Eat less land animal fat and more fish, nuts, and seeds
  Eat a lot of colorful fruits and vegetables
  Vitamin E: 400 iu per day
  Vitamin C: 2,000 mg per day

- *To directly decrease inflammation:*
  Quercetin: 500 mg twice a day
  Flaxseed, evening primrose or fish oil: 2–4 grams a day

Inflammation is a normal, and important, body function. Through inflammation, the body removes damaged cells, eliminates toxins, fights invading microorganisms, and begins the repair process. Unfortunately, our modern lifestyle often causes the inflammatory process to go seriously awry. Instead of an effective, controlled process, many experience an excessive and, at times, misdirected inflammatory response that results in chronic swelling and pain and, if allowed to continue unchecked, progressive damage to the essential tissues and organs of our bodies. When the inflammatory processes are out of balance, not only are abnormal cells and toxins removed, but healthy tissues are also damaged and, for some, a self-perpetuating, progressively destructive, inflammatory process can ensue. This contributes to the development of chronic inflammatory diseases (such as rheumatoid arthritis) and autoimmune diseases (such as multiple sclerosis and systemic lupus erythematosis).

This imbalance shows up in three ways: excessive inflammatory response to damage, inadequate quenching of the inflammation process when the job is done, and/or excessive activation of the inflammatory process. In general, each of these has a specific cause: excessive animal fats in the diet result in too many inflammatory chemicals being produced, lack of critical nutrients in the diet (such as essential fatty acids and antioxidants) weakens the anti-inflammatory processes, and high exposure to several unfortunately common environmental toxins chronically activates the inflammatory processes, even when they are not needed. Finally, if our healing and regenerative processes are not working adequately, the inflammatory process may continue to run, even though nothing is being accomplished.

Real-Life Messages from an Inflammatory System Out of Balance

Arthritis

Jane was 32 and had been recently diagnosed as having the early stages of rheumatoid arthritis. While her morning pain and stiffness weren't too bad and easily relieved by two aspirin, she was quite distraught. Her mother and all her aunts suffered from severe forms of the disease; several were so bad that their hands were quite deformed. She was not willing to accept her family physician's prognosis of having to live with a disease that would relentlessly progress.

Fortunately, she came to see me before her disease had progressed very far. I explained to her that I thought her joint inflammation was being caused by a combination of a leaky gut due to food allergies and an over-reactive inflammatory system. While she had never heard of such an explanation for rheumatoid arthritis, she was desperate enough to try anything. I immediately started her on a water fast for four days. We then reintroduced foods, one each day, looking for those that caused a reaction. She was easy to diagnose because her joints flared up anytime she ate a food to which she was allergic. (Often the reaction to a food is so delayed—as long as three days in some people—that it can be very difficult to make the connection.) As is typical of most people, her problem foods were wheat and dairy products.

I then helped her design a diet that not only avoided all grains (she had to also avoid rye, oats, corn, and rice since those with allergies to wheat also tend to be allergic to the other grains) and dairy products; we also decreased her meat and fat consumption. Basically, her diet now consisted of fish, fruits, vegetables, beans, nuts, and seeds. I also had her take 1 gram of eicosapentaenoic acid from fish oils, 1,000 iu of vitamin E, and 2,000 mg of vitamin C daily.

By the end of her fast, her symptoms had already decreased 50%. After one month of carefully following her diet and supplement prescription, she had no further pain in her joints. After three months, all her lab tests had returned to normal!

Not all of my rheumatoid arthritis patients respond so well. I still vividly remember with great sadness a 55-year-old woman who had had the disease for over 20 years. Her hands were so deformed she could hardly hold a pen, and she was having chronic stomach problems from all the aspirin she was taking. Although I applied exactly the same therapy, all we could accomplish was to decrease her dosage of aspirin. Sometimes diseases do progress past the point of the body's ability to heal.

■ *The message:* The body has a tremendous ability to heal even "incurable" diseases if given a chance. But don't wait too long. The earlier the underlying problem is corrected, the better the outcome.

A Dramatic Recovery

For most people, taking care of oneself and using natural medicine results in progressive improvement in health rather than the dramatic "cures" so widely publicized by conventional medicine. However, sometimes even simple nutritional therapies can have immediate and dramatic results. Shortly after we opened the teaching clinic at Bastyr University in 1980, we helped a boy with a serious chronic disease who responded so well to our treatment that the local

CBS television affiliate filmed a special on it, which was aired both locally and nationally.

Mary brought her very sick nine-year-old son Justin to our teaching clinic. He was suffering from a rare condition diagnosed as Schöenlein-Henock purpura by the medical specialists she had taken her son to see. This is a terrible, totally out-of-control inflammatory disease. The child suffers from chronic abdominal pain, skin rashes, arthritis, and kidney damage. In addition, Justin also had serious problems with his immune system and was always sick with one infection or another. His mother related that every week over the past two years, her son had either seen a doctor or been hospitalized for one health problem after another.

At that time, our chief medical officer in the teaching clinic was Dr. Ed Madison, a conscientious physician who spent a lot of time in the library. (Unfortunately Dr. Madison no longer practices or teaches at Bastyr, a great loss.) While studying a medical research journal a few months before, Dr. Madison had read about this condition and a team of researchers who had treated it with two nutrients—vitamin C and the bioflavonoid quercetin. The researchers reported a complete cure in several cases, and we decided to try this treatment with Justin.

Within a week of starting the supplements, his symptoms improved and within a few weeks, all the symptoms he had suffered from for years had totally resolved! An "incurable" disease was cured by simple anti-inflammatory nutrients.

- *The message:* When needed, vitamin C and the bioflavonoids can be potent anti-inflammatory nutrients.

How the Inflammatory System Works

Our tissues are regularly damaged in many ways: trauma, infection, ischemia (very poor blood supply that results in degeneration), poisons, foreign particles (such as asbestos), radiation, and so on. Even normal wear and tear causes damage that needs to be repaired. Regardless of the cause, the inflammatory process is essentially the same. When a cell or tissue is damaged, an orderly sequence of events occurs that eventually results in repair.

When the damage to a cell is minor, a special organ within the cell, called the lysosome, ruptures, releasing enzymes. These enzymes immediately begin to digest the damaged parts of the cell. As long as the damage is slight, only a portion of the cell is removed, and the cell is repaired and normal function restored. If the damage to the cell is severe, the entire cell is digested (a process called autolysis), and the process for regeneration of a new cell is initiated.

When many cells are involved, a much more extensive process ensues. As shown in Figure 6-1, when cells are killed (1), either by the trauma or autolysis, two classes of chemicals are released (2) into the surrounding tissues where they initiate the inflammatory process. The first class of these are called vasoactive mediators (3). They include such chemicals as histamine, leukotrienes, and

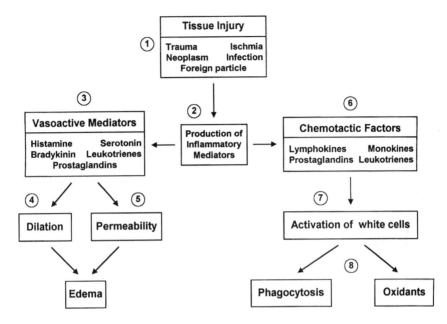

Figure 6-1 *The Inflammatory Response*

pro-inflammatory prostaglandins. These inflammatory chemicals cause the local blood vessels to dilate (4), which is why the area becomes hot and red, and the capillaries to become more permeable (5), which is why the area becomes swollen. The end result is a great increase in the flow of blood to the area, allowing easier migration of white cells and needed nutrients through the capillaries and into the damaged areas.

The second class of inflammatory chemicals are called chemotactic factors (6). They include such chemicals as lymphokines and, once again, the leukotrienes and pro-inflammatory prostaglandins. When released, they attract white cells (7) to the area and stimulate them to digest and remove the damaged tissues (8), a process called phagocytosis. In addition, the white cells release powerful oxidizing agents to destroy any pathogens that might be in the area. The greater the damage or the more serious the invasion, the greater the activation of these inflammatory processes.

This inflammatory process can become quite involved, with toxic chemicals flying everywhere, highly activated white cells trying to eat everything in sight, and any pathogen in the area fighting back with its own chemicals. If the process is not limited, the surrounding healthy tissues can be unwillingly pulled into the fray. They protect themselves by releasing chemicals that limit the spread of the inflammation. They secrete anti-inflammatory prostaglandins to neutralize the pro-inflammatory prostaglandins, antioxidants to neutralize the inflammatory chemicals, anti-chemotactic chemicals to tell the white cells

"Stop, your job is done," and proteolytic enzymes to break down the digestive enzymes released by the white cells. As the damaged tissues are removed, fewer pro-inflammatory chemicals are released and these anti-inflammatory processes progressively quench the inflammatory process until all is back to normal.

Once inflammation is finished, the repair processes begin. As long as there has not been too much damage, either from the original insult or the inflammatory process, the body regenerates the destroyed tissues and normal function is restored. However, if too much tissue is irreversibly injured, scar tissue forms.

Normally, this process works fine. In fact, a low level inflammation/ removal/repair process is always ongoing throughout the body because all of our tissues are, over time, broken down and regenerated as part of the normal maintenance process of the body. Without this repair process, we would quickly become dysfunctional; cells and tissues are delicate and need considerable maintenance. However, our modern lifestyle often causes this crucial process to go awry.

How Inflammation Becomes Imbalanced

As is typical of many of the body's normal physiological processes, the inflammatory system represents a balance of several processes. As shown in Table 6-1, this balance can go awry in several ways. The body can overreact to damage, the inflammatory process might not be stopped when it should be, or chemicals and drugs in the body may excessively stimulate or inappropriately activate the inflammatory reaction. The body needs to maintain a delicate balance between limiting the inflammation only to where it needs to be, so other tissues are not unnecessarily damaged, while allowing the inflammatory process to get its work done, whether that's killing off bacteria or removing damaged tissues.

Table 6-1 Causes of Inflammation Dysfunction

Cause	Description
Excessive inflammatory response to damage	A diet high in animal fats and low in essential fatty acids revs up the pro-inflammatory prostaglandin pathways, while the essential fatty acids found in vegetable and fish oils that support the anti-inflammatory prostaglandin pathways are deficient.
Poor inflammation quenching	A deficiency in bioflavonoids and antioxidants allows normal inflammatory process to proceed out of control.
Excessive inflammatory stimulation	Several drugs, many food additives (colorings, flavorings, preservatives, and emulsifiers), and environmental poisons either increase sensitivity to inflammatory reactions or directly cause inflammation.

Excessive Inflammatory Response to Damage

The intensity and duration of the inflammatory process is governed by the degree of tissue injury and the balance between the strength of the inflammatory response and the anti-inflammatory response. Much of the pro- and anti-inflammatory activity is determined by the ratio of inflammatory and anti-inflammatory prostaglandins. The ratio of these chemicals is greatly affected by genetic and dietary factors.

Prostaglandins

Prostaglandins are a group of regulatory molecules synthesized in the body from fatty acids. While there are several families of prostaglandins, in general only three impact the inflammatory process: series 2 pro-inflammatory prostaglandins (PG-2) and series 1 and 3 anti-inflammatory prostaglandins (PG-1 and PG-3). The ratio of these prostaglandin classes is determined by the availability of the fatty acids from which they are made and how well the enzymes that make the conversion are working.

As shown in Figure 6-2, each of these classes of prostaglandins is made from different fatty acids. Since these fatty acids are either not synthesized (which is why they are called "essential") or poorly synthesized by humans, they must be obtained from the diet, just like vitamins and minerals. As might be expected, the types of fatty acids a person has in his or her cells is virtually totally determined by the diet because different foods contain different fatty acids. For example, a diet rich in land-animal fats results in high levels of pro-inflammatory arachidonic acid in the blood and cell membranes, while a diet rich in fish results in a high level of anti-inflammatory EPA.

As can be seen in Figure 6-2, the anti-inflammatory series 1 prostaglandins are made by an enzyme called cyclooxygenase from the essential fatty acid dihomogammalinolenic acid (DGLA). DGLA is found in human milk and is made in the body from gammalinolenic acid. GLA is found in foods such as evening primrose, borage, and black currant oils and is synthesized from linoleic acid by the enzymes delta-6-desaturase and elongase. We get linoleic acid in our diet from almost all nuts and seeds and their oils, e.g., brazil, peanut, pecan, safflower, sesame, sunflower, and corn.

The pro-inflammatory series 2 prostaglandins are made from the fatty acid arachidonic acid by the cyclooxygenase enzyme. Arachidonic acid is also converted by lipoxygenase and other enzymes to several other potent mediators of inflammation, including leukotrienes, thromboxanes, and prostacylins. The only dietary source of arachidonic acid is land-animal fats. Arachidonic acid can be made from DGLA by the enzyme delta-5-desaturase. However, this enzyme doesn't work very well in humans, so virtually all of our arachidonic acid comes from our diet.

Finally, the series 3 prostaglandins are made, again using the cyclooxygenase enzyme, from the essential fatty acid eicosapentaenoic acid (EPA).

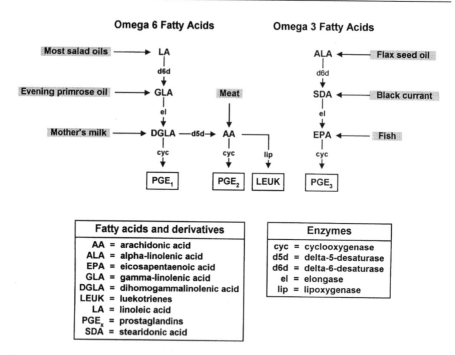

Figure 6-2 *The Synthesis of Prostaglandins from Fatty Acids*

EPA comes to us in our diet from fish oils or is synthesized from linolenic acid (ALA) by delta-6-desaturase and elongase. Linolenic acid is obtained in our diet principally from flax seed (linseed) oil while black currant seed oil contains a small amount of stearidonic acid, which is useful if delta-6-desaturase isn't working very well. (Fish oils also contain docosahexaenoic acid (DHA), which has similar effects. For simplicity, throughout this book we will only refer to EPA.

While I have noted only a few examples of foods rich in certain essential fatty acids, it is important to recognize that many foods are mixtures of several fatty acids. For example, soybean, walnut, and canola oils have mixtures of linoleic and alpha-linolenic acid.

How prostaglandins and other mediators
of inflammation become imbalanced
The alert reader will have noted that many of the steps of conversion of fatty acids to prostaglandins, whether inflammatory or anti-inflammatory, share the same enzymes. This means that a relative excess of one fatty acid will tend to hog an enzyme system, resulting in decreased conversion of the other fatty acids.[1] Conversely, a deficiency of one fatty acid will result in excessive conversion of the others. Therein lies a significant problem.

Several research studies have clearly documented that the more animal fats an animal or human eats, the more arachidonic acid they have in their blood and cell membranes, and the higher their level of inflammatory chemicals.[2] Conversely, a diet high in fish or supplemented with fish, flax seed, or borage seed oils results in substantially less arachidonic acid in the cell membranes, a lower level of the inflammatory chemicals, and higher levels of the anti-inflammatory chemicals.[3]

We are not simply talking about subtle effects. The levels of pro- and anti-inflammatory prostaglandins and other mediators of inflammation can be altered by a factor of two to three, simply by modifying dietary consumption of fatty acids! For example, in one study of patients with ulcerative colitis (a painful, progressive, inflammatory disease of the bowels, which often eventually results in the bowels being surgically removed), simple supplementation with fish oils resulted in a dramatic 65% drop in the patients' levels of inflammatory leukotrienes and a 75% decrease in their clinical symptoms.[4] Unfortunately, in the U.S. over the past century, we have dramatically increased our consumption of arachidonic-acid rich animal fats while greatly decreasing our consumption of fish and seed oils. I believe this is a major cause of the serious increase in the incidence of chronic inflammatory diseases that are now running so rampant in our society.

Finally, alcohol consumption inhibits the production of anti-inflammatory prostaglandins. Some research suggests that 10% of adult Americans are alcoholics, so this may be another common cause of excessive inflammation.

Essential fatty acid deficiencies are common

Recent research indicates that the prevalence of fatty acid deficiencies may be far greater than suspected.[5] However, this deficiency is largely unrecognized since the measures of fatty acid status have lacked sensitivity, and conventional physicians have not been taught how to recognize when a patient is suffering from such a deficiency. According to Dr. Ed Siguel, a pioneer researcher in fatty acid deficiencies, at least 10% of the population is deficient in essential fatty acids as measured by fatty acids in their blood and cell membranes.

We are commonly deficient in the essential fatty acids crucial for the production of anti-inflammatory prostaglandins for several reasons: excessive consumption of arachidonic acid (land-animal fats) in the diet, low amounts of essential fatty acids in the diet (aggravated by a lowfat diet), and destruction of essential fatty acids by hydrogenation, cooking, and oxidation of vegetable oils.

Table 6-2 Diseases Commonly Associated with Essential Fatty Acid Deficiency[5]

Cancer
Cardiovascular disease
Diabetic complications
Inflammatory disorders such as arthritis, eczema, and multiple sclerosis

Table 6-3 Unhealthful Effects of Trans-Fatty Acids[9,10]

Poison the delta-6-desaturase enzyme needed for production of anti-inflammatory
  prostaglandins
Lower HDL cholesterol (the good type)
Raise LDL cholesterol (the bad type)
Raise apolipoprotein B (a bad type of blood fat)
Increase risk of myocardial infarction and coronary disease

In nature, the unsaturated essential fatty acids in food are found in what is call the "cis" formation. This means the hydrogen molecules are all on same side of the molecule, making it easier for the body to process. Hydrogenation (the process used to make margarine and shortening out of vegetable oils) and cooking transform some fatty acids into what are called trans-fatty acids and other abnormal forms. Trans-fatty acids have their hydrogens on opposite sides, which makes them appear to the body to be the same as saturated fatty acids. Not only are they not able to be converted to needed prostaglandins, they actually interfere with prostaglandin synthesis and inhibit delta-6-desaturase, the enzyme critical for the production of anti-inflammatory series 1 and 3 prostaglandins.[6] Even worse, they increase the risk of cardiovascular disease.[7]

Unfortunately, trans-fatty acids comprise a large portion of the standard American diet since we eat so much margarine and shortening. Interestingly, wide variations exist in the amount of trans-fatty acids in European and American margarines. Of total fatty acid content, German margarines contain an average of 1.2 to 1.4% trans-fatty acids; a United Kingdom product named Flora contains 0.5%; while U.S. stick-form corn oil margarine contains 18.6%![8] Table 6-3 lists a few of the well-documented problems with the consumption of trans-fatty acids.

Cooking foods with high dietary levels of dietary arachidonic acid also aggravates the problem. At high temperatures, arachidonic acid is oxidized to form a variety of compounds, many of which, when chronically or excessively consumed, not only increase inflammation, but also increase the rate of atherosclerosis and the formation of blood clots.

The bottom line is that we must eat a diet rich in nuts and seeds and their uncooked oils and low in land-animal fats if we want our prostaglandins, and thus our inflammatory process, to function properly.

Some of us have poorly functioning enzymes

As shown in Figure 6-2, several enzymes are required to convert dietary fatty acids into needed prostaglandins. However, for some of us, these enzymes don't work very well due to genetic weakness, environmental toxins, age, disease, or a deficiency of the vitamins and minerals needed to activate the enzyme.

Cortisone: Not the Best Way to Treat Eczema

Lauri brought her three-year-old son Jeremy to see me for the eczema he had had since infancy. For years, she'd faithfully applied cortisone cream to the lesions behind his ears, in the folds of his arms, and between his fingers. While the cortisone worked just fine, as soon as she stopped using it, his itchy, oozing rash would quickly return, seemingly worse than ever. She knew there had to be a better way. After learning that he had not been breast fed and that asthma, eczema, and allergies were common in his family, I easily recognized his problem.

His family history suggested that he had a weak delta-6-desaturase enzyme, which was doing a poor job of converting his dietary fatty acids into the forms needed for the production of the anti-inflammatory prostaglandins. In addition, being bottle fed seriously aggravated the situation because infant formulas, until just recently, were grossly deficient in essential fatty acids. The cow's milk alternative wasn't helping much either because it wasn't supplying him with enough zinc. While cow's milk is richer in zinc than human milk, the zinc in cow's milk is not nearly as easily absorbed.

His treatment program was simple: 1 gm a day of evening primrose oil to directly supply the anti-inflammatory prostaglandins, 10 mg a day of zinc picolinate (just like the form found in mother's milk) to increase the activity of his weak enzyme, and the addition to his diet of raw nuts and seeds, which are good sources of zinc and essential fatty acids.

Fortunately, Jeremy's disease was not too far advanced, and within a few weeks, Jane reported his eczema was improving. When I saw him six months later, his skin had totally returned to normal. In addition, Lauri commented that she thought he seemed in better spirits and was more interested in games and intellectually stimulating activities. This was not surprising because essential fatty acid abnormalities and a zinc deficiency impair brain development.

An example of a genetic weakness can be found in the chronic inflammatory skin disease, atopic eczema. This disease commonly starts in childhood and is medically treated, sometimes for life, with corticosteroids. While their diet typically contains the same amount of essential fatty acids as those without the disease, in people suffering from this disease, the delta-6-desaturase enzyme doesn't work very well. This results in inadequate production of the anti-inflammatory prostaglandins, while the inflammatory prostaglandin pathways continue to work, resulting in chronic, unbalanced inflammation. Supplementing them with evening primrose oil (a rich source of gammalinolenic acid) bypasses the weak enzyme and supports the natural anti-inflammatory prostaglandins, resulting in a reversal of the disease. In addition, providing extra zinc helps stimulate the weak enzyme to do its job better.[11]

Some diseases, while not due to an essential fatty acid deficiency, can cause problems with fatty acid metabolism. For example, the high blood sugar levels found in diabetics tend to block the delta-6-desaturase enzyme resulting in decreased production of anti-inflammatory prostaglandins. This may be a large part of the reason diabetics develop the neurological damage that can lead to blindness and loss of sensation in their hands and legs. The administration of gamma-linolenic acid from evening primrose oil has been shown to reverse the nerve damage in human diabetics because it bypasses the inhibited enzyme.[12]

Inadequate Inflammation Quenching

In addition to the anti-inflammatory prostaglandins discussed above, several nutrients, hormones, chemicals, and enzymes limit the intensity and duration of the inflammatory reaction. Antioxidants, such as vitamins C and E, inhibit the synthesis of pro-inflammatory prostaglandins and help quench the inflammatory process. Several bioflavonoids limit the production of leukotrienes and stabilize the cells that secrete the inflammatory chemicals, so they won't react quite so vigorously. Unfortunately, many of these important nutrients are deficient in the typical U.S. diet.

Perhaps the most important of the inflammation quenching nutrients are the antioxidants. When the normal cells surrounding the area or inflammation have adequate amounts of antioxidants in their cell membranes (such as vitamin E and the carotenoids) they are better able to protect themselves from the highly damaging oxidizing chemicals released during the inflammatory process.

The carotenoids represent the most widespread group of naturally occurring pigments in nature. Although the term carotene is typically used synonymously with provitamin A, only a few of the more than 600 identified carotenoids are believed to have vitamin A activity. Current research shows that carotenes are much more than just vitamin A precursors, e.g., carotenes are very potent quenchers of free radicals, many times more potent than vitamin E.[13] Although most of the research has focused on beta-carotene, other carotenes are more potent in their antioxidant activity.

Carotenoids' antioxidant properties are especially important in protecting the body from the free radicals (for a full discussion of these noxious but necessary chemicals, see Chapter Five) released during inflammation and created by environmental toxins. These free radicals cause widespread inflammation and damage throughout the body and accelerate the degeneration of tissues and organs, resulting in more rapid aging. This may explain the research showing that tissue carotenoid content has a better correlation with the maximal lifespan potential of mammals, including humans, than any other factor that has been studied.[14] In other words, the higher the carotenoid level, the slower the aging process.

The flavonoids are another group of plant pigments (4,000 have now been identified) that provide remarkable protection against free radical and inflammatory damage. These compounds are largely responsible for the colors of fruits and flowers. However, they also serve other than aesthetic functions. In plants, flavonoids serve as protection against environmental stress. In humans, they limit inflammation, quench free radicals, and slow down the synthesis of pro-inflammatory prostaglandins.

The bioflavonoids directly protect the healthy cells by stabilizing the membranes of the inflammatory cells, so they don't overreact to local damage. For example, flavonoids such as quercetin (very high in onions) powerfully limit the secretion of histamine and other inflammatory chemicals. The anthocyanidins and proanthocyanidins are the flavonoids responsible for the red to blue colors of blueberries, blackberries, cherries, grapes, hawthorn berries, and many flowers. By increasing intracellular vitamin C levels, decreasing capillary permeability, and neutralizing free radicals, they modulate the inflammatory process.[15]

An extremely interesting aspect of flavonoids and carotenoids is their tendency to preferentially concentrate in specific tissues. For example, the carotenoid lutein, found in spinach, concentrates in the macula, the part of the eye responsible for acute vision. This is also the part of the eye suffering the most oxidative damage, since the light entering the eye is concentrated on this tiny spot. Macular degeneration, the leading cause of blindness in the elderly, is largely caused by uncontrolled inflammatory damage to the macula, usually from ultraviolet light. Research has shown an inverse correlation between the levels of antioxidants and the incidence of macular degeneration. Since it concentrates its antioxidant activity where most needed, lutein appears to be especially important in protecting us from macular degeneration.[16]

As another example, the flavonoid anthocyanidins concentrate in the collagen, where they inhibit its destruction. Collagen is destroyed during inflammatory conditions involving bones, joints, and cartilage, i.e., rheumatoid arthritis, osteoarthritis, and periodontal disease, so these flavonoids are especially important.

As might be expected, a whole-foods, vegetarian diet contains far more flavonoids and carotenoids than the typical animal-foods based diet.

Excessive Inflammatory Stimulation

Several drugs, food additives, and environmental toxins either increase the activity of our inflammatory processes or activate them when not needed. Unfortunately, the primary drugs that cause problems are commonly used. They include allopurinol (used for treating gouty arthritis), barbiturates (used as sedatives), eucalyptus (an herb used to help clear congestion), fluorides (added to water and toothpaste to control cavities), iodine (when used in large dosages to inhibit an overactive thyroid), and some antibiotics. Interestingly, some drugs that normally do not cause inflammation can become a real problem due to additives used in their formulation to preserve them or make them more attractive or easier to swallow. The most notorious example is the addition of sulfite preservatives to inhalants that asthma sufferers take to relax their lungs during an attack. Due to an enzyme defect, about 10% of these poor people have an asthma attack 10 to 20 minutes after exposure to sulfites![17] In some, the reaction can be so severe that it is life-threatening.

Food and drug additives, including coloring agents, flavorings, preservatives, and emulsifiers, have been shown in several studies to cause inflammatory problems, especially among those with such chronic inflammatory diseases as asthma and eczema.[18] The dyes causing the most trouble are the yellow ones made from tartrazine. They are commonly added to foods ranging from cheddar cheese to cheese puffs to candy.

Many chemicals, called flavoring agents, are added to foods to improve their taste (to make up for the loss of quality caused by the synthetic fertilizers used in modern agriculture). Those causing the most trouble are made from monosodium glutamate (MSG), salicylates, and aspartame (an artificial sweetener).

Several preservatives cause problems, especially the benzoates, nitrites, and sorbic acid. While antioxidants are a good idea to keep food from spoiling, unfortunately, many of the most commonly used ones cause problems. The worst are hydroxytoluene, sulfites, and propyl gallate. Sulfites (usually in the form of sodium or potassium bisulfite) are widely used in restaurants to keep salads and uncooked vegetables looking fresh and as a whitener for potatoes, grapes, and shrimp.

Finally, several emulsifiers and stabilizers are often added to give food more bulk. A few of these, the polysorbates and vegetable gums (especially carrageenan) increase sensitivity to inflammatory reactions and are associated with chronic inflammatory bowel disease in some individuals. Table 6-4 lists some common food additives known to cause inflammatory problems, the typical sources, and the reactions they cause.

Recognizing When the Inflammatory System Is Out of Balance

Considering the large percentage of us suffering from chronic inflammatory diseases, the typical high meat/low essential fatty acid diet, and prevalence of pro-inflammatory chemicals in our food, I think it very likely that almost everyone is suffering from some degree of inflammatory imbalance. Table 6-5 lists the common signs and symptoms, and Table 6-6 lists the typical diseases associated with inflammatory imbalance.

Reestablishing Inflammatory Balance

Reestablishing inflammatory balance requires normalizing the inflammatory prostaglandins, optimizing the level of anti-inflammatory nutrients, and avoiding chemicals that overstimulate the pro-inflammatory pathways.

Table 6-4 Common Food Additives Known to Cause Inflammatory Problems

Food Additive	Common Sources	Reaction
Sulfites	Wine Beer Salad bars Frozen french fries Dried fruit Lemon concentrates Some baked goods	Asthma attack, a reaction, abdominal pain (intestinal inflammation), urticaria (hives), edema, rhino-conjunctivitis (red eyes and runny nose), seizure (from brain swelling), death
Monosodium glutamate	Chinese meals Soups Stews	Asthma, Chinese restaurant syndrome (a combinaton of facial flushing, perspiration, dizziness, and headache)
Benzoates, butylated hydroxytoluene, butylated hydroxyanisole	Some soft drinks Pickles Jams Jellies Cakes	Chronic hives (urticaria)
Tartrazine	Jams Some butters Cheddar cheese Candies Cakes Tablets	Asthma, urticaria (hives)
Aspartame	Artificially sweetened foods	Urticaria (hives), edema

Table 6-5 Typical Signs and Symptoms of Inflammation Dysfunction

Chronic red eyes and runny nose
Dry skin, especially behind the ears, around the nose and eyebrows
Environmental allergies
Fluid retention
Food allergies
Pain and stiffness in the morning
Swollen ankles
Unexplained abdominal pain

Normalizing Prostaglandins

The best way to normalize the prostaglandins is to eat less land-animal fat and more fish, nuts, and seeds. Arachidonic acid, derived almost entirely from dietary animal fats, contributes greatly to the inflammatory process through its conversion to inflammatory prostaglandins and leukotrienes. Vegetarian diets are often beneficial in the treatment of inflammatory conditions, presumably

Table 6-6 Typical Diseases Associated with Inflammatory Dysfunction

Asthma
Autoimmune diseases, e.g., multiple sclerosis, systemic lupus erythematosis
Chronic inflammatory conditions, e.g., eczema, osteoarthritis, rheumatoid arthritis
Cystic acne
Hay fever
Inflammatory bowel disease, e.g., Crohn's disease, ulcerative colitis
Migraine headaches
Seborrheic dermatitis

because they decrease the availability of arachidonic acid for conversion to pro-inflammatory prostaglandins and leukotrienes and provide more of the essential fatty acids needed to make the anti-inflammatory prostaglandins.[19,20]

However, diet alone will take a long time to correct the imbalance since not only are the fatty acids of the blood and the cell membranes out of balance, but so are all the fat stores of the body. Given that the average adult weighs about 150 pounds of which 30% is typically fat, this means he or she is carrying around 45 pounds of imbalanced fatty acids! Therefore, for those suffering from significant chronic inflammatory problems, I recommend supplementation with modest amounts (about 2 tablespoons a day depending on the person's size and severity of disease) of flax seed, evening primrose, and fish oils for several months. The need for essential fatty acids is increased for those who must repair or create a large number of cells (e.g., growing children, pregnant women, patients with burns or infection, etc.) or those who have malabsorption or increased losses (e.g., cystic fibrosis and Crohn's disease).[21]

Eating a Diet Rich in Antioxidants

The best way to ensure that inflammatory processes are quenched when they need to be is to eat a diet high in antioxidant nutrients. This means lots of carotenoid, flavonoid, and vitamin-C rich fruits and vegetables, organically grown if possible. In general, the more colorful the fruit or vegetable, the higher its concentration of antioxidant nutrients. Vitamin-E rich foods are also quite important. This important nutrient is found in whole grains, nuts, and seeds. Unfortunately, processing and cooking rapidly destroy vitamin E, so few can get enough from their diet alone. I recommend supplementation with 600 iu per day of natural, mixed tocopherol vitamin E.

Avoiding Chemicals

Finally, decrease exposure to oxidizing chemicals and ultraviolet light. This means eating foods that are organically grown and have no chemical additives and avoiding contact with household and industrial chemicals. It also means either limiting your sun exposure or making sure you take plenty of vitamin E and other antioxidants when going for that suntan.

Quenching the Inflammatory Reaction

Several nutrients and herbs are safe and effective for quenching an out-of-control inflammatory reaction. However, they should not be used in excess or to cover up inappropriate behavior. Remember, we need the inflammatory process to fight infections and to perform the body's normal repair processes.

Anti-Inflammatory Nutrients

Vitamin C

Historically, vitamin C supplementation has been a foundation of nutritional medicine. Vitamin C's value in inflammation control is through its antioxidant activity as a direct neutralizer of free radicals, its ability to increase superoxide dismutase (an enzyme that scavenges free radicals), and its antihistamine effects.[22] As might be expected, the white cell and plasma concentrations of vitamin C are significantly decreased in patients with chronic inflammatory diseases such as rheumatoid arthritis.[23]

The antihistamine activity of vitamin C is well-documented, even in healthy people. For example, one study looked at the impact of vitamin C supplementation for four weeks in five women and four men who were not smokers and not taking any medications. Initially, they reduced their vitamin-C rich foods to one serving or less per day. In a double-blind, placebo-controlled protocol, the patients then consumed a single placebo capsule during the initial week of the study, and then during the second and third weeks they consumed 500 mg of vitamin C daily in a single dose. At weeks 4 and 5, the daily dose was increased to 2,000 mg as a divided dose. During the final week of the study, two placebo capsules were taken daily. Total vitamin C plasma values rose 46% over baseline after two weeks of vitamin C at 500 mg per day, and did not really differ from the 2,000 mg dose or the one week withdrawal period. (This means that blood histamine values were not significantly altered by the 500 mg dose of vitamin C.) However, after two weeks of the 2,000 mg dose, the blood histamine level fell 40%. The effect appears to last since the blood histamine levels did not rise significantly during the week-long, placebo-controlled withdrawal period.[24]

- *Dosage:* 2,000 to 4,000 mg per day in divided dosages; use less if diarrhea or bloating develops (this means you are taking more vitamin C than your intestines can absorb)

Vitamin E

Vitamin E, another cornerstone in nutritional medicine, is the term used for eight naturally occurring fat-soluble nutrients called tocopherols. Its anti-inflammatory activity comes primarily from its antioxidant properties. As discussed in more detail in Chapter Five, vitamin E is a potent quencher of many types of free radicals. It also inhibits the production of pro-inflammatory chemicals from arachidonic acid.[25] It has been used alone with modest success in several inflammatory conditions such as osteoarthritis, rheumatoid arthritis (especially in conjunction with selenium), periodontal disease, gout and psoriasis, and in helping prevent such diseases as cancer, atherosclerosis, and heart attacks. However, it is best used, like vitamin C, in conjunction with other anti-inflammatory nutrients. Supplementing with vitamin E is especially important when also supplementing with fish and seed oils because they are very susceptible to oxidation and rancidity, which is prevented by vitamin E.

Vitamin E can even be applied topically for inflammation of the skin. In animal experiments, hairless mice were given a sunburn by irradiating them with ultraviolet light. Applying vitamin E to the burn decreased the degree of redness by 40 to 55% and prevented the swelling and thickening of the mice's skin normally seen a week after the sunburn.[26]

- *Dosage:* 400 iu per day; apply topically for skin inflammation

Quercetin
Quercetin and many other flavonoids have been shown to be potent quenchers of several aspects of the inflammatory response. Quercetin neutralizes several inflammatory chemicals, inhibits the release of histamine from mast cells and basophils, and tunes down activated neutrophils.[27,28] These actions are probably due to its ability to stabilize cell membranes, neutralize free radicals, and inhibit some of the enzymes that produce inflammatory chemicals. Quercetin also inhibits inflammation by decreasing white cell secretion of the enzymes used to digest the surrounding matter.

Quercetin (high in onions) has been shown to inhibit many steps in the production of pro-inflammatory prostaglandins and leukotrienes. Probably of most significance is its inhibition of phospholipase A_2 and lipoxygenase enzymes.[29] The net result of quercetin supplementation is a significant reduction in the formation of these potent inflammatory chemicals. Excessive formation of these chemicals has been linked to such inflammatory diseases as asthma, psoriasis, eczema, gout, and the inflammatory bowel diseases.[30] The importance of the leukotriene reduction cannot be overstated; leukotrienes are 1,000 times as potent as histamine in promoting inflammation.

- *Dosage:* 500 mg per day

Flax seed, borage, black currant, and evening primrose oils
The most effective fatty acids for inflammation control are those that bypass early steps (i.e., the desaturation enzymes) needed to prepare them for conversion to prostaglandins. Examples of these fatty acids include eicosapentaenoic acid (EPA) and docosahexanoic acid (DHA) from fish oils, and gamma-linolenic acid (GLA) from plant oils such as evening primrose, borage, and black currant.

For example, supplementing with gamma-linolenic acid is very effective in helping relieve pain and inflammation for patients suffering from rheumatoid arthritis. In a double-blind, placebo-controlled study of 37 patients, supplementing for six months with 1.4 gm per day of gamma-linolenic acid from borage seed oil reduced the number of sore joints by 36%, joint tenderness by 45%, swollen joint count by 28%, and swollen joint score by 41%, all with no side effects.[31] However, lower dosages (480 to 540 mg per day) do not show such good results. Impressive effects on rheumatoid arthritis have been obtained using 1.4 gm of gamma-linolenic acid from black currant seed oil and from evening primrose oil.[32]

Supplementation with gamma-linolenic acid has proven beneficial to several inflammatory diseases, including asthma, allergies, dermatitis, eczema, ulcerative colitis, seborrheic dermatitis, other forms of arthritis, and even high blood pressure.[33,34,35]

- *Dosage:* 1 gm per day of gamma-linolenic acid

Fish oils

Another effective way of decreasing the inflammatory response is the consumption of cold-water fish such as mackerel, herring, sardines, and salmon. These fish are rich sources of eicosapentaenoic acid (EPA), which competes with arachidonic acid for enzymes and provides the precursors for the anti-inflammatory prostaglandins. The net effect of consumption of these fish is a significantly reduced inflammatory/allergic response.

Supplementation with 3.2 and 4.0 gm of eicosapentaenoic acid to healthy human volunteers increased the EPA content of cells more than seven-fold. This results in significant anti-inflammatory effects since EPA (1) decreases the release of arachidonic acid from cell membranes thereby decreasing the production of the arachidonic acid cascade of inflammatory chemicals; (2) forms less potent leukotrienes and other eicosanoids (the leukotriene formed from EPA [LTB5] is a much less potent mediator of inflammation than the leukotriene that is derived from arachidonic acid [LTB4]); and (3) decreases leukotriene synthesis by 48% (via inhibition of 5-lipoxygenase) and leukotriene potency by nearly 100-fold.[36,37] EPA is used by the same enzymes as arachidonic acid, but instead of producing highly inflammatory chemicals, EPA is converted to anti-inflammatory chemicals, which uses up the enzymes, so none are left for the arachidonic acid to be converted to inflammatory forms.

Supplementation with fish oils is very effective in treating inflammatory diseases, especially rheumatoid arthritis. For example, a double-blind study of patients with rheumatoid arthritis demonstrated that a diet rich in polyunsaturated fats and low in saturated fat, which was supplemented daily with 1.8 gm of eicosapentaenoic acid, brought about significant improvement.[38] Additional studies have repeatedly demonstrated the beneficial effects of fish oils; a 24-week double-blind, placebo-controlled trial showed a dose-dependent response.[39] In other words, the more fish the subjects ate and the more fish oils they supplemented with, the better the results. A very early study performed almost 40 years ago found that supplementation with cod liver oil also resulted in significant clinical improvement.[40] Cod liver oil is much less expensive than other fish oils.

- *Dosage:* 1 gm per day of eicosapentaenoic acid

Selenium

The trace mineral selenium is effective in reducing inflammation and has shown some benefit in the treatment of rheumatoid arthritis in patients with low selenium levels. Selenium appears to modulate the inflammatory response through three mechanisms: stimulating the activity of glutathione peroxidase (an enzyme that neutralizes free radicals), improving the phagocytic activity of white cells, and decreasing the production of pro-inflammatory prostaglandins.

Oxygen free radicals are a serious problem for those with joint inflammation since they damage the synovial tissues (the tissues that surround the joint) and destroy the hyaluronic acid that provides lubrication for the joint. These oxygen radicals are released by white cells into the joint space whenever the white cells are called in to repair damage. In a variety of studies, decreased selenium levels have been seen in rheumatoid arthritis. In one small four-month trial, supplementation with either sodium selenite at 160 mcg per day, selenomethionine at 100 mcg per day, or selenium-enriched yeast at 200 mcg per day improved approximately 40% of a group of rheumatoid arthritic patients.[41]

- *Dosage:* 200 mcg a day

Anti-Inflammatory Herbs

Many herbs have demonstrated anti-inflammatory activity. The following are those that have been researched with good results and are consistently successful in my clinic.

Hamamelis virginiana (Witch hazel)

It may be dismissed by some as an old wives' tale, but witch hazel really is effective for the relief of skin inflammation. Topical application of witch hazel is especially effective for eczema (atopic dermatitis) and hemorrhoids, with essentially no side effects.[42] Both water-alcohol and water extracts are effective. The anti-inflammatory activity of witch hazel distillate has been compared with other anti-inflammatory herbs and drugs. In one study using ultraviolet-induced superficial skin burns, 1% hydrocortisone cream was found most effective, followed closely by witch hazel and then chamomile cream. Adding the nutrient phosphatidylcholine to a witch hazel cream made it even more effective in relieving skin inflammation.[43]

- *Dosage:* apply distillate locally several times a day

Curcuma longa (Turmeric)

Turmeric is the major ingredient of curry powder and is also used in prepared mustard. It is extensively used in foods both for its color and flavor. In addition, turmeric is used in both the Chinese and Ayurvedic (from India) systems of medicine as an anti-inflammatory agent.

The volatile oil fraction of *Curcuma longa* has been demonstrated to possess potent anti-inflammatory activity in a variety of experimental animal models.[44] Even more potent in acute inflammation is curcumin, the yellow pigment of turmeric. Used orally, curcumin exhibits many direct anti-inflammatory effects including inhibiting leukotriene formation, inhibiting white cell response to inflammatory chemicals, and stabilizing white cell lysosomal membranes so they don't release inflammatory chemicals[45] (which also inhibits the formation of leukotrienes). Curcumin has been found to be as effective as cortisone or phenylbutazone in models of acute inflammation, but only half as effective in chronic models.[46] However, while phenylbutazone and cortisone are associated with significant toxicity, curcumin displays virtually no toxicity. It has also been shown to be more potent than the common anti-inflammatory drug ibuprofen. At low levels, curcumin inhibits prostaglandin synthesis, while at high levels, it stimulates the adrenals to secrete more cortisone.[47]

- *Dosage:* turmeric herb used liberally as a spice; 400 mg of curcumin three times a day

Bromelain

Bromelain refers to a mixture of proteolytic enzymes obtained from the stem of the pineapple plant. A large amount of research has demonstrated its usefulness for a wide variety of inflammatory conditions. Its anti-inflammatory activity appears due to its inhibition of the production of pro-inflammatory prostaglandins, induction of the production of anti-inflammatory series 1 prostaglandins, and inhibition of the increase in capillary permeability that causes edema.[48]

It has been used with success to treat a wide variety of inflammatory diseases including arthritis, athletic injuries, cellulitis (an infection in the deep tissues, typically in the legs), edema, sinusitis, and thrombophlebitis (blood clots in the legs). Bromelain is especially helpful in decreasing the pain and swelling caused by surgical trauma and even appears to speed the rate of healing.[49]

- *Dosage:* bromelain (standardized at 1,800 to 2,000 m.c.u.) 125 to 450 mg three times a day on an empty stomach

Tanacetum parthenium (Feverfew)

Feverfew has been used for centuries in Europe as an anti-inflammatory herb for the treatment of migraines and arthritis. Recent research has documented its efficacy and elicited its mechanism of action, which is due to its inhibition of the synthesis of inflammatory prostaglandins, leukotrienes, and thromboxanes, and activity of white cells.[50] It has been shown to be clinically effective in treating rheumatoid arthritis and migraine headaches.[51]

- *Dosage:* dried leaves (in capsules)—25 mg twice a day; tincture—30 to 40 drops three times a day

  Note: Feverfew is best used as an extract or in capsules because chewing the leaves results in ulcerations of the tongue and swelling in the mouth in about 10% of users.

Glycyrrhiza glabra (Licorice root)

Licorice root is one of the most extensively researched botanical medicines. It has been used for thousands of years in both Eastern and Western natural medicine to treat viral infections and inflammatory diseases. Its major active component is glycyrrhizin, which is converted in the body to glycyrrhizic acid. It is found in the root in concentrations ranging from 6 to 14%.

Licorice root has significant anti-inflammatory and anti-allergy activity.[52] It appears to accomplish this though two mechanisms: cortisol-like activity and inhibition of the production of pro-inflammatory prostaglandins and leukotrienes.[53,54] It appears to be clinically useful in most inflammatory conditions.

- *Dosage:* Powdered root   1 to 4 gm a day
             Fluid extract   1 tsp before meals
             Solid extract   ½ tsp before meals

  Note: Licorice root should not be taken for more than a few weeks at a time; it can cause an elevation of blood pressure in some susceptible patients. It should not be used by those with a history of high blood pressure, kidney problems, or when using digitalis.

How to Treat Common Inflammatory Diseases

Rheumatoid Arthritis

Rheumatoid arthritis is a complex disease that affects a lot of people, about 3% of adults in the U.S. It appears to be due to some kind of initial damage to the synovium (the tissues surrounding the joints), followed by an overactive inflammatory reaction, which continues the damage. When the damage gets bad enough, the body starts producing antibodies to the tissues of the joints, resulting in a continuing escalation of the disease. Fortunately, natural medicine has some answers for those suffering from this painful and frustrating disease.

Our approach consists of removing all known factors that may be damaging the joints and damping down the inflammatory process so that the self-destructive cycle can be stopped. Food allergies appear to be a very significant initiator of the rheumatoid arthritis process. This is apparently due to the damage inflicted on the intestinal membranes when the body has an allergic reaction to a food. This results in leakage of toxins, immune complexes, bacterial poisons, and other noxious substances into the body. Some of these toxins appear to be especially damaging to the joints. Elimination of allergenic foods from the diet has been shown to offer significant benefit to some individuals with rheumatoid arthritis.[55] Strict fasting has been even more effective, however. Water fasting not only results in total avoidance of all allergens, it also allows the intestines to heal and intestinal permeability to return to normal.[56]

One of the reasons those with rheumatoid arthritis develop food allergies is that many with the disease are deficient in stomach acid and other digestive factors.[57] Taking betaine HCl (hydrochloric acid) with meals greatly aids digestion (especially of protein), and improved digestion helps reduce food sensitivities.

The second step is to aggressively quench the excessive inflammatory response. This can be accomplished in several ways; supplementation with antioxidants, fish oils, and borage or evening primrose oil appears to be the most effective. I supplement arthritis patients with large dosages of antioxidants (vitamins C and E and the trace mineral selenium) and encourage them to eat colorful fruits and vegetables as much as possible since these foods are rich in the anti-inflammatory flavonoids and carotenoids.

As discussed above, supplementing the diet with fish oils or cod liver oil is very effective in reducing inflammation in rheumatoid arthritis and other inflammatory conditions.[58,59] In general, if the only therapy is fish oil (2 to 3 gm per day of eicosapentaenoic acid), significant clinical improvement takes about four months to manifest. Interestingly, at the time of improvement, measurements of several inflammatory chemicals in the studies reviewed showed a drop ranging from 19% to a remarkable 54.7%.[39] Clearly fish oils are excellent anti-inflammatory nutrients. Those with mild cases may find that fish oil supplementation is not necessary if they eat a serving of cold-water fish at least once a day.

Also effective is supplementation with the fatty acid gamma-linolenic acid (GLA). Found in evening primrose, black currant, and borage seed oils, GLA also decreases pain and inflammation in arthritis.[32] These oils, however, do not work quite as reliably for some people as the fish oils since they need to go through an additional enzyme before being converted to anti-inflammatory prostaglandins. Please note that fatty acid supplementation works best when total fat consumption, especially of land-animal fats, is decreased.

Allergies and Hay Fever

Allergies are an increasingly common health problem for Americans. An allergic reaction occurs because a person is overly sensitive to something in the environment. While allergies have many causes, overreaction of the pro-inflammatory prostaglandins is an important one. The natural medicine approach is to decrease exposure to triggering substances, tune down the inflammatory response, and directly inhibit the symptoms when needed.

Avoiding the trigger is not always easy because triggers can occur in the air we breathe, the food we eat, and the world we come in contact with. However, we don't need to control everything. Sometimes, just avoiding the worst or most frequently encountered allergens will be enough to allow our general allergic reactivity to decrease.

The idea here is that with every contact with an allergen, histamine, prostaglandins, and other inflammatory chemicals are released. This not only activates the local inflammatory process, but also results in higher blood levels of these mediators of inflammation, which then make all other parts of our bodies more reactive to other allergens. Therefore, every time we decrease our exposure to an allergen, we decrease our general level of reactivity. By far, the allergens most people encounter most frequently and in the largest dosages are those found in the foods they eat every day. So my first approach is to help people identify and avoid their major food allergens. (See Chapter Five for a full discussion of how to do this.)

The next step is to decrease the amount of inflammatory chemicals a person has circulating in the blood and concentrating in the tissues. As noted above, supplementing with large dosages of vitamin C significantly decreases blood levels of histamine. Eating lots of onions is also helpful because they are high in quercetin, which also helps decrease histamine levels. The levels of pro-inflammatory prostaglandins can be decreased by lowering the intake of land-animal fats, and eating more fish and raw nuts and seeds. This effect can be further enhanced by taking flax seed, borage, evening primrose, or fish oil supplements.[60] One to two grams a day of gamma-linolenic acid or eicosapentaenoic acid is usually sufficient to significantly reduce symptoms within a few weeks.

Finally, the herb *Ephedra sinica* (also known as Mormon tea, ephedra, and Ma Huang) is very useful for relieving symptoms of the *acute* allergic attack. However, it does not in any way cure the disease and is contraindicated in people with heart disease, high blood pressure, thyroid disease, diabetes, or prostate enlargement.

Asthma

Asthma is essentially an allergic reaction that occurs in the airways of the lungs. In asthma, white cells in the bronchi secrete histamine, and the smooth muscle cells of the lung airways contract more readily. The combination of airway swelling and bronchial contraction results in much smaller passages for air to enter and leave the lungs, which is why asthma patients have trouble breathing. The natural medicine approach is the same as for allergies, but applied with more intensity because this is a serious, even life-threatening disease.

As noted above, as many allergens as possible, both dietary and environmental, need to be identified and eliminated. Once again, lack of hydrochloric acid in the stomach appears to significantly contribute to the development of food allergies and the disease. This has been known for over half a century. In

Solving a Dietary Puzzle

Emily was basically a healthy young woman, except for experiencing sporadic but very severe attacks of asthma. The drugs she used were effective in stopping the attacks, but she was worried; over the previous year they seemed to be coming more often. Despite considerable detective work, she had not been able to determine what triggered her attacks; there was no discernible pattern. She had heard of my natural approach to medicine and came to me hoping to find an answer to her puzzling problem.

At first I was perplexed. She ate a healthy vegetarian diet, lived in a relatively clean environment, and had not had any allergy problems as a child. Her physical exam was equally clean except for mild rales in her lower lungs (a sign of mucus in the lungs). Further questioning revealed the surprising fact that her attacks actually started a few months after she had become a vegetarian! Before that she had essentially eaten only fish and vegetables. She had become a vegetarian by replacing fish with peanut butter and grains. I immediately suspected the wheat since it is such a common allergen, but a trial period of abstinence had no effect. I then had her stop eating peanuts, and the results were a dramatic drop in the frequency of her attacks. Finally, I recommended that she start eating cold-water fish again (the type of fish with the highest concentration of the anti-inflammatory fatty acids). She then had no further attacks, unless she ate peanut butter.

I think her asthmatic reaction was a combination of an idiosyncratic allergic reaction to peanuts and poorly functioning fatty acid conversion enzymes, which made her unable to convert the vegetable oils to anti-inflammatory prostaglandins. This had not been a problem for her before because the fatty acids she got from fish bypassed the faulty enzymes.

- *The message:* Don't let dietary prejudice keep you from recognizing that almost any food, no matter how healthy, can cause an allergic reaction. Also, eating cold-water fish appears to be a very effective way of establishing normal inflammatory balance.

1931, Dr. G. W. Bray performed gastric analyses on 200 asthmatic children and found that 80% of them had gastric acid secretions below normal levels.[61]

After eliminating allergic foods and improving digestion, I then modify the diet to significantly lower total fat, especially land-animal fat, while increasing the consumption of cold-water fish. Supplementation with substantial amounts of flax seed, black currant, borage, and fish oils is a very important part of the therapy. Many researchers have now demonstrated that decreasing fat intake and enriching the diet with seed and fish oils has a very beneficial impact on asthma.

For example, in one experiment in France, 12 asthma patients were given, on a double-blind basis, either placebo or 1 gm per day of eicosapentaenoic acid from fish oil for a period of one year. The health of the subjects' respiratory system was evaluated by measuring their ability to breathe. This is a very good measure since, as their airways swell, asthma patients have progressively more difficulty getting a full breath. The researchers found that simply providing the fish oil supplement opened the subjects' airways by an average of 23% at 9 months, with the airways continuing to improve at 12 months when the study ended.[62] It is very important to note that the objective improvement did not start until after 6 months. This is probably how long it took to significantly change the balance of fatty acids in the cell membranes and also explains why there have been a few negative studies. The negative studies were virtually all of short duration, typically ten weeks, which is just not long enough. As useful as fish oils are, there is one note of caution. About 10% of asthma patients experience an aggravation of their disease when they take aspirin. Some research suggests that these asthma patients also show a similar aggravation when they take fish oil supplements.

Several herbs are very useful in helping decrease the incidence of attacks, while others help stop the acute attack when it occurs.

Although onions and garlic are not normally thought of as herbs, eating large amounts of either is very helpful for asthmatics since they contain several substances that help quench the inflammatory processes. Specifically, they both inhibit lipoxygenase and cyclooxygenase, the enzymes that generate the inflammatory prostaglandins and leukotrienes.[63] Onion also contains quercetin, which may account for some of its anti-histamine effect, but its major protective actions appear to be related to its content of benzyl- and other isothiocyanates (mustard oils). Although the relative importance of onion's constituents is unknown, it has been proven to be clinically useful for asthma patients.[64]

Extracts of the herb *Coleus forskohlii* appear to be particularly useful in asthma because they help relax the bronchial muscles and relieve respiratory symptoms. Forskolin, the primary active component, has been shown to have remarkable effects in relaxing constricted bronchial muscles in asthmatics.[65,66] This antispasmodic action of forskolin supports the folk medicine use of C. *forskohlii* in the treatment of not only asthma, but also intestinal colic, menstrual cramps, angina, and hypertension. In addition to forskolin's ability to relax smooth muscle, its other anti-allergic activities, such as inhibiting the release of histamine and synthesis of allergic compounds, are also of benefit in the treatment of asthma.[67]

One double-blind clinical study sought to compare the anti-asthmatic effects of forskolin with the drug fenoterol. Sixteen patients with asthma were studied using three different preparations: single inhalation doses of fenoterol as dry powder capsules (0.4 mg), metered doses of fenoterol (0.4 mg), and forskolin dry powder capsules (10.0 mg). All three caused a significant improvement in respiratory function and bronchodilation. However, while the fenoterol preparations caused tremors and decreased blood potassium levels, no such negative effects were seen with forskolin.[68] The typical oral dose of the standardized extract (18% forskolin) is 50 mg two to three times a day.

For stopping an acute attack, ephedra (Ma Huang, Mormon tea) has been used successfully for centuries in both Eastern and Western natural medicine. It contains 0.75 to 1.0% ephedrine and variable quantities of pseudoephedrine, both of which are potent dilators of the bronchi. These components have been synthesized and are still widely prescribed in the treatment of asthma, particularly in chronic cases.

Since this can be a difficult condition to treat, simply supplementing with one nutrient or herb, no matter how valuable, is not nearly as effective as using a comprehensive program.

Chronic Obstructive Pulmonary Disease (Chronic Bronchitis and Emphysema)

Chronic obstructive pulmonary disease (COPD), a collective term used to describe chronic bronchitis and emphysema, is a serious, life-threatening disease of the lungs seen in life-long smokers. It is caused by chronic inflammation in the lungs from the irritating toxins in cigarette smoke. Over the years of smoking, the chronic inflammation progressively destroys the lungs until there is so little functional lung tissue left that the patient suffocates. While smoking is a very health damaging practice and not recommended, studies have now shown that at least some of the damage to the lungs can be decreased by eating fish. Comparing smokers who ate fish four times a week with those who ate fish less than once a week showed that the high fish consumers cut their incidence of COPD by an incredible 45%.[69] Don't smoke. But if you do or did, eat cold-water fish!

Eczema

Eczema (also known as atopic dermatitis) is a very common inflammatory condition of the skin, affecting about 5% of the population. It can be described as a severe allergic reaction occurring in the skin, but not from things the skin comes into contact with (that condition is called contact dermatitis). In other words, it's an allergic reaction coming from within.

Once again, the causes are similar to those found in rheumatoid arthritis and asthma: food allergies, inadequate hydrochloric acid in the stomach, and an imbalance in the inflammatory chemicals. This inflammatory chemical imbalance is now known to be due to an impairment in the enzymes needed to convert dietary essential fatty acids into the form needed for conversion to anti-inflammatory prostaglandins.

As early as 1933, researchers had shown that children with eczema have lower levels of essential fatty acids in their blood.[70] Later research found that the enzyme delta-6-desaturase, the enzyme necessary for preparation of fatty acids for conversion to anti-inflammatory prostaglandins (see Figure 6-2) is deficient in eczema patients. Current studies of infants have shown that those with lower levels of dihomogammalinolenic acid in their blood and umbilical cord have a greater risk of developing eczema in childhood.[71] These observations led to several clinical trials of supplementation with various oils to determine if they could help relieve the inflammation.

Several studies have shown that supplementation with either eicosapentaenoic acid from fish oils or gamma-linolenic acid from evening primrose oil (and presumably from borage and black currant oils) markedly improves the condition.[72,73] As with other fatty acid supplementation studies, the clinical effects take several months to develop.

Supplementation with seed oils even helps dogs with inflammatory skin conditions! Providing dogs with these rich sources of essential fatty acids has been shown to help atopic dermatitis and seborrheic dermatitis. In general, it took four to nine weeks of supplementation for the dogs' symptoms to improve.[74]

Inflammatory Bowel Disease (Ulcerative Colitis and Crohn's Disease)

Inflammatory bowel disease is the general term for a group of chronic inflammatory disorders of the bowel. It is divided into two major categories: Crohn's disease and ulcerative colitis. Those with these conditions suffer from recurrent inflammatory attacks in various parts of their intestines. It can become so severe that parts of these patients' intestines are surgically removed. Once again, these chronic inflammatory conditions can be simply described as allergic reactions in the intestines. Inflammatory prostaglandin levels are greatly increased in the intestinal lining, serum, and stools of patients with these conditions, apparently due to a combination of chronic damage and an over-reactivity of the inflammatory system.

Inflammatory bowel disease is a complex condition requiring the expert care of a physician. For example, one of the reasons for the chronic inflammation in ulcerative colitis appears to be a defect in the mucus secreted by the intestinal lining to protect itself from the toxic constituents in the intestines. In addition, these patients appear to have much higher levels of toxic bacteria in their intestines (see Chapter Five).[75]

Even with all these abnormalities, supplementation with fish oils appears to help. In a double-blind, placebo-controlled, multi-center research trial, supplementation with 18 capsules of fish oil a day (3.24 gm of eicosapentaenoic acid and 2.16 gm of docosahexaenoic acid) resulted in an average 65% drop in the level of inflammatory chemicals in the intestines, an 80% drop in the level of cellular abnormalities in the intestine, and a weight gain of 4 pounds after four months.[76] Excellent results for a tough condition.

Summary

An effective yet balanced inflammatory system is crucial for health and longevity. If our inflammatory system is underactive, we can't fight off infections as well as we need to and aren't able to replace cells and tissues when they wear out. When this system is overactive, inflammation goes out of control, damaging healthy tissues and promoting chronic inflammatory diseases.

The best way to maintain a well-balanced inflammatory system is to eat a diet rich in nuts, seeds, and fish and limited in land-animal fat. Equally important is the consumption of the more colorful fruits and vegetables, at least five servings a day.

Those suffering from chronic inflammatory problems should avoid all drugs and chemicals known to increase inflammation (see Table 6-4) and greatly limit their consumption of land-animal fats. In addition, supplementation with substantial amounts of antioxidants and essential fatty acids from evening primrose, flax seed, borage, black currant, and fish oils will, after several weeks, significantly decrease the pain and swelling.

Chapter Seven

Optimizing Metabolic Function

You need to study this chapter if you suffer from any of the following:

- *Symptoms*

  Abdominal bloating

  Bed wetting

  Chronic constipation

  Chronic diarrhea

  Chronic fatigue

  Dark circles under eyes

  Passing gas

  Poor hair and nails

  Puffiness under eyes

  Rectal itching

- *Diseases*

  Anemia

  Asthma

  Autoimmune diseases

  Candidiasis

  Canker sores

  Celiac disease

  Dermatitis herpetiformis

  Diabetes mellitus

  Eczema

  Failure to thrive (in children)

  Food allergies

  Hives

  Intestinal parasites

  Irritable bowel syndrome

  Osteoporosis

  Vitiligo

Behaviors that increase risk:

- Chronic use of antibiotics
- Eating commercially versus organically grown foods
- Excessively large meals
- Excessively high levels of sugar, fat, or refined foods
- Not regularly taking a good multivitamin and mineral supplement
- Taking antacids

Thumbnail: Quick Help to Improve Nutritional Status and Digestion
- *To improve nutritional status:*
  Eat organically grown foods
  Take a high quality multivitamin and mineral supplement with a
  formula similar to the recommendations in Table 7-3
- *To improve digestion:*
  Take herbal bitters with meals
  Take one or two 10-grain tablets of betaine hydrochloride with pepsin
  during meals
  Have your stools tested for parasites if you have been to a Third World
  country or are in close contact with someone who has
  Supplement with acidophilus (such as HMF or Eugalin Forte) once a
  day between meals

The body's processes all depend on enzymes, which catalyze the chemical reactions that make our cells work. The better they function, the healthier and more energetic we feel. Unfortunately, for most of us, many of our enzymes do not work as well as they should. This occurs for several reasons: lack of the micronutrients needed for the enzymes to function, environmental toxins that poison enzymes, and genetic weaknesses resulting in poorly formed enzymes. Fortunately, most of these problems are correctable.

In general, enzymes are composed of a special protein (called an apo-enzyme) combined with a cofactor. These cofactors are typically a vitamin or mineral, which is why these micronutrients are called "essential." These essential micronutrients are commonly deficient because most people eat foods that are low in micronutrients. Modern agriculture produces foods that look nice, but which have gradually become deficient in the essential trace minerals because synthetic fertilizers do not add them back to the soil. What micronutrients foods contain are further reduced by refining, storage, and cooking. Not only are many diets micronutrient poor, but maldigestion further aggravates the problem; poor digestion results in poor absorption of micronutrients from food.

Compounding the problem is the high level of toxins people are exposed to in their food, water, and air. These toxins damage our health in many ways (as discussed in Chapter Five), one of the most important of which is that they can displace the micronutrients from our enzymes, effectively turning them off. As discussed in Chapter Five, there are many effective ways to decrease our exposure to toxins and eliminate them from our body. Although not technically toxins, excessively high intakes of some foods, e.g., sugar, animal fats, and cholesterol, also can damage or alter the activity of some enzymes.

Another factor in malabsorption is genetic weakness. While there is little we can do to change our genetic character (although there is certainly a lot we can do to optimize our children's genetic potential), we can optimize what we have. For example, if the protein structure of an enzyme is not made well, providing extra amounts of its cofactors can help it work better.

This is the underlying justification for a therapeutic approach called "orthomolecular medicine" or "megavitamin therapy." It emphasizes the extreme importance of establishing optimal nutritional status to ensure the best opportunity for even weak enzymes to work adequately. Almost all chronic diseases include some component of enzyme dysfunction.

Real-Life Messages About Malnutrition and Maldigestion

Gas and Bloating

Gas and bloating had troubled Helen most of her life. She'd seen her family doctor several times and all he could recommend were antacids. They had helped some, but the problems continued. In addition, she couldn't understand why she was tired all the time and having trouble losing weight; she ate a healthful, whole-foods diet, although she tended to eat too much. Further questioning revealed that as a child, she had suffered from asthma and eczema, but had supposedly "grown out of them."

Helen's problem was immediately obvious to me. Gas and bloating are common symptoms of low hydrochloric acid in the stomach, and low stomach acidity is found in about 80% of children with asthma.[1] I began her on a simple program of taking tablets of hydrochloric acid with meals, starting with one a meal and every day increasing by one a meal until her symptoms improved. Four tablets a meal did the job. Not only did her gas and bloating improve, but she also began feeling more energetic and, to her great surprise, she lost some of her excess weight.

She felt more energetic because she was finally absorbing the critical nutrients she needed. For the same reason, she was having less trouble with her appetite because she was losing her cravings for difficult-to-absorb nutrients such as zinc, which some researchers believe is one of the key nutrients the body uses to regulate the appetite. Interestingly, zinc is a critical nutrient for the enzyme that produces hydrochloric acid in the stomach and is commonly deficient in those suffering from asthma and eczema. Her use of antacids was one of the worst things she could have done; it actually made the problem worse by neutralizing what little hydrochloric acid she had left.

- *The message:* A healthful diet does little good if we can't digest and absorb all the nutrients it contains.

Indigestion

Intermittent episodes of indigestion brought Maria, a 45-year-old Mexican-American mother of three, to my office. She described the indigestion as an upper abdominal fullness associated with gurgling noises and gas. The discomfort came one to several hours after meals, lasted for several hours, and then gradually disappeared. Occasionally, it was associated with diarrhea. Over the prior few months, the symptoms had become more frequent and were lasting longer. Other than being substantially overweight, she had no other health problems.

Maria had not made any changes in her diet, and the antacids her family doctor had recommended had not helped. Her symptoms and nationality led me to suspect lactose intolerance, a condition in which people are unable to digest the milk sugar in dairy products. Maria doubted that this was the problem, saying that she had eaten dairy products all her life. However, because she was desperate, she agreed to take my advice. She was quite surprised when all of her symptoms disappeared after four days of scrupulously avoiding all dairy products. But just to be sure, after a week she drank a glass of milk and suffered the worst symptoms she had ever had!

Although mother's milk is a natural food for infants, lactose intolerance is very common in adults, especially those of African, Mexican, or Mediterranean descent. Once we leave infancy, most people's intestinal cells stop producing the lactase enzyme needed to digest milk sugar. Sometimes, people continue to produce lactase into their adult lives, but then lose it later in life. This can be difficult to recognize because people don't expect foods they normally eat to suddenly become a problem.

- *The message:* As people age, their digestive systems do not work as well, resulting in marginal foods becoming a problem.

A Lucky Man

About six months before coming to see me, Lawrence, a 39-year-old attorney, had had an episode of sharp, stabbing, left chest pain immediately after concluding a successful malpractice suit. The frightening pain lasted until he sat down for several minutes. He immediately went to the local emergency room where the attending physicians could find no problem with his heart; neither his EKG nor his blood showed any abnormalities.

Over the ensuing five months, he had six similar episodes, each lasting 30 to 60 seconds. There was no pattern to the attacks. Several occurred when he was sitting at his desk, while others occurred when he was walking home from work. Several visits to his family doctor produced no answers to his recurrent pain because his doctor could find no signs of heart-threatening atherosclerosis. After experiencing three attacks in the past month, Lawrence was desperate for a solution.

His diet was quite poor—he ate lots of red meat and refined foods and very few fresh fruits and vegetables—and he smoked one pack of cigarettes a day. He did, however, exercise religiously and was an avid tennis player. His only other health problem was gastritis (burning pain in the stomach), which he treated with antacids.

After some thought, I realized that he might be suffering from spasming of the cardiac arteries due to transient deficiencies of magnesium. Although such transient magnesium deficiency is considered rare in conventional medical circles, those of us specializing in nutritional medicine believe it is a very common cause of heart attacks. This belief is supported by several observations: (1) epidemiological research shows heart attacks are more common in communities with low amounts of magnesium in their food and water, (2) putting a piece of a normal artery in a magnesium-deficient solution will cause it to spasm, and (3) giving magnesium to men having a heart attack, or immediately afterwards, decreases their mortality rate by 50%.[2]

I deduced that Lawrence's magnesium levels were very low because his diet was deficient in magnesium, the antacids he was taking were blocking the absorption of the little magnesium that was in his diet, and his heavy exercise was further depleting his magnesium stores (magnesium is lost when we sweat). While I could have performed a sophisticated test to determine his actual magnesium status, I realized that people with such a deficiency are at high risk of sudden death from a heart attack. I immediately began him on 600 mg of magnesium (in the form of magnesium citrate) spread out in four doses throughout the day. He had no further symptoms of chest pain.

Although he has not improved his diet and lifestyle as much as I would have liked, he continues to take a maintenance dose of 400 mg once a day.

■ *The message:* Simple nutrients can save your life.

Optimal Nutrition

For total wellness, we need optimal nutrition. This requires a foundation of eating whole, organically grown, properly prepared foods. In addition, we need to add nutritional supplements to our diets to ensure that all our enzymes are functioning at their best. But, do we really need to eat organically grown foods to be healthy? Are nutritional deficiencies really that common? How much of these vitamins and minerals do we need to be optimally healthy? And can we take too much; aren't some vitamins dangerous?

Organically Grown Foods

Although little research has directly compared the level of pollutants and nutrients in organically versus conventionally grown foods, the research that has been done is very compelling in favor of organically grown foods. For example, the results of one such study, which evaluated 4 to 15 samples of organically and commercially grown foods (apples, wheat berries, pears, and potatoes) in one community, are reproduced in Table 7-1. As you can see, not only are the heavy metal pollutants significantly lower (except cadmium for some inexplicable reason) in the organically grown foods, but they also contain

Table 7-1 Comparison of Mineral Content of Organically Versus
Conventionally Grown Foods[3]

Mineral	Organic Higher	Conventional Higher
Toxic minerals		
Aluminum		40%
Cadmium	5%	
Lead		29%
Mercury		25%
Nutritional minerals		
Boron	70%	
Calcium	63%	
Chromium	78%	
Cobalt	Same	Same
Copper	48%	
Iodine	73%	
Iron	59%	
Lithium	118%	
Magnesium	138%	
Manganese	170%	
Molybdenum	68%	
Nickel	66%	
Phosphorous	91%	
Potassium	125%	
Rubidium		28%
Selenium	390%	
Silicon	86%	
Sodium	159%	
Strontium	133%	
Sulfur	20%	
Vanadium	8%	
Zinc	60%	

much higher concentrations of essential minerals, especially manganese, which is 1.7 times higher, and selenium, which showed a remarkable 4 times higher concentration. The message is clear: Organically grown foods are safer and much more nutritious.

Nutritional Deficiencies Are Very Common

The research is clear: Few of us eat very well, and frank and marginal nutritional deficiencies are very common. This is especially a problem for the elderly and hospitalized patients. Even many supposedly "normal" people have been found to be nutritionally deficient. For example, in a 30-month study of 800 patients in two U.S. hospitals, who were admitted for conditions not normally associated with malnutrition (pneumonia, hip fracture, etc.), blood tests found 55% to be malnourished.[4] The malnourished surgical patients stayed in the hospital an average of five days longer than the adequately nourished, with hospital food possibly compounding their problem.

In a study of 402 elderly Europeans living at home, the nutrient content of their diet was found to be low: folic acid intake was low in 100% of those studied, zinc in 87%, vitamin B_6 in 83%, and vitamin D in 62%.[5] Table 7-2 summarizes science's current best understanding of the frequency of specific nutrient deficiencies and the more common symptoms and diseases that are caused by these deficiencies.

Why the Recommended Daily Allowances Are Not Adequate

While the recommended daily allowances (RDAs) have been used as the standard nutrition guide for several decades, they simply aren't an adequate guide for total wellness. The RDAs have many limitations, probably the most important of which is that they were developed for healthy people under normal circumstances (i.e., no illness, no genetic weaknesses, no environmental toxin exposure) to prevent the development of overt deficiency diseases. They were *not* developed to serve as a guide to determining optimal nutritional needs.

In addition, the studies that were used to determine the level of a nutrient sufficient to prevent a nutritional deficiency were typically conducted for six to nine months, only about 1% of the average human life span. Nutritional studies with animals have shown that the amounts of some nutrients sufficient to provide health and the prevention of a deficiency disease for short periods of time may be totally inadequate to maintain the health of the animal over its entire lifespan.

The Suggested Optimal Daily Nutritional Allowances (SONAs)

The suggested optimal daily nutritional allowances (SONAs) developed by Alex Schauss, Ph.D., provide a far better guideline to optimal health. Schauss developed his recommendations primarily from the extensive work of Emanuel Cheraskin and W. M. Ringsdorf Jr. of the University of Alabama School of Medicine.[8] Over a 15-year study, these two pioneering nutrition researchers conducted comprehensive health evaluations (health status questionnaires, physical exams, laboratory measures, and cardiac function and blood sugar regulation tests) and collected nutrient intake data on 13,500 male and female adults living in six regions of the United States. The data from their $2 million study were recorded in 49,000 bound pages in 153 volumes and have resulted in the publication of over 100 research articles during the last 20 years.

Table 7-2 Nutritional Deficiencies[6,7]

Nutrient	Incidence of Deficiency	Typical Symptoms and Diseases
Biotin	Uncommon	Dermatitis, eye inflammation, hair loss, loss of muscle control, insomnia, muscle weakness
Calcium	Average diet contains 40 to 50% of RDA*	Brittle nails, cramps, delusions, depression, insomnia, irritability, osteoporosis, palpitations, periodontal disease, rickets, tooth decay
Chromium	90% of diets deficient	Anxiety, fatigue, glucose intolerance, adult-onset diabetes
Copper	75% of diets deficient; average diet contains 50% of RDA*	Anemia, arterial damage, depression, diarrhea, fatigue, fragile bones, hair loss, hypothyroidism, weakness
Essential fatty acids	Very common	Diarrhea, dry skin and hair, hair loss, immune impairment, infertility, poor wound healing, premenstrual syndrome, acne, eczema, gall stones, liver degeneration
Folic acid	Average diet contains 60% of RDA*; deficient in 100% of elderly in one study; deficient in 48% of adolescent girls; requirement doubles in pregnancy	Anemia, apathy, diarrhea, fatigue, headaches, insomnia, loss of appetite, neural tube defects in fetus, paranoia, shortness of breath, weakness
Iodine	Uncommon since the supplementation of salt with iodine	Cretinism, fatigue, hypothyroidism, weight gain
Iron	Most common mineral deficiency	Anemia, brittle nails, confusion, constipation, depression, dizziness, fatigue, headaches, inflamed tongue, mouth lesions
Magnesium	75 to 85% of diets deficient; average diet contains 50 to 60% of RDA*	Anxiety, confusion, heart attack, hyperactivity, insomnia, nervousness, muscular irritability, restlessness, weakness
Manganese	Unknown, may be common in women	Atherosclerosis, dizziness, elevated cholesterol, glucose intolerance, hearing loss, loss of muscle control, ringing in ears
Niacin	Commonly deficient in elderly	Bad breath, canker sores, confusion, depression, dermatitis, diarrhea, emotional instability, fatigue, irritability, loss of appetite, memory impairment, muscle weakness, nausea, skin eruptions and inflammation
Pantothenic acid (B$_5$)	Average elderly diet contains 60% of RDA*	Abdominal pains, burning feet, depression, eczema, fatigue, hair loss, immune impairment, insomnia, irritability, low blood pressure, muscle spasms, nausea, poor coordination

Table 7-2 Nutritional Deficiencies (*continued*)

Nutrient	Incidence of Deficiency	Typical Symptoms and Diseases
Potassium	Commonly deficient in elderly	Acne, constipation, depression, edema, excessive water consumption, fatigue, glucose intolerance, high cholesterol levels, insomnia, mental impairment, muscle weakness, nervousness, poor reflexes
Pyridoxine (B_6)	71% of male and 90% of female diets deficient	Acne, anemia, arthritis, eye inflammation, depression, dizziness, facial oiliness, fatigue, impaired wound healing, irritability, loss of appetite, loss of hair, mouth lesions, nausea
Riboflavin	Deficient in 30% of elderly Britons	Blurred vision, cataracts, depression, dermatitis, dizziness, hair loss, inflamed eyes, mouth lesions, nervousness, neurological symptoms (numbness, loss of sensation, "electric shock" sensations), seizures, sensitivity to light, sleepiness, weakness
Selenium	Average diet contains 50% of RDA	Growth impairment, high cholesterol levels, increased incidence of cancer, pancreatic insufficiency (inability to secrete adequate amounts of digestive enzymes), immune impairment, liver impairment, male sterility
Thiamin	Commonly deficient in elderly	Confusion, constipation, digestive problems, irritability, loss of appetite, memory loss, nervousness, numbness of hands and feet, pain sensitivity, poor coordination, weakness
Vitamin A	20% of diets deficient	Acne, dry hair, fatigue, growth impairment, insomnia, hyperkeratosis (thickening and roughness of skin), immune impairment, night blindness, weight loss
Vitamin B_{12}	Serum levels low in 25% of hospital patients	Anemia, constipation, depression, dizziness, fatigue, intestinal disturbances, headaches, irritability, loss of vibration sensation, low stomach acid, mental disturbances, moodiness, mouth lesions, numbness, spinal cord degeneration
Vitamin C	20 to 50% of diets deficient	Bleeding gums, depression, easy bruising, impaired wound healing, irritability, joint pains, loose teeth, malaise, tiredness
Vitamin D	62% of elderly Danes' diets deficient	Burning sensation in mouth, diarrhea, insomnia, myopia, nervousness, osteomalacia, osteoporosis, rickets, scalp sweating

Table 7-2 Nutritional Deficiencies *(continued)*

Nutrient	Incidence of Deficiency	Typical Symptoms and Diseases
Vitamin E	23% of male and 15% of female diets deficient	Gait disturbances, poor reflexes, loss of position sense, loss of vibration sense, shortened red blood cell life
Vitamin K	Deficiency in pregnant women and newborns common	Bleeding disorders
Zinc	68% of diets deficient	Acne, amnesia, apathy, brittle nails, delayed sexual maturity, depression, diarrhea, eczema, fatigue, growth impairment, hair loss, high cholesterol levels, immune impairment, impotence, irritability, lethargy, loss of appetite, loss of sense of taste, low stomach acid, male infertility, memory impairment, night blindness, paranoia, white spots on nails, wound healing impairment

*RDA = recommended daily allowance

Using all this data, Cheraskin and Ringsdorf correlated the intake of specific nutrients with health status and tried to find a truly ideal level of intake for each nutrient. Interestingly, more was not always better. Table 7-3 tabulates the nutritional recommendations gleaned by Schauss from intensive study of this remarkable work and an incredible 500 other references.

Can We Take Too Much of a Supplement?

Yes. While most nutrients are safe, some can be dangerous and too much of anything can be toxic. Table 7-4 lists the known toxic levels of most nutrients and the symptoms and diseases that excessive supplementation may cause. The acute toxicity usually results from one or two large doses, while chronic toxicity usually refers to months of supplementation or excessive exposure in water or food. Unless otherwise noted, all the data in the table refer to chronic adult dosages. The nutrient with the greatest risk of toxicity is vitamin A, especially for children and pregnant women.

Under no circumstances should dosages near those noted as toxic in the table be taken without the expert guidance of a physician skilled in nutritional medicine. While some people can take more of a nutrient than the toxic dosage and experience no ill effects, some can experience a toxic effect at even lower dosages. You are your own best advisor of your individual reactions to any supplement. Even at lower dosages, always monitor yourself carefully and respect the feedback your body provides.

Table 7-3 The Suggested Optimal Daily Nutritional Allowances (SONA)*

Nutrient	Men RDA	Men SONA	Women RDA	Women SONA
Fat-soluble vitamins				
Vitamin A (RE, 1 RE = 1 µg = 3.33 iu)	1,000	2,000	800	2,000
β-carotene (mg)	n/a	100	n/a	80
Vitamin D (µg, 1µg = 40 iu)	5	24	5	24
Vitamin E (iu, 1 iu α tocopherol equivalent to 1 mg α tocopherol)	10	800	8	800
Vitamin K (mg)	80	80	65	65
Water-soluble vitamins				
Vitamin C (mg)	60	800	60	1,000
Vitamin B_{12} (µg)	2	3	2	3
Folic acid (µg)	200	2,000	180	2,000
Niacin (mg)	15	30	15	25
Pyridoxine (B_6) (mg)	2	25	1.6	20
Riboflavin (B_2) (mg)	1.4	2.5	1.2	2
Thiamin (B_1) (mg)	1.2	9.2	1	9
Minerals				
Boron (mg)	n/a	2.5	n/a	3
Calcium (mg)	800	700	800	1,200
Chromium (µg)	50–200	300	50–200	300
Copper (mg)	1.5–3	1.5–4	1.5–3	1.5–4
Iodine (µg)	150	150	150	150
Iron (mg)	10	20	15	20
Magnesium (mg)	350	600	280	550
Manganese (mg)	2–5	10	2–5	10
Phosphorous (mg)	800	800	800	800
Potassium (gm)	2	3	2	3
Selenium (µg)	70	250	55	200
Sodium (mg)	500	400	500	400
Zinc (mg)	15	20	12	17

* *While these are for all adults, they are most accurate for those aged 51 and above.*

Digestion and Nutrient Absorption

Eating an optimal diet does little good if we are unable to extract the nutrients we need. This requires good digestion to break apart the food and then efficient absorption to bring the released nutrients into the body. Unfortunately, this process often works poorly and maldigestion and/or malabsorption occur in many people, especially those with chronic diseases and the elderly.

As people age, many aspects of gastrointestinal function become impaired: sense of taste decreases, appetite decreases, hydrochloric acid secretion in the

Table 7-4 Potentially Toxic Dosages and Side Effects of Nutrients[6,7,8,9]

Nutrient	Toxic Dosage	Symptoms and Diseases
Biotin	n/a	No side effects from oral administration at therapeutic doses have been reported
Boron	>10 mg	No side effects reported
Calcium	>2,000 mg	No side effects reported, reduces iron absorption if taken with meals
Carotene	>300 mg	Orange discoloration of skin, weakness, low blood pressure, weight loss, low white cell count
Chromium	>50 mg	Dermatitis, intestinal ulcers, kidney and liver impairment
Copper	15 mg	Fatigue, poor memory, depression, insomnia, increased production of free radicals, may suppress immune function
Fluoride		
acute	500 mg	Poisons several enzymes, (5,000 mg lethal)
chronic	5 mg	Fluorosis (white patches on teeth), bone abnormalities
Folic acid	15 mg	Abdominal distention, loss of appetite, nausea, sleep disturbances, may interfere with zinc absorption, may prevent recognition of vitamin B_{12} deficiency
Iodine	2 mg	Thyroid impairment
Iron	25 mg	Intestinal upset, interferes with zinc and copper absorption, loss of appetite, not safe for those with iron storage disorders such as hemosiderosis, idiopathic hemochromatosis, or thalassemias
Magnesium	n/a	No toxicity reported except in those with kidney failure, diarrhea at large dosages of poorly absorbed forms (like Epsom salts)
Manganese	75 mg	Toxicity only reported in those working in manganese mines or drinking from contaminated water supplies, which results in loss of appetite, neurological damage, loss of memory, hallucinations, hyperirritability, elevation of blood pressure, liver damage
Niacin		
acute	100 mg	Transient flushing, headache, cramps, nausea, vomiting
chronic	3 gm	Anorexia, abnormal glucose tolerance, increased plasma uric acid levels, gastric ulceration, elevated liver enzymes
Pantothenic acid (B_5)	High dose	Occasional diarrhea
Phosphorous	High dose	Can reduce calcium absorption
Potassium	High dose	Mental impairment, weakness
Pyridoxine (B_6)	300 mg	Sensory and motor impairment
Riboflavin	n/a	No toxic effects have been noted

Table 7-4 Potentially Toxic Dosages and Side Effects of Nutrients *(continued)*

Nutrient	Toxic Dosage	Symptoms and Diseases
Selenium	750 µg	Diabetes, garlic-breath odor, immune impairment, loss of hair and nails, irritability, pallor, skin lesions, tooth decay, nausea, weakness, yellowish skin
Thiamin	n/a	No toxic effects noted for humans after oral administration
Vitamin A		
acute (infant)	75,000 iu	Anorexia, bulging fontanelles, hyperirritability, vomiting
acute (adult)	2 million iu	Headache, drowsiness, nausea, vomiting
chronic (infant)	10,000 iu	Premature epiphyseal bone closing, long bone growth retardation
chronic (adult)	50,000 iu	Anorexia, headache, blurred vision, loss of hair, bleeding lips, cracking and peeling skin, muscular stiffness and pain, severe liver enlargement and damage, anemia, fetal abnormalities (pregnant women must be very careful)
Vitamin B_{12}	n/a	No side effects from oral administration have been reported
Vitamin C		
acute	10 gm	Nausea, diarrhea, flatulence
chronic	3 gm	Increased urinary oxalate and uric acid levels in rare cases, impaired carotene utilization, chelation (binding of vitamin C with minerals) and resultant loss of minerals may occur, sudden discontinuation can cause rebound scurvy
Vitamin D		
acute	70,000 iu	Loss of appetite, nausea, vomiting, diarrhea, headache, excessive urination, excessive thirst
chronic	10,000 iu	Weight loss, pallor, constipation, fever, hypercalcemia, calcium deposits in soft tissues (pregnant women must be careful)
Vitamin E	1,000 iu	The safe dose is probably over 2,000, but some people experience weakness, fatigue, exacerbation of hypertension, increased activity of anticoagulants at 1,000 iu, while some research shows that as little as 300 iu can slow down the immune system. A small amount of immune suppression is probably a reasonable trade off for vitamin E's much needed antioxidant activity.
Vitamin K	n/a	No known toxicity with natural (phylloquinone); synthetic (menadione), while relatively safe, when administered to infants may cause hemolytic and liver enlargement
Zinc	75 mg	Gastrointestinal irritation, vomiting, adverse changes in HDL/LDL cholesterol ratios, impaired immunity

stomach decreases, and blood flow through the liver decreases.[10] These add up to decreased availability and absorption of virtually all nutrients, especially vitamin B_{12}, calcium, iron, zinc, and protein. In 20 to 30% of older adults (37% of those 80+), this gastrointestinal dysfunction progresses to gastric atrophy, a condition in which few functional cells are left in the stomach and nutrient absorption is greatly impaired.

Nutrients are not well-absorbed for essentially three reasons: inadequate secretion of hydrochloric acid in the stomach, inadequate secretion of enzymes by the pancreas, and damage to the intestinal lining, which impairs the absorption of nutrients.

While the digestive process deals with the daily dietary intake (approximately 100 gm of fat, 75 gm of protein, 350 gm of carbohydrates, and 3.5 quarts of water), it must in addition digest, absorb, or eliminate intestinal secretions of up to 100 gm of protein (primarily from sIgA), 30 gm of fat, and over 7 quarts of water! This is why the wasting diseases seen in advanced AIDS are so devastating and can progress so rapidly. Not only do the AIDS sufferers have trouble digesting and absorbing the nutrients from the food they eat, but they are also unable to reabsorb the nutritionally important molecules they secrete as part of the normal digestive process. They literally waste away through their intestinal tract.

How the Digestive System Works

In the mouth, chewing breaks up the food and mixes it with saliva. Saliva performs many important functions: It makes the chewed food easier to swallow, protects the throat from the abrasive effect of the food, coats the throat with secretory IgA antibodies to keep bacteria in the food from invading, and contains enzymes (lipase, amylase, and ptyalin) that initiate fat and starch digestion. Saliva even helps to remineralize the teeth with calcium salts and tags food molecules for better protein digestion.

The stomach continues the digestive process by producing 1 to 2 quarts of gastric juices containing hydrochloric acid, intrinsic factor, and pepsin. Hydrochloric acid (secreted by the parietal cells) begins the digestion of proteins, frees many minerals from the food, and helps kill bacteria in ingested matter. Mucus is secreted by the stomach cells, forming an acid- and pepsin-resistant coating for the stomach. Intrinsic factor binds with vitamin B_{12}, protecting it from digestion and improving its absorption in the intestine. Finally, the stomach secretions contain several digestive enzymes such as pepsin (protein digestion), rennin (clots milk), and lipase (partial fat digestion).

Most of the digestion and absorption takes place in the small intestine through the action of enzymes secreted by the pancreas, intestinal cells, and liver. The primary enzymes are summarized in Table 7-5.

The intestinal lining of the small and large intestines finishes the digestive process and absorbs needed nutrients, while keeping unwanted substances out

Table 7-5 The Digestive Enzymes of the Small Intestine

Enzyme	Source	Action
Bicarbonate	Pancreas	Neutralizes stomach acid
Trypsin and chymotrypsin	Pancreas	Digest proteins to polypeptides and amino acids
Amylase	Pancreas	Splits starch to disaccharides (double sugars)
Lipase	Pancreas	Splits fats to monoglycerides and free fatty acids
Bile	Liver	Emulsifies fats to allow the action of water-soluble lipases
Lactase, sucrase, and maltase	Intestinal lining cells	Digest specific disaccharides

of the body. To accomplish this, the gastrointestinal tract has a huge surface area (when stretched out flat it would be about the size of two tennis courts). This is 600 times as much surface area as might be expected from a simple cylinder the length of the intestines. This increased surface is due to the intestinal folds—villi and microvilli (villi are like little fingers of cells sticking into the intestines).

Absorption is largely controlled by the membranes of the cells lining the intestine. Molecules penetrate this protein/lipid membrane by various mechanisms such as simple passive diffusion, facilitated diffusion, active transport, or pinocytosis (in which the cells engulf the molecule and transport it into the blood). One of the ways the intestinal system keeps toxins and other undesirable molecules out of the body is by secreting the immunoglobulin sIgA. Secretory IgA binds to bacteria and undesirable molecules, blocking their penetration of the intestinal lining cells.[11]

The large intestine finishes the absorption of water (about a quart daily) and provides a controlled route for excretion of waste products and toxic substances. The large intestine also provides an environment for microbial fermentation and degradation of carbohydrates that results in the production of short chain fatty acids which are the main energy source for colonic epithelial cells.

Intestinal Microecology

The microflora of the gastrointestinal tract constitute an enormously complex ecosystem of microorganisms, some of which are health-promoting and some of which are toxic. The typical person harbors at least 400 to 500 species of intestinal flora.[12] The normal human is composed of over 10^{14} cells, 90% of which are microbial cells, and most of these reside in the gastrointestinal tract. In other words, there are more bacteria in the gut alone than the total number of human cells in the body, and these bacteria are more metabolically active than we are.[13]

Flora content is surprisingly stable within an individual over time.[14] In many ways, the gut flora can be viewed as an organ of the body in its own right because these microbes profoundly influence many of our physiological processes. The microflora in the gut play a role in metabolizing nutrients, vitamins, drugs, hormones, and carcinogens; synthesizing short chain fatty acids; preventing the growth of pathogens in the intestines; and stimulating maturation of the normal immune response.[15]

A special property of colonic bacteria is their fermentation of carbohydrates to short chain fatty acids (acetate, propionate, butyrate, and valerate).[16] In the healthy intestine, these short chain fatty acids provide up to 70% of the energy for lining cells.[17]

Maldigestion

Maldigestion often begins simply with inadequate chewing of food. Because digestion is entirely a chemical process, it only works when the hydrochloric acid and digestive enzymes come into contact with the food molecules. Large food molecules result in the nutrients in the middle being undigested because the enzymes can't get to them before they are excreted in the feces. Not only are their nutrients lost, but sometimes these undigested particles provide inappropriate nutrients to the bacteria of the large intestine, allowing them to overgrow and cause problems.

One of the old-time natural therapies was called "Fletcherization" after a Dr. Fletcher who advised his patients to chew each mouthful 100 times! This was probably excellent advice since analysis of the stools of most people reveals large amounts of unchewed food particles. This might explain why putting fruits and vegetables through a juicer before eating them is of such great value in promoting optimal nutrition.

Hypochlorhydria (Insufficient Stomach Acid)

Gastric acid secretion is a fundamental step in digestion and assimilation, particularly of proteins and minerals. Although much has been said about hyperacidity, little attention has been paid to hypochlorhydria. This deficiency of stomach acid is a significant health problem; far more health problems are caused by too little stomach acid than too much stomach acid. As can be seen in Table 7-6 and Table 7-7, many symptoms, signs, and diseases are associated with low gastric acidity, particularly several autoimmune diseases. The problem with low stomach acid is that not only does the first step in digestion not work well, but the second step, pancreatic enzyme digestion, doesn't work as well either because the dumping of acid from the stomach into the small intestine is a major signal for the pancreas to secrete its enzymes.

Table 7-6 Common Signs and Symptoms of Low Gastric Acidity[18]

Bloating, belching, burning, and flatulence immediately after meals
A sense of fullness after eating
Indigestion, diarrhea, or constipation
Systemic reactions after eating
Nausea after taking supplements
Rectal itching
Weak, peeling, or cracked fingernails
Dilated capillaries in the cheeks and nose (in nonalcoholic individuals)
Post-adolescent acne
Iron deficiency
Chronic intestinal infections: parasites, yeast, bacteria
Undigested food in stool

Table 7-7 Diseases Associated with Low Gastric Acidity[18]

Addison's disease	Hepatitis
Asthma	Lupus erythematosis
Celiac disease	Myasthenia gravis
Chronic autoimmune disorders	Osteoporosis
Chronic hives	Pernicious anemia
Dermatitis herpetiformis	Rosacea
Diabetes mellitus	Sjogren's syndrome
Eczema	Thyrotoxicosis
Food allergies	Hyper- and hypothyroidism
Gallbladder disease	Vitiligo
Gastric carcinoma	

Many studies have shown that our ability to excrete stomach acid decreases with age; low stomach acidity has been found in over half of those over age 60.[19] One study of elderly people found that their tissue nutrient levels could be saturated only with intramuscular supplementation because oral supplementation was ineffective.[20] The authors speculated that this was due to atrophy of various digestive organs.

Pancreatic Insufficiency

Inadequate delivery of pancreatic lipase, proteases, and bicarbonate to the small intestine can also result in maldigestion. Pancreatic insufficiency leads to impaired absorption of dietary fat and protein with potential major negative systemic effects. The absorption of carbohydrates and water-soluble vitamins, however, is only partially impaired. Pancreatic insufficiency appears to be relatively uncommon except in those with cystic fibrosis or low levels of stomach acid.

The Problem with Antacids

Many people take antacids for heartburn and gastric ulcers. Unfortunately, not only are antacids not particularly effective for healing stomach ulcers, they seriously interfere with digestion. By neutralizing the acid in the stomach, they block the extraction of minerals from food and inhibit the stimulation of pancreatic enzyme secretion by the pancreas. Even worse, many of them are salts of aluminum. As discussed in Chapter Five, aluminum is toxic to the brain, and high levels in the body have been associated with Alzheimer's disease.

Malabsorption

Malabsorption results when food isn't digested enough to free the needed nutrients or when the intestinal lining is damaged. When the intestines are damaged, the surface area becomes smaller, so there is less opportunity for nutrients to diffuse into the blood. In addition, damaged cells are not as able to facilitate the absorption of nutrients, which can only be absorbed by active processes. Aging and accumulated damage result in a progressive decrease in nutrient absorption.[21]

Amino acids, carbohydrates, fats, vitamins, and trace elements are all absorbed by different processes, so malabsorption for one nutrient does not necessarily imply malabsorption of others. However, most people with malabsorption have problems absorbing most nutrients. In the case of fat malabsorption, besides the loss of the highest source of dietary calories, essential fatty acid deficiency may result. As noted in Chapter Six, essential fatty acids are crucial precursors for prostaglandins, leukotrienes, and other compounds involved in the inflammatory process.

The signs and symptoms of malabsorption vary depending on the type and level of deficiency. Table 7-8 lists the common signs and symptoms of malabsorption. Also included is the typical reason for each symptom.

Malabsorption has many causes (listed in Table 7-9). Unabsorbed carbohydrates from the small intestine are rapidly broken down in the large intestine by colonic bacteria. This degradation liberates hydrogen and other gases, which, if excessive, result in bloating and passing gas.

Food Allergy

Without a doubt, one of the most common causes of malabsorption (and of many common diseases) is the intestinal damage caused by food allergies. This is not a new problem. It has been recognized at least since Hippocrates, who observed that milk could cause intestinal upset and hives. He wrote, "To many this has been the commencement of a serious disease when they have merely taken twice in a day the same food which they have been in the custom of taking once."[22]

Table 7-8 Signs and Symptoms of Malabsorption

Signs and Symptoms	Possible Explanations
Abdominal bloating, gas	Undigested carbohydrates resulting in excess gas production by bacteria in colon; lactose intolerance; excess unabsorbed small molecules, such as too much vitamin C or indigestible sugar (sorbitol in "sugarless" candies)
Abdominal cramps	Intestinal inflammation; excessive gas (as above); candidal overgrowth
Chronic diarrhea	Chronic inflammation; chronic infection; unabsorbed small molecules; candidal overgrowth
Constipation	Accumulation of undigested materials
Greasy stools	Fat maldigestion
Easy bruisability	Abnormal microflora resulting in malabsorption of vitamin K needed for blood clotting
Chronic fatigue	Impaired vitamin or mineral absorption
Poor quality hair and nails	Impaired protein absorption
Food allergies	Maldigestion; damaged intestinal lining allowing food particles to leak into the body
Unexplained weight loss	Malabsorption of needed nutrients
Anemia	Hypochlorhydria; deficiency of intrinsic factor
Chronic intestinal infections	Hypochlorhydria; abnormal intestinal microflora
Chronic autoimmune diseases	Maldigestion; damaged intestinal lining allowing food particles and microbial toxins to leak into the body
Poor growth rate and failure to thrive in children	Damage to the small intestine mucosa resulting in decreased ability to absorb needed nutrients

Table 7-9 Causes of Malabsorption

Cause	Effect
Insufficient concentrations of digestive enzymes	Nutrients not removed from foods and therefore not absorbable
Food allergies	Damage intestinal mucosa
Bacterial and viral infections	Damage intestinal cells; decrease intestinal cell enzymes; compete for nutrients
Inadequate absorptive surface	Decreased absorption efficiency
Drugs (cholestyramine, neomycin, colchicine, irritant laxatives)	Damage intestinal lining; block absorption of specific nutrients
Some diseases (Crohn's disease, lactose intolerance, Sprue, Whipple's disease)	Intestinal damage

The incidence of food allergies and the number of individuals suffering from diseases caused by or aggravated by food allergies (e.g., asthma, eczema, hives) has increased dramatically during the last 25 years. Nutritionally oriented physicians believe that food allergies are the leading cause of most undiagnosed symptoms and contribute to most chronic diseases. Others maintain that at least 60% of all Americans, both "healthy" and sick, suffer from symptoms associated with food reactions.

Theories of why the incidence has increased include: poor digestion, increased stresses on the immune system (such as increased chemical pollution in the air, water, and food), less breast feeding, earlier weaning and earlier introduction of solid foods to infants, genetic manipulation of plants resulting in food components that cross-react with normal tissues, and increased ingestion of fewer foods. Probably all of these and more have contributed to the increased frequency and severity of symptoms.

While it is easy to recognize a food allergy when an immediate reaction occurs after a food is eaten (such as hives or an asthma attack), most food allergies don't manifest that way. One reason food allergies are so difficult to recognize is that the reactions are often delayed several hours, so it is hard to recognize the correlation. There are even reports in the research literature of reactions occurring as late as three days after a food is eaten. The food groups most frequently involved in food allergies are grains (wheat, rye, barley, oats, rice, corn), dairy (milk, cheese, yogurt), eggs, peanuts, beef, the tomato family (tomato, potato, red and green peppers, pimento, cayenne) and shellfish (oysters, shrimp, clams).

The mechanisms by which food allergies damage the intestines are pretty well understood:

1. A person eats a food to which he or she has become sensitive
2. The food is inadequately digested in the stomach and small intestine so that
3. Intact proteins come into contact with the intestinal lining cells and
4. Antibodies in and on the intestinal mucosa combine with the food protein, initiating an inflammatory reaction
5. The inflammatory reaction damages the surrounding cells
6. Continued exposure results in progressive damage to the intestinal lining
7. The damaged intestinal lining decreases the surface area of the intestines decreasing absorption of needed nutrients while paradoxically allowing undesirable toxins to leak into the body through the areas of damage

The end result is a progressively worsening malnutrition combined with increased absorption of disease-causing toxins. Table 7-10 lists the common signs and symptoms of food allergies. Food allergies are discussed in more detail in Chapter Five, including methods for determining which foods cause problems for you.

Table 7-10 Common Signs and Symptoms of Food Allergies

Dark circles under eyes	Bed wetting
Puffiness under eyes	Chronic infections
Horizontal creases in the lower lid	Excessive mood swings
Chronic diarrhea	Asthma
Chronic fatigue	Canker sores
Chronic swollen glands	Hives
Chronic, non-cyclic fluid retention	Eczema
Irritable bowel syndrome	

Intestinal Infections

Every day, our intestines are exposed to many microorganisms (bacteria, yeasts, parasites, and viruses), some of them pathological. Normally, we are protected from infection by our stomach acid, pancreatic enzymes, secretory IgA antibodies, microflora, antibacterial enzymes, peristalsis (i.e., the excretion of feces), and competitive growth inhibition by normal flora. The healthier the composition of our intestinal microflora, the greater our resistance to intestinal infections.[23]

Besides the acute symptoms of abdominal cramps and diarrhea, intestinal infections can cause a wide range of systemic and chronic effects stemming from inflammation of the intestines, disruption of normal flora, and increased intestinal permeability, which allows entry of intestinal toxins. These effects can cause malabsorption of nutrients. Pathogens produce toxins that can lead to reactions which contribute to chronic systemic inflammatory conditions (e.g., psoriasis and lupus). There is also evidence that some microflora have proteins on their surfaces that are so similar to normal tissues that when the body forms antibodies against these organisms, the antibodies also attack our normal tissues. This disconcerting interaction is discussed in more detail in Chapter Five. Research and clinical experience highlight the profound relation between gastrointestinal tract infections, malabsorption, permeability changes, and health.

Candida albicans

In the last few years, *Candida albicans* has attracted considerable attention and controversy as a possible cause of chronic illness.[24] Many investigators have suggested that an intestinal overgrowth of *Candida albicans* (and other intestinal yeast) may be an etiologic factor in food allergy, migraine headaches, irritable bowel syndrome, asthma, indigestion and gas, depression related to PMS, vaginitis, and chronic fatigue.

While the normal gastrointestinal tract harbors small amounts of yeast, overgrowth of yeast appears to be more common now as a consequence of several decades of widespread use of antibiotics, corticosteroids, and birth control pills, and increased amounts of sugars in the diet. Nutritionally oriented physicians believe that it is not yeast's presence but rather its overgrowth and its effects on systemic processes in patients that cause the problems. Over 20 research studies have shown that patients with intestinal infections have C. *albicans* in their feces over twice as often as normal controls.[25] One article reported that chronic diarrhea and abdominal cramps may be caused by large numbers of dead or damaged yeast found in feces.[26] See Chapter Five for how to treat chronic intestinal yeast overgrowth.

Parasites

Parasites (worms in the intestines) are a surprisingly common cause of intestinal damage and nutrient malabsorption. Parasitic infections chronically activate the immune system, damage the intestinal mucosa, and consume several nutrients, making them unavailable for absorption. Different organisms cause malabsorption of different nutrients such as iron and vitamins A and B_{12}. The tapeworm *Diphyllobothrium latum* causes a vitamin B_{12} deficiency. The hookworms trichuris and chistosoma can cause significant blood loss, which elevates iron needs and contributes to anemia. The very common large worm *Ascaris lumbricoides* reduces fat absorption and interferes with the absorption of vitamin A and beta-carotene.[27]

Parasite infections are far more common than previously thought. One leading physician of nutritional medicine, Leo Galland, M.D. (who practices in New York City), reported a high frequency of giardiasis (infection with *Giardia lamblia*) in patients with chronic digestive complaints. Out of 197 consecutive patients with a variety of gastrointestinal symptoms, an incredible 95 were found to have giardiasis, and 98% of those experienced clinical improvement after successful irradication of the parasite. Typical symptoms included diarrhea, abdominal bloating, chronic fatigue, food intolerance, abdominal pain, and constipation. Many of his patients had traveled outside the country.[28] Galland also found giardiasis in 61 of 218 patients whose chief complaint was chronic fatigue. Treatment resulted in 13 of 48 patients experiencing complete remission of their chronic fatigue with an additional 29 experiencing partial to marked improvement in symptoms.[29] *Giardia lamblia* is a protozoan parasite that is transmitted by contaminated water or food, or from person-to-person contact.

The problem is not limited to giardiasis. In one 1987 study, state diagnostic laboratories evaluated over 200,000 stool specimens. Parasites were found in 20.1% of the stools. The researchers found *Giardia lamblia* in 7.2%, *Entamoeba coli* and *Endolimax nana* in 4.2%, *Blastocystis hominis* in 2.6%, hookworm in 1.5%, *Trichuris trichiura* in 1.2%, *Entamoeba histolytica* in 0.9%, *Ascaris lumbricoides* in 0.8%, and lesser percentages of several other parasites. The incidence of *Giardia lamblia* had increased significantly from the 4% found in 1979.[30] The incidence of parasitic infection in undeveloped countries is even higher, with some researchers estimating an incidence as high as 99%. Thus, those who travel to Third World countries need to have their stools checked if they experience any sign of intestinal upset.

Some Unwanted Stowaways

Jed walked into my office one day with an unusual complaint—every month for the past ten years he had suffered from two- to three-day long bouts of a mysterious fever combined with severe worsening of his chronic fatigue and intestinal upset. He had gone to dozens of medical specialists and hospitals, and spent over $10,000, to no avail. After asking Jed for a detailed history, I learned that his problems had started a few months after a trip to South America. I immediately suspected parasites. He dismissed this possibility because one of the doctors he had seen had tested his stools and had found no worms or other pathogens.

Fortunately, I was able to talk him into repeating the test, but this time at a laboratory I knew to be reliable. I explained to him that looking for parasites in stools is, at best, a particularly unpleasant task. As a result, most lab technicians perform a cursory examination of stools. The lab I worked with was run by an unusually conscientious lab technician who was particularly skilled in the recognition and diagnosis of parasites. As it turned out, Jed had not one, but two different intestinal parasites. The periodicity of his symptoms was due to the reproductive cycles of the parasites.

I put him on a special parasite-unfriendly diet and used anthelmintic herbs to kill off the parasites. (I am being purposely vague about my therapy because parasites are not a self-treatable condition and require the expertise of a physician.) He responded very well to treatment and immediately started feeling better. However, it took several months of heavy nutritional supplementation before we could fully reestablish his nutritional status and sense of well-being. We repeated the parasite tests after two weeks, two months, and six months to be sure that we took care of both the parasites and their eggs, which can be much more difficult to eradicate.

- *The message:* Chronic, unexplained fatigue and gastrointestinal upset is often due to unrecognized parasitic infection.

The most common symptom of parasitic infection is diarrhea, followed by chronic abdominal pain. Other typical symptoms include: intestinal gas, foul-smelling stools, intestinal cramps, loss of appetite, nausea, weight loss, belching, heartburn, headache, constipation, vomiting, fever, chills, bloody stools, mucus in the stools, and fatigue. Parasites should not be self-treated; consult a physician if you suspect that you have parasites.

How to Improve Digestion and Nutrient Absorption

There are many ways to improve digestion and heal the damaged intestines. Because a damaged intestine is a significant source of toxins, some ways to heal the damaged intestines are discussed in Chapter Five. In general, the best way to improve digestion is to stimulate the normal digestive processes, so that the stomach secretes the needed hydrochloric acid, and the pancreas secretes the needed enzymes. However, at times, this is too slow a process, so supplementation with hydrochloric acid and pancreatic enzymes is necessary.

Reestablishing Stomach Acid Production

As long as the stomach has not totally atrophied (a condition called atrophic gastritis), hydrochloric acid secretion can be increased, even to normal levels. Interestingly, zinc deficiency appears to be a major cause of hypochlorhydria. (Another common cause of stomach dysfunction is infection with *Helicobacter pylori*, which is discussed in Chapter Five.)

Zinc

The first step in reestablishing stomach hydrochloric acid production is supplementation with zinc. The typical signs and symptoms of zinc deficiency include loss of appetite, loss of taste sensation, and impaired secretion of hydrochloric acid.[31] Several studies have found that the elderly have both inadequate dietary consumption of zinc and impaired absorption of zinc, with an estimated 25 to 30% suffering from at least a mild zinc deficiency.[32] This leads to a vicious cycle: Decreased zinc consumption results in decreased production of hydrochloric acid, which results in impaired ability to absorb zinc from food, causing a further drop in zinc status. Much of the age-related decrease in digestion may simply be due to chronic zinc deficiency. The good news is that zinc supplementation reverses these problems. Whole grains, nuts, and vegetables are good sources of zinc.

- *Dosage:* 25 mg zinc picolinate per day

Herbal bitters

The next step is to stimulate the stomach to produce hydrochloric acid through the use of herbal bitters. These have been used for centuries by virtually all cultures of the world to stimulate digestion. When a bitter substance is tasted, it sends a message to the digestive system to increase the secretion of saliva in the mouth, acid in the stomach, and enzymes by the pancreas. My favorite herbal bitter is a tincture made of gentian root and wormwood. A few drops in a small amount of water can be quite effective. Several good bitters products are available in health food stores.

Hydrochloric acid supplements

If a you do not respond to the herbal stimulant, it is time to use supplemental hydrochloric acid. The following are the directions I've given countless patients suffering from low stomach acid:

1. Begin by taking one hydrochloric acid capsule (10 grains of betaine HCl) at your next large meal. At every meal after that of the same size take one more capsule. (One capsule at the first meal, two at the meal after that, then three at the next meal.)
2. Continue to increase the dose until you reach six capsules or when you feel a warmth in your stomach, whichever occurs first. A feeling of warmth in the stomach means that you have taken too many capsules for that size meal. Take one less next meal. However, it is a good idea to try the larger dose again at another meal to make sure that it was the hydrochloric acid that caused the warmth and not something else.
3. After you have determined the largest dose that you can take at your large meals without feeling any warmth, maintain that dose at all meals of similar size. Take fewer capsules with smaller meals.
4. When taking several capsules, it is best to take the capsules throughout the meal, rather than all at once.
5. As your stomach begins to regain the ability to produce the amount of hydrochloric acid needed to properly digest your food, you will notice the warm feeling again and will have to cut down the dose level.

After a few months, you should no longer need to supplement with hydrochloric acid.

Enzymes

Normally, once adequate hydrochloric acid secretion is reestablished, the pancreas will secrete adequate amounts of enzymes. However, people with diseases such as cystic fibrosis and chronic pancreatitis secrete very small amounts of enzymes, while others with chronic maldigestion for unknown reasons simply don't secrete enough. Fortunately, supplementing with digestive enzymes can reestablish normal digestive function. There are two types of enzyme products commercially available, those extracted from animal sources (such as the pancreas of hogs) and those extracted from fungal sources (typically *Aspergillus oryzae*). They contain varying ratios of lipases, proteases, and amylases. Both types appear to be effective.

For example, a 1985 cross-over (meaning the patients received all the therapies, but at different times) study compared the effectiveness of regular pancreatic enzymes, enteric-coated pancreatic enzymes (meaning the enzymes were coated with a substance to protect them from stomach acid), and fungal enzymes in patients with chronic pancreatitis or severe pancreatic insufficiency. All suffered from steatorrhea, meaning they had a lot of undigested fat and other nutrients in their stools.[33] Seventeen patients in the study were divided into two treatment groups based on surgical status. Nine patients had had part of their intestines surgically removed 3 to 8 months prior to the study (group A). This group's pancreatic secretion was less than 10% of normal. In

Table 7-11 Stool Weight and Fecal Fat in Patients with Steatorrhea

	Fecal fat gm/day		Stool weight gm/day	
Treatment Protocol	Group A	Group B	Group A	Group B
Placebo	180	82	906	675
Enteric-coated pancreatin	75	39	494	324
Pancreatin	55	48	437	345
Fungal lipase	87	48	519	316

The upper limit of the normal range for fecal fat excretion is 7 gm/day and for stool weight is 250 gm/day

the remaining eight non-surgical patients (group B), pancreatic enzyme secretion was down to between 4% and 28% of normal. This poor level of pancreatic functioning resulted in these patients suffering from chronic abdominal pain and a tendency to lose weight. All measures of their stools were abnormal, i.e., their stools were loose, in too great a volume, and contained too much fat.

All patients were placed on a diet containing 100 gm of fat per day and stools were collected for 72 hours, five days after discontinuing all medications (e.g., pancreatic enzymes, antacids, and hydrogen receptor antagonists). Thereafter, each group was placed on identical two-week periods of treatment using enteric-coated pancreatin first, then conventional pancreatin, and, finally, acid-stable fungal enzymes. Stools were collected for the last three days of each treatment period and analyzed for stool weight, fat concentration, and total fecal fat excretion.

All three treatment protocols led to a significant reduction in total daily stool weight and total daily fecal fat excretion as compared to controls in both groups. Perhaps more importantly, all patients in both groups became virtually symptom-free on each of the three treatment protocols. Table 7-11 shows fecal fat excretion and stool weight for group A and group B. As can be seen, all three of the enzyme preparations substantially improved digestion and absorption of needed nutrients.

Healing Metabolic Disorders in Real Life

Men at Risk for Heart Attacks and Pregnant Women Suffering Pre-eclampsia Share the Same Problem

Perhaps one of the most important and commonly deficient minerals is magnesium, particularly for men. It is a cofactor in over 300 enzyme systems throughout the body, especially those associated with energy production and utilization. It is also particularly important for maintaining neurological and muscular tone. It is estimated to be deficient in the diet of over 50% of the population (see Table 7-2). Since magnesium is an intracellular element, measurement of serum levels (the way most doctors measure magnesium levels) does not reflect a person's actual magnesium status. In fact, serum levels don't drop until a person is so deficient that he or she is manifesting such symptoms as cardiac arrhythmias, seizures, pre-eclampsia in pregnant women, and high blood pressure.[34]

Women who suffered pre-eclampsia, eclampsia, or hypertension during pregnancy may be at risk for low magnesium levels. These problems are largely relieved when the pregnant women are supplemented with magnesium, or, if their problems are serious, when magnesium is injected intramuscularly.[35]

Magnesium is particularly important for men, especially those who have had or are suffering from a heart attack. Low magnesium levels are commonly found in cardiac surgery patients, and low magnesium levels after cardiac surgery is strongly associated with morbidity. Epidemiological studies show a higher rate of heart attacks in men living in areas with lower amounts of magnesium in their food and water.[36] Magnesium administration greatly decreases the post-operative morbidity.[37]

- *Dosage:* for men, 400 mg magnesium citrate per day; for women, 350 mg magnesium citrate per day

Chromium, Diabetes, and Hypoglycemia

Maintaining balanced blood sugar levels is essential for good health because the brain is totally dependent on blood sugar for energy, as are many other enzymatic processes. However, most people have trouble maintaining normal sugar metabolism. This can manifest as hypoglycemia (fluctuating blood sugar levels resulting in irritability, cravings for sugar, fatigue, etc.) which then often progresses to adult-onset diabetes, a problem that affects 4.5% of the population. While many factors contribute to its incidence, a deficiency of the trace mineral chromium is a significant cause. Adequate chromium levels are needed to maintain normal glucose levels, utilize insulin effectively, and keep blood lipid levels down.[38]

Supplementation with chromium, even without dietary change (much better results are obtained when all refined carbohydrates are also removed from the diet), improves both hypoglycemia and diabetes, with most diabetics being able to reduce, and even eliminate, their need for insulin. Several studies have shown a 50% reduction in insulin requirements after a few months of supplementation with 200 to 500 µg per day.[39]

For supplemental purposes, chromium picolinate is the best form because it is very well absorbed by the body.[40]

- *Dosage:* 200 µg chromium picolinate per day

Stomach Ulcers

Many people consume antacids to relieve stomach pain due to stomach ulcers. This is *not* a good idea—most antacids contain aluminum, a known brain toxin. Equally important, many people with ulcers do not produce excessive stomach acid and, in fact, need their acid for proper digestion. Stomach ulcers are generally not caused by excessive stomach acid. Rather they are caused by an imbalance between the rate of healing and regeneration of the stomach cells and the amount of trauma to which they are exposed. Without question, one source of trauma is hydrochloric acid. However, the normal stomach is well-designed to protect itself from the acid it secretes.

The other primary source of damage is from infection with *Helicobacter pylori*. This has become recognized as a significant cause of hypochlorhydria, stomach ulcers, gastric atrophy, and even stomach cancer.[41] Virtually all patients with ulcers are infected with *H. pylori*. However, 30% of those without ulcers also are infected with *H. pylori*, and only 5 to 10% of the population has ulcers.[42] In other words, only one-third of those infected with *H. pylori* have ulcers. This means that, like other infectious agents, it only produces ulcers in those who are susceptible.

Elimination of this bacteria and stimulation of healing are both effective therapies. Several herbs and nutrients have been found to be consistently effective in stimulating healing of stomach ulcers. Unfortunately, no research has been reported on the efficacy of these natural medicines in eliminating the bacteria. Since rates of recurrence are very low in ulcers that have been healed with natural medicines, especially as compared to antacids and H_2-blockers (which block the secretion of stomach acid), these approaches probably also help the body eliminate *H. pylori*.

Raw cabbage juice

Raw cabbage juice has been well-documented as having remarkable success in treating peptic ulcers.[43] One liter per day of the fresh juice, taken throughout the day, resulted in total ulcer healing (confirmed by x-rays) in an average of only ten days. Further research has shown that the high glutamine content of cabbage juice is probably responsible for its efficacy. In a double-blind clinical study of 57 patients, 1.6 gm of glutamine a day was compared to conventional therapy (antacids, antispasmodics, milk, and bland diet). Glutamine proved to be the more effective treatment. Half of the patients in the glutamine-treated group showed complete healing (according to x-rays) within two weeks, and 92% showed complete relief and healing within four weeks.[44] Although the mechanism for these results is not known, the authors postulated that glutamine increased the biosynthesis of the mucoproteins that protect the stomach lining.

Licorice root

Glycyrrhiza glabra (licorice root) has historically been regarded as an excellent natural medicine for stomach ulcers, and its effectiveness has been documented in several dozen animal and clinical studies. However, one of licorice root's constituents, glycyrrhizinic acid (GA), can increase blood pressure in susceptible individuals. Therefore, a manufacturing procedure was developed to remove GA from licorice to form deglycyrrhizinated licorice (DGL). The result is a very successful anti-ulcer agent without any known side effects.[45] DGL is so safe and effective that it has been shown to be far superior to cimetidine, the drug which was for years the primary medical treatment.[46] DGL has been shown to increase the blood supply to the damaged mucosa, increase the number of cells producing the mucus that protects the stomach, and increase the amount of mucus the cells produce.[47]

Full resolution of stomach ulcers requires the assistance of a physician. First, if there is Helicobacter pylori in the stomach, it must be eliminated. Then, the herbs and nutrients can be used to stimulate repair of the damaged stomach lining.

- *Dosage:* DGL, 250 mg three times a day; glutamine 1,000 mg per day

Summary

Total wellness starts with optimal nutrition, and the research, though limited, is clear: Unprocessed, organically grown foods are much higher in essential nutrients and lower in environmental pollutants than commercially grown foods. However, even the best diet does little good if nutrients are not properly extracted from the food and absorbed into the body, a process which requires an effective digestive system. Total wellness often requires supplementation to ensure adequate levels of nutrients for optimal enzyme function, especially when some of our enzymes do not work as well as they should.

Chapter Eight

Balancing Regulatory Systems

You need to study this chapter if you suffer from any of the following:

- *Symptoms*

  Abdominal obesity
  Depression
  Fatigue
  Impotence
  Insomnia

  Irritability
  Loss of sexual drive (both men
    and women)
  Uncomfortable menopause
  Menstrual irregularities

- *Diseases*

  Allergies
  Autoimmune diseases (e.g.,
    lupus erythematosis,
    rheumatoid arthritis)
  Frequent infections
  Dermatitis herpetiformis
  Hair loss
  High cholesterol levels

  Hyperthyroidism
  Hypothyroidism
  Infertility
  Loss of muscle mass and strength
  Obesity
  Osteoporosis
  Premenstrual tension

Behaviors that increase risk:

- Consumption of alcohol
- Poor diet (refined and/or commercially grown foods)
- Smoking
- Chronic physical or emotional stress

Thumbnail: Quick Help for the Regulatory System

- *To increase thyroid activity*
  Limit brassica family foods (e.g., cabbage, broccoli, brussels sprouts) to
    three servings a day
  Kelp or other sea vegetables: 3 tablets a day
  Copper: 5 mg per day
  Selenium: 150 µg per day
  Zinc: 25 mg per day
  Thyroid gland extract from which the thyroid hormones have been
    removed: 3 tablets a day

- *To increase DHEA levels*
  Stop smoking
  Engage in a regular stress reduction program
  Exercise five days a week
  Eleutherococcus senticosus (Siberian ginseng): 2 to 16 ml fluid extract or
    100 to 200 mg standardized extract

- *To improve female hormone balance*
  Eat at least three ounces of soy foods a day
  Zinc (picolinate best): 20 mg per day
  Vitamin A: 5,000 iu per day
  Vitex agnus-castus: 40 drops tincture a day

- *To improve male hormone function*
  Avoid environmental estrogens
  Stop smoking
  Limit saturated fat intake
  Zinc (picolinate best): 25 mg per day
  Panax ginseng: 10 mg of ginsenosides three times a day

All the major functions of the body are regulated by two major control systems: the nervous system (discussed in Chapters Nine and Ten) and the hormonal or endocrine system. In general, the endocrine system controls the metabolic functions of the body, such as the level of energy production, the rate of enzyme activity in the cells, and absorption and transport of some minerals. Hormones also control our growth, sexual function, and blood pressure. The primary endocrine organs are the pituitary gland, adrenal cortex, thyroid gland, islets of Langerhans in the pancreas, ovaries or testes, and parathyroid gland. In addition, the placenta in pregnant women functions as an endrocine gland. Imbalances in any of our hormones can cause widespread dysfunction.

A complete discussion of the extremely complex endocrine system is, of course, beyond the scope of this book. However, brief overviews of the primary activities of all of the endocrine glands are provided in this chapter. The endocrine glands exert their influence through the secretion of hormones. Hormones are a wide range of chemical substances that affect other tissues, either locally or at a distance. Some, such as adrenocorticotropin (a pituitary hormone that activates the adrenal gland), affect only specific tissues, while others, such as thyroid hormone, impact all the cells and tissues of the body.

The pituitary gland (located in the middle of the brain) is considered the master endocrine gland of the body because it generally controls the activity of most of the other endocrine glands. The front part of the pituitary secretes growth hormone, which controls the growth rate of almost all cells and tissues, plus hormones that impact the activity of the adrenal cortex, thyroid, breasts, and ovaries. The back part of the pituitary regulates blood pressure and the retention of water by the kidneys.

The adrenal cortex (located on top of the kidneys) controls the metabolism of proteins, carbohydrates, and fats, and blood pressure. The thyroid gland (located just below the larynx) regulates the rate of chemical reactions in almost all cells, thus controlling our rate of metabolism. The thyroid gland also works with the parathyroid gland (located in the thyroid) to regulate calcium absorption. Through insulin and glucagon, the islets of Langerhans in the pancreas regulate the level of sugar in our blood. The ovaries and testes regulate our fertility and our sexual characteristics.

Many health problems and diseases are due to inadequate or excessive secretion of one or more hormones. However, only a handful (hypothyroidism and low sex hormones) occur commonly and all are amenable to improvement through nutrition, herbs, and lifestyle modification. Since our hormones affect so many aspects of our health, reestablishing normal function has remarkable health-promoting results.

Real-Life Messages About Hormone Imbalance

The Frustration of Infertility

As one of the few licensed male midwives in the country, I have many wonderful memories of helping to bring new lives into the world. There is little to compare with sharing the joy of a family as a new baby is the welcomed into their home. I readily understand the frustration of couples unable to conceive. Surprisingly, I've helped a remarkable number of couples become pregnant through simple nutritional and herbal remedies.

Marilyn's case was typical. She and her husband, John, had been trying for four years to conceive. After numerous unsuccessful visits to fertility specialists, they were considering one of the experimental fertility drugs. Then they decided to consult with me.

A bit of questioning revealed that although Marilyn was healthy, she had experienced menstrual irregularities ever since she had stopped taking birth control pills. I've seen many women who've experienced the same menstrual problems after stopping the pill. Rather than focusing on her infertility, I decided to start by trying to reestablish a healthy cycle. Birth control pills work by turning off the pituitary gland's secretion of hormones that stimulate the ovaries to work. Although I can't quote any hard research, I've observed that some women's pituitaries seem to have trouble resuming normal function after they've been suppressed by birth control pills for several years.

I recommended a combination of herbs: squaw vine (*Mitchella repens*), heloniasis (*Chamaelirium luteum*), and black haw (*Viburnum opulus*), which have historically been used to help women reestablish their hormonal balance, apparently by stimulating the pituitary. I also worked with Marilyn to optimize her nutrition. By her third menstrual cycle, she was regular, by her fourth, she was pregnant.

■ *The message:* You can't mess with mother nature with impunity.

Weight Problems

Claudia was fat. She had had problems with her weight all her life. She had lost over 300 pounds and gained 400. Her family doctor could find no metabolic reasons for her weight problems; all her blood tests were normal.

While many diet plans and schemes are widely touted for their weight loss prowess (it's a $6 billion a year market), most fail. My own experience has shown that the only successful weight loss program is one that incorporates all four of the following: (1) an unprocessed, whole-foods diet, (2) regular significant exercise, (3) support for the thyroid, and (4) psychological counseling.

I had Claudia do a self-test for thyroid function by measuring her basal body temperature when she awoke in the morning (this test is discussed below). As I'd expected, hers was only 96.0, which is quite low. I then started her on a program of unprocessed whole foods, one hour of brisk walking three times a week, and nutritional support to stimulate her thyroid. The program worked, and she lost 1 to 2 pounds a week for the next six months.

■ *The message:* Functional tests are often more useful than blood tests because they measure how the body is really responding.

Unfortunately, Claudia had another message for me. After losing forty pounds, she was feeling and looking good. Then disaster struck. While at a bar with some friends, a man made a pass at her. Claudia gained twenty pounds in the next two weeks. This is when I learned that weight problems aren't always only metabolic in nature and that I really should practice what I preach, i.e., treat the whole person.

I immediately referred her to a counselor with whom I regularly worked. As is all too common, a childhood history of abuse had been sabotaging her efforts to establish an intimate adult relationship. Once she worked through this, she was able to maintain a healthful weight (not as Ms. Twiggy either).

(Please do not take this as an assertion that all overweight men and women are obese because they are afraid of intimate relationships. While that is certainly true for some, for most, uncontrolled weight gain is a normal physiological response to excessive calories and inadequate physical activity, magnified by hormonal imbalances.)

- *The message:* We sometimes have an emotional reason for being sick. Optimal wellness requires that all aspects of our being—physical, mental, emotional, and spiritual—be in healthful harmony.

Systemic Lupus Erythematosis

One of the first graduates of Bastyr University, Dr. Davis Lamson practices in Kent, Washington. As an associate of the brilliant holistic medical doctor Jonathan Wright, Lamson has worked with many patients suffering from complex and difficult diseases. He recently related to me a particularly gratifying case history of Chloe, a woman with severe systemic lupus erythematosis (SLE). While drug therapy had provided some relief early in her disease process, the SLE continued to relentlessly progress to such a degree that she was desperate for another solution. The drugs were not helping much anymore, and she was experiencing significant side effects.

Lamson provided the usual nutritional advice for improving Chloe's health and supplied a relatively large daily dose (100 mg per day—*not recommended without the direct supervision of a physician*) of steroid hormone precursor dehydroepiandrosterone (DHEA). The results were remarkable: her severe facial rash and debilitating arthritis totally resolved. Her blood work even improved. As of the publication of this book, she has been asymptomatic for one year.

- *The message:* Even severe "incurable" diseases can be alleviated by reestablishing normal hormone balance.

The Thyroid Gland

The thyroid gland provides the primary control of the rate of our metabolic activity. A person with no thyroid hormone production will experience a 40% fall in metabolic activity, while excessive secretion of thyroid hormones can increase metabolic activity up to 100% above normal. Apparently this control of metabolic rate is exerted through the impact of thyroid hormones on the mitochondria, the energy generating organelles within our cells. In general, the higher the amount of thyroid hormone, the greater the number, size, and ATP (energy) production of mitochondria. Thyroid hormones also have a great impact on how quickly molecules are transported across the cell membranes. The amount of thyroid hormone secretion is largely determined by the pituitary gland, which secretes a hormone called thyroid stimulating hormone (TSH). The hormones secreted by the thyroid are primarily thyroxin (T_4) plus a smaller amount of triiodothyronine (T_3).

In addition to controlling our metabolic rate, the thyroid has a direct impact on the rate at which we grow and metabolize carbohydrates and fats. It also affects our cholesterol levels, the rate at which we convert beta-carotene to vitamin A, our heart rate and contraction strength, blood pressure, rate of respiration, appetite, mental acuity, reflexes, and libido.

Thyroid Dysfunction

Thyroid deficiency is surprisingly common, affecting 1 to 10% of adults according to blood tests. However, if one uses a functional test of thyroid function, such as that developed by Dr. Broda Barnes (a medical doctor who specialized in evaluating hormonal status through functional testing rather than blood levels), the incidence is estimated to be an incredible 25%. Since the thyroid regulates the metabolic activity of virtually every cell, a deficiency affects virtually every bodily function.

The common symptoms of low thyroid function include lethargy, fatigue, weight gain, depression, low body temperature, dry skin, headaches, menstrual problems, recurrent infections, constipation, and sensitivity to cold.

There are several reasons functional tests show a far greater incidence of low thyroid than blood tests. The most important is that blood tests measure thyroxine (T_4), which accounts for 90% of the hormone secretion by the thyroid. However, the form that affects the cells the most is T_3 (triiodothyronine), which our cells make from T_4. Thus, a person can have normal levels of thyroid hormone in the blood, yet be thyroid deficient if the cells aren't able to convert it to the more active T_3. Blood tests for T_3 were popular for awhile, but research found that they missed low thyroid function in 50% of patients.

A better way of assessing thyroid function is to measure its effects on the body. This is done by measuring a person's resting metabolic rate, which is controlled by the thyroid gland. Dr. Barnes found that measuring basal body temperature was a good way of assessing basal metabolic rate and thus the body's response to thyroid hormones, regardless of their blood level. This finding is important because some people have plenty of thyroid hormone in their blood, but for various reasons their cells don't respond to it adequately. (However, Barne's approach can also be in error because a low basal metabolic rate can indicate nutritional deficiencies, inadequate physical activity, and so on, just as fever from an infection or other disease can result in an inaccurately high body temperature.)

Even just using blood tests, thyroid function is commonly low in older adults. One study evaluated 370 elderly subjects, 60 to 97 years of age. About 18.1% of the patients already had an established history of past or current thyroid disease. Another 5.4% had a history of thyroid surgery. Of the remaining 283 patients with no history of thyroid disease, 14.6% of the women and 15.4% of the men had subclinical hypothyroidism, according to blood tests. In other words, 40% of these elderly had current or past problems with their thyroid [1]

Table 8-1 Low Thyroid Function[3]

System	Signs and Symptoms
Brain	Depression, mental fatigue, irritability, anxiety, poor memory and concentration, difficulty sleeping, headaches
Nerves	Dizziness, hearing loss, Meniere's disease, poor vision, night blindness, slow speech
Gastrointestinal	Constipation, gas and/or bloating, poor appetite, poor digestion
Female	PMS, menstrual cramps, irregular menses, multiple miscarriages, infertility, fibrocystic breast pain
Male	Erectile dysfunction, decreased numbers and mobility of sperm
Male and female	Diminished libido, reduced sexual sensations
Metabolism	Fatigue, exhaustion, poor stamina, weight gain, hypoglycemia, high blood cholesterol levels, water retention, decreased tolerance to cold, cold hands and feet
Cardiovascular	Slow heartbeat, congestive heart failure later in life, abnormal heart rhythm, palpitations, increased atherosclerosis
Immune	Increased susceptibility to infections, prolonged length of infection, decreased white cell count
Musculoskeletal	Muscular weakness, cramps and pains, stiff or painful joints, loose ligaments, low back pain, carpal tunnel syndrome
Skin, hair, and nails	Coarse or dry skin or hair, easy bruising, hair loss, pale skin or lips, cool skin, adult acne, slow wound healing, nail ridges, decreased sweating

Several diseases have been shown to be associated with low thyroid function, even some that seem to have no apparent relationship. For example, one study compared the thyroid function of 56 patients suffering from dermatitis herpetiformis (a skin disease with very itchy little blisters on the scalp, base of the spine, elbows, and knees) with 26 control subjects. The patients with dermatitis herpetiformis had significantly increased abnormalities of thyroid function tests (32% versus 4%), with hypothyroidism being the most common abnormality and affecting 12 of the 56 patients.[2]

How to Determine If Your Thyroid Is Underactive

There are two ways you can recognize a low level of thyroid activity: symptoms and basal body temperature.

Symptoms of an underactive thyroid

Table 8-1 lists the typical signs and symptoms of low thyroid activity. As can be seen, low thyroid activity results in a surprisingly wide range of health problems.

Table 8-2 Interpretation of Basal Body Temperature

Temperature	Interpretation	Common Signs and Symptoms
97.6° to 98.2°	Normal	
<97.2°	Possible low thyroid	Depression, difficulty losing weight, dry skin, headaches, lethargy or fatigue, menstrual problems, recurrent infections, sensitivity to cold (also see Table 8-1 above)
>98.6°	Possible high thyroid	Fast pulse, hyperactivity, inability to gain weight, insomnia, irritability, menstrual problems, nervousness, bulging eyeballs (if severe)

Obviously, no one would have all these signs and symptoms, but more than one or two symptoms in most of the categories is highly suggestive of poor thyroid activity.

Measuring your basal temperature
A more objective way of determining thyroid activity is by measuring your basal body temperature. All that is needed is a basal thermometer, which is easily available from a drug store. The procedure is as follows:

1. Shake down the thermometer to below 95°F and place it by your bed before going to sleep at night.
2. On waking, place the thermometer in your armpit for a full ten minutes. It is important to make as little movement as possible. Lying and resting with your eyes closed is best. Do not get up until the ten-minute test is completed.
3. After ten minutes, read and record the temperature and date.
4. Record the temperature for at least three mornings (preferably at the same time of day). Menstruating women must perform the test on the second, third, and fourth days of menstruation. Men and postmenopausal women can perform the test at any time of the month.

Interpretations of the results are listed in Table 8-2.

Ways to Increase Thyroid Function

Iodine
As noted above, low thyroid activity is a common problem and much can be done to help reestablish adequate thyroid function. The first step in improving thyroid function is to ensure that the body is producing enough thyroid hormone. This requires an adequate intake of iodine because this mineral is used to form the thyroid hormones. Deficiencies of iodine intake are rare since the

Goiter

George came to my office complaining of chronic tiredness. He couldn't understand it since he ate a very good vegetarian diet, exercised regularly, and had a low stress job and good family environment. Further questions revealed no clues to his problem. However, during the physical examination, I noticed a slight swelling of his thyroid, a condition called goiter. While very common in the last century, iodination of table salt has resulted in dramatic lowering of the incidence of this condition. At this point, I asked more detailed questions about George's diet and discovered that he was eating over a pound of raw cabbage, cauliflower, and broccoli a day! Upon becoming a vegetarian three years earlier, he had discovered a real taste for these foods and now couldn't eat a meal without them.

While these are certainly very healthful foods, especially considering their support for liver detoxification, they also contain substances called goitrogens. Goitrogens bind iodine so that it can't be used by the thyroid, which results in low thyroid hormone levels. The thyroid becomes enlarged because the pituitary oversecretes hormones trying to stimulate the thyroid to produce more hormones.

George's therapy was simple: less cabbage, more foods rich in iodine (kelp, sea vegetables, and seafood), and supplementation with iodine (150 µg per day). It took several weeks, but finally George noticed a gradual improvement in his energy.

- *The message:* Too much of anything, no matter how healthful, can cause an imbalance.

addition of iodine to table salt. However, some foods, called goitrogens, can induce an iodine deficiency by combining with the iodine and making it unavailable to the thyroid. These foods include foods of the brassica family (turnips, cabbage, rutabagas, mustard greens, radishes, horseradishes), cassava root, soybeans, peanuts, pine nuts, and millet.[4] This is not to suggest that these foods not be eaten, but rather that they not be eaten in excess. In general, cooking inactivates these goitrogens. Good sources of iodine include saltwater fish, sea vegetables (kelp, dulse, arame, hijiki, nori, wakame, kombu) and iodized salt.

Other nutrients

Even though iodine levels may be adequate, iodine still needs to be attached to the amino acid tyrosine. Several nutrients are needed to accomplish this, including zinc, copper, and vitamins A, B_2, B_3, B_6, and C. Good sources of zinc include seafood (especially oysters), beef, oatmeal, chicken, liver, spinach, nuts, and seeds. Copper is found in liver and other organ meats, eggs, yeast, beans, nuts, and seeds. The best sources of the B vitamins are yeast, whole grains, and liver.

Another way to increase thyroid hormone secretion is to take desiccated thyroid from which the thyroid hormones have been removed. The idea here is that this supplies all the known, and unknown, nutrients needed to ensure proper functioning of the thyroid. These products are pretty safe to use and are available in health food stores.

The next step is to ensure that the cells are responding appropriately to the thyroid hormones. This requires providing the nutrients needed for cellular conversion of thyroid hormones to the more active form. The trace minerals zinc, copper, and selenium are the required co-factors for iodothyronine iodinase, the enzyme that converts T_4 to the far more active T_3. There are several different forms of this enzyme, each requiring a different trace mineral. Supplementation with zinc (the second most common mineral deficiency) has been shown to reestablish normal thyroid function in hypothyroid patients who were zinc deficient, even though they had normal serum T_4 levels.[5]

Similarly, selenium supplementation may be important because those living in areas of the world where selenium is deficient have a greater incidence of thyroid disease.[6] While a selenium deficiency does not decrease the conversion of T_4 to T_3 in the thyroid or the pituitary, it does result in a great decrease in this conversion in the other cells of the body.[7] People with a deficiency of selenium often have elevated levels of T_4 and TSH (the hormone secreted by the pituitary to stimulate the thyroid to secrete more T_4). That is, selenium deficiency results in low thyroid activity in the cells even though hormone levels are normal or even elevated. The body does not try to correct this problem because the thyroid and pituitary are not affected by a selenium deficiency as much as other cells, so the regulatory feedback system fails. This is another reason why blood measurement of thyroid hormone levels is not a very reliable measure of *functional* thyroid activity. Supplementation with selenium has been found to result in a decrease in T_4 and TSH and normalization of thyroid activity.[8]

As discussed in Chapter Seven, selenium is deficient in about 50% of people's diets, which may account for the large number of people with low thyroid activity. (Yet another reason to eat organically grown foods; they contain almost four times as much selenium as commercially grown foods.)

The impact of selenium deficiency on thyroid dysfunction was a major insight for me. Prior to this discovery, the frequent occurrence of low thyroid function had been puzzling to me because I couldn't understand why the pituitary gland wasn't secreting more TSH to correct the problem. Now I understand how, once again, a common nutritional deficiency derails the body's normal self-regulatory function.

Even if enough thyroid hormone is produced and converted to the more active form in the cell, the thyroid-hormone dependent enzymes also need to be functioning properly. For example, when 10 iron-deficient women were compared to 12 controls, they were found to have lower rectal temperatures, lower rates of oxygen consumption, and lower plasma thyroid hormone levels. Iron supplementation (78 mg for 12 weeks) resulted in reversal of the anemia and improvement of their rectal temperatures, suggesting improved response to thyroid hormones. The women even experienced a partial normalization of their thyroid hormone levels.[9]

- *Dosage:* Copper: 5 mg per day; iron: 10 mg per day; selenium: 150 µg per day; zinc: 25 mg per day

Exercise

Interestingly, exercise not only increases thyroid secretion of hormones, it also increases cellular response to the hormones. It even helps prevent the drop in thyroid hormone production that normally occurs during weight loss.[10] The exercise need not be intense, but it does need to be regular and substantial. Walking several miles, bicycling for an hour, or jogging four miles three or more times a week will do the job.

Thyroid medications

If following the above recommendations is not adequate to relieve your symptoms and restore normal metabolic rate as measured by basal body temperature, see a nutritionally oriented doctor for possible thyroid medications. While I prefer to not use drugs, establishing normal thyroid function is so important for total wellness, and thyroid medications are so safe, that I would not hesitate to take prescription thyroid. But remember, taking prescription thyroid is not nearly as effective when you are deficient in the zinc and selenium required for its utilization by the cells.

The Great Precursor: Dehydroepiandrosterone

Dehydroepiandrosterone (DHEA) is the most abundant steroid hormone circulating through our bodies. Most of it is made by the adrenal glands, although some is synthesized in the brain and skin. As shown in Figure 8-1, DHEA is used to make several hormones, especially the sex hormones, estrogen and testosterone. Some DHEA researchers have suggested it be referred to as a "buffer hormone," since it is only used by the body when needed. Its effects vary according to a person's hormonal milieu, having either an estrogen-like or androgen-like effect, depending on the need.

As important as DHEA is to maintaining normal sex hormone levels, many of its beneficial results appear due to its inhibition of the damaging

Chronic Stress and Low DHEA

Sean took good care of himself: He ate well (he had been a health-conscious vegetarian for 25 years), exercised regularly, drank alcohol rarely, and had never smoked. However, at 45, he was chronically tired, losing muscle mass, slowly gaining fat weight, losing his sex drive, and having problems with allergies, both to foods and the environment. Every spring he suffered from hay fever severe enough to require antihistamines, and every fall he developed a severe respiratory infection, which often progressed to pneumonia.

Further questioning and a physical examination revealed little wrong with him, except a very high level of job stress, which had plagued him for almost 20 years. Realizing that long-term stress can result in the adrenal glands producing stress hormones such as cortisol instead of DHEA (which is the precursor for testosterone and other important functions), I decided to check his 24-hour urinary excretion of dehydroepiandrosterone (DHEA). Sean's was only 3 mg, far below the normal range of 5 to 20 mg per day.

I helped him develop better ways of reducing his stress and prescribed 5 mg of DHEA twice a day. The results were remarkable: His environmental allergies cleared (although he continued to have to avoid his food allergens), he lost 10 pounds of fat, his immune system improved so much he didn't have even one cold for over a year, his muscle mass increased, and he experienced a modest increase in libido.

- *The message:* Chronic stress devastates the normal metabolic processes of the body.

effects of stress, especially on the immune system. This is probably why it appears to play an important role in fighting AIDS and cancer. DHEA also plays other important roles. It increases cellular sensitivity to insulin, increases fat metabolism, increases the synthesis of antioxidant enzymes in the liver, and helps scavenge free radicals. Low DHEA levels are found in many people with chronic diseases.

Research has shown that DHEA protects against viral infection in animal models and is an inhibitor of the human immunodeficiency virus 1 *in vitro.* One very interesting study compared 41 HIV-negative controls with 41 asymptomatic HIV-positive patients who did not progress to AIDS during the study and 41 initially asymptomatic HIV-positive subjects who did progress to AIDS within five years after entering the study. From the start, DHEA levels were highest in the HIV-negative group and lowest in those who eventually progressed to AIDS. This longitudinal study clearly demonstrated a relationship

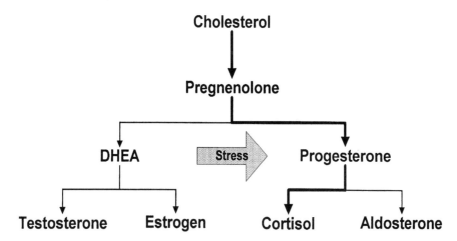

Figure 8-1 DHEA, The Hormone Precursor

between low serum DHEA levels in HIV-infected men and more rapid progression to AIDS. The reason for the decline in DHEA levels before AIDS development is unknown but it could be a combination of impaired adrenal function, mild inhibition of the HIV virus, and enhancement of interleukin-II synthesis, which is deficient in advanced HIV infection. Two small studies on DHEA administration in HIV-infected subjects have demonstrated possible effects on immune function without clear anti-HIV effects.[11]

DHEA may be especially important in helping to prevent cancers, especially those induced by chemical carcinogens. This protection has been shown in both animal research and human epidemiological studies. One study prospectively compared DHEA levels in 35 individuals who subsequently developed bladder cancer (the type of cancer most commonly due to chemical carcinogens) with 69 matched controls. Pre-diagnosis levels of DHEA were significantly lower in the bladder cancer cases than in the controls. As the bladder cancers developed there was a subsequent decrease in DHEA levels.[12]

The average male produces 31 mg of DHEA per day, while the average female produces 19 mg per day. However, the highest levels of DHEA are found in women during pregnancy.[13] DHEA is primarily detoxified by the liver.

Although only recently coming to the attention of the public, this important hormone has been the subject of over 5,500 research studies since 1966.

Why DHEA Levels Become Inadequate

DHEA levels become low for several reasons, the most important being stress, aging, and smoking. When we are under stress, the body shifts adrenal metabolism

Table 8-3 Common Stressors

Type	Examples
Physical	Broken bones, burns, cold exposure, intense exercise, surgery, pain, lack of sleep
Metabolic	Hypoglycemia, infection, toxins, chronic inflammation
Psychological	Anxiety, anticipation of stressful situations (e.g., college exams, surgery), death of spouse, divorce, jail term, new marriage, change in work, new mortgage or large loan

away from the production of DHEA, producing instead more stress steroids (i.e., cortisol). Acute anxiety and hypoglycemia appear to be the strongest stimulants of adrenal production of cortisol. Table 8-3 lists common stressors. As might be expected, people with Type A (high stress) personalities have lower levels of DHEA.

While our metabolic response to acute stress is an important part of maintaining health in the face of life's challenges, chronic stress results in metabolic imbalances that progressively rob us of our vitality. As can be seen in Table 8-4, during the early stages of chronic stress, the adrenal glands respond by synthesizing excessive levels of cortisol at the expense of DHEA. This causes problems with blood sugar utilization, the replacement of muscle with fat, water retention, and inhibition of several aspects of the immune system. In the late stages of stress, the adrenal glands become exhausted and not only are DHEA levels low, but so are cortisol levels. This end stage of adrenal exhaustion manifests as decreased energy production with the concomitant symptoms one would expect, i.e., chronic fatigue, muscle weakness, and depression.

We synthesize less DHEA as we age, about 20% less every decade. This means that those in their 80s produce only 10 to 20% as much as they did in their 20s! The decline in DHEA is even greater in those suffering from Alzheimer's disease. These patients have typically half the levels found in healthy age-matched controls. Whether this is a result or cause of the disease is unknown at this time.

Finally, smoking depresses DHEA. Nicotine and conitine (a breakdown product of nicotine) inhibit 11-beta-hydroxylase, an enzyme required for the manufacture of DHEA.[14]

How to Determine If Your DHEA Levels Are Low

Table 8-5 lists the common signs and symptoms of low levels of DHEA as well as the diseases that are associated with low DHEA levels. As can be seen, many chronic diseases, especially autoimmune diseases, dominate the list. It is not clear whether the low DHEA levels found in these chronic diseases are

Table 8-4 The Health-Damaging Effects of Chronic Stress

Stage	Hormone Levels	Metabolic Effects	Signs and Symptoms
Early (adrenal adaptation)	High cortisol Low DHEA	Decreased insulin sensitivity Decreased glucose utilization Increased blood sugar Increased calcium loss Increased fat accumulation at waist Increased protein breakdown Increased water retention Decreased secretory IgA Decreased natural killer cell activity Decreased interleukin Decreased T lymphocytes	Increased incidence of infections Chronic viral infections (e.g., CMV, herpes) Yeast overgrowth Allergies Insomnia Reduced vitality Reduced sex drive Inexplicable hunger Premenstrual tension
Late (adrenal exhaustion)	Low cortisol Low DHEA	Low blood sugar Decreased energy production Depressed immune function	Alcohol intolerance Allergies Chronic fatigue Chronic inflammation Degenerative diseases Depression Headaches Hypoglycemic Inexplicable hunger Irritability Loss of ability to concentrate Muscle weakness Poor memory Premenstrual tension Reduced sex drive

caused by or are the result of low DHEA levels. However, supplementation with DHEA results in substantial improvement, especially in the autoimmune diseases, which do not respond very well to other therapies.

While symptoms and diseases can provide an indication of low DHEA, according to Dr. Davis Lamson, diagnosing by symptoms alone frequently gives the wrong answer and thus objective tests must be performed. Objective determination of DHEA levels can be done either by measuring 24-hour urinary excretion or by measuring salivary DHEA. Salivary DHEA measurement has the advantage of being collected several times a day, which allows a better understanding of how adrenal function varies during the day, especially when cortisol levels are measured at the same time.

Table 8-5 Low Levels of DHEA

Signs and Symptoms	Dry skin, low sex drive, increased fat weight, high blood pressure, muscle wasting
Conditions and Diseases	AIDS, allergies, asthma, autoimmune diseases (e.g., systemic lupus erythematosis, rheumatoid arthritis, ulcerative colitis, Crohn's disease, multiple sclerosis), burns, chronic fatigue syndrome, impaired immunity, most chronic illnesses, high levels of stress, osteoporosis

How to Increase DHEA Levels

The first step, of course, is to eliminate the causes of low DHEA. While little can be done about aging, smoking can be stopped, stress controlled, a regular exercise program adopted, nutrition optimized, and herbs supplemented. Decreasing your stress reaction does not mean avoiding all stressors—you can't (even in a monastery you can *feel* stressed out). You can, however, change the way you respond to stress. Interestingly, people's self-assessment of their level of psychological stress and objective measures of physical fitness correlate well with serum DHEA levels, i.e., the lower the perceived level of stress and higher the level of fitness, the higher the serum DHEA.[15]

Lifestyle changes

Exercise is great for relieving stress. During exercise, the levels of stress hormones decrease, emotions such as anxiety are alleviated, and the adrenal overresponse to stress found in men with Type A personalities normalizes.[16,17] In addition to decreasing stress hormone levels, exercise also slightly increases serum DHEA levels.

The health-promoting effects of transcendental meditation (TM) have received a considerable amount of research attention. Many of TM's benefits appear to be due directly to its calming effects. One study compared DHEA levels in the blood of 423 people who practiced TM with 1,253 healthy people who did not. They found that the TM practitioners had DHEA levels comparable to those five to ten years younger.[18] Other methods of stress reduction also work. For example, one study compared 20 army officers participating in a stress reduction program with 17 other officers. While the untreated group showed a marked reduction in DHEA-S levels during the study, the stress reduction group experienced a small increase.[19]

Nutritional moderation of the stress response

Nutrition appears to be very important in helping to prevent an overreaction to stressful events. For example, vitamin C has been recommended for decades by nutritional doctors for those under stress. Apparently, it helps by reducing the adrenal gland's secretion of cortisol in response to stress.[20] Low magnesium levels substantially increase the adrenal output of cortisol in response to stress. This further aggravates the problem because the stress hormones increase urinary excretion of magnesium, and the fatty acids released by stress bind to magnesium, making it less available. These combinations of effects partly explain the additional risk of heart attack seen in magnesium-deficient patients when exposed to stress.[21]

Herbal support

While I was unable to find any research that evaluated the impact of the ginsengs on DHEA levels, a large amount of research does document their positive effects on our ability to handle stress. *Panax ginseng* (Korean ginseng) appears to help by relieving anxiety and improving the body's response to stress by strengthening the adrenal glands.[22] However, *Panax ginseng* may not be useful when a person is overproducing cortisol, since it increases pituitary stimulation of the adrenals to produce even more. While this mechanism is beneficial for short episodes of severe stress (such as found in the common experiment of mice swimming in ice-cold water), under conditions of chronic stress, it may be counterproductive.

Eleutherococcus senticosus (Siberian ginseng) may be a better choice because it moderates the stress response. Specifically, eleuthero has been shown to reduce activation of the adrenal cortex in response to stress (alarm-phase reaction) and prevent stress-induced damage to the thymus and lymph glands.[23] Eleuthero supplementation results in an increased sense of well-being, ability to withstand stress, more mental alertness and work output, and improved athletic performance. It is a very safe herb with virtually no known toxicity.

- *Dosage:* 2 to 16 ml fluid extract or 100 to 200 mg standardized extract of *Eleutherococcus senticosus* one to three times daily

Supplemental DHEA

If the above lifestyle, nutritional, and herbal therapies aren't adequate, synthetic DHEA can be taken. As shown in Table 8-6, supplementation with DHEA has been shown to have a wide range of beneficial results, all of which are due to three actions: its improvement in the production of sex hormones, its improvement of liver detoxification, and its modulation of the damaging effects of stress, especially those mediated by the glucocorticoids. This latter effect explains most of its benefits for the immune system which, as discussed in Chapter Four, can be so devastated by stress.

One of the most immediate and consistent effects of DHEA supplementation is an increased sense of physical and psychological well-being.[25] While the mechanism is unknown, it may be due to DHEA's stimulation of increased REM sleep, the portion of sleep that is so important for memory storage and regeneration.[26]

Table 8-6 The Beneficial Effects of DHEA Supplementation[24]

System	Effects
Immune	Enhances resistance to viral and bacterial infections, increases T and B cell activity, increases rate of recovery from infection, inhibits HIV damage to the immune system, may have some direct anti-viral activity
Stress	Protects the thymus from stress-induced damage, reverses stress-induced inhibition of interleukin production, improves resistance to cold-induced stress
Aging	Reverses skin degeneration, improves memory, improves libido in men
Cancer	Inhibits activation of some carcinogens
Metabolism	Increases lean muscle mass, decreases fat, increases liver phase I detoxification, increases scavenging of free radicals in liver, reverses some aspects of low thyroid function
Specific diseases that have responded to treatment with DHEA	AIDS, congestive heart failure, diabetes, lupus erythematosis, multiple sclerosis, Parkinson's disease, obesity

As noted above, DHEA supplementation appears to be especially beneficial for those suffering from autoimmune diseases. This is well-demonstrated by a study of ten patients with mild-to-moderate systemic lupus erythematosis and various other diseases. After three to six months of supplementation with 200 mg of DHEA per day, all disease measures for systemic lupus erythematosis activity improved and corticosteroid drug requirements were decreased. Of three patients with significant proteinuria (a sign of advanced kidney damage from the disease), two showed a marked and one a modest reduction in protein excretion.[27]

A dose of 50 mg of synthetic DHEA per day will restore blood levels to those seen in 20 year olds. While DHEA is now available in health food stores, I strongly recommend it only be taken under the guidance of a physician, as the side effects can be subtle, but very significant.

- *Dosage:* 5 to 25 mg DHEA twice a day

Possible side effects of DHEA supplementation
At normal dosages (5 to 50 mg per day), DHEA appears quite safe. However, larger dosages (150 to 300 mg per day) can produce reversible hirsutism (abnormal hair growth) in women (probably from overproduction of testosterone), acneiform dermatitis, increased abdominal obesity in women, liver damage, bloating, and carpal tunnel syndrome.[24] Very large dosages produce liver cancer in rats. Since DHEA is an androgen precursor, there is concern

over possible increased risk for prostate cancer. However, in animal research DHEA actually inhibits prostate cancer induction, and no increase in prostate cancer has been seen in men using high dosages.[28]

The Male Hormones

The testes produce several male sex hormones, which are collectively called androgens. These include testosterone, dihydrotestosterone, and androstenedione. The testes produce a large amount of testosterone that is converted in the target tissue to the more physiologically active dihydrotestosterone. The adrenal glands also produce a small amount of androgens. Not only is testosterone responsible for the distinguishing characteristics of the masculine body, it also plays several other important roles in both men and women. For example, it is important for libido, muscle growth, and calcium deposition in the bones.

As one would expect, low testosterone levels in men results in lowered libido, loss of muscle mass, decreased size of sexual organs (if the deficiency is severe), difficulty establishing an erection, and infertility. However, low testosterone also results in other less obvious problems: atherosclerosis and hip fractures. Testosterone levels start to decrease slowly at age 30, and then drop rapidly beginning at age 60, declining to levels comparable to those found in prepubescent boys by the age of 80.

Some recent research shows that testosterone may protect men from the atherosclerosis that leads to a heart attack, exactly the opposite of what many have believed for years. Men who suffer a heart attack tend to have abnormally low levels of testosterone. In one study, men who had a low concentration of testosterone in their blood were significantly more likely to have serious coronary artery disease than those with higher levels in the blood. The researchers postulate testosterone possibly helps to prevent heart disease in men in a manner similar to the way estrogen helps prevent heart disease in females.[29]

Another interesting study, this one conducted in an in-patient orthopedic service, compared serum testosterone levels in 17 men who had a hip fracture after simple falls over a 10-month period, 11 men with a history of hip fracture in the preceding 25 months, and 25 matched controls at a mean age of 73 years. Serum testosterone was significantly lower in the hip-fracture groups than the control group, with frank testosterone deficiency found in 71% of the men with hip fractures versus 32% of the controls.[30]

Why Male Hormone Dysfunction Occurs

The testes' metabolic processes are sensitive to stress, smoking, environmental toxins, estrogens, and nutritional deficiencies. The increase of these factors has resulted in a growing incidence of male infertility (male sperm counts are half what they were at the turn of the century), a doubling of testicular cancer in this century, and a decrease in male sexual function.

Lifestyle

It is hard to find a system of the body not adversely affected by stress, including the testes. In a study of 439 men, all 51 years old, chronic psychosocial stress was shown to be associated with elevated insulin levels, low testosterone levels, and compensatory high luteinizing hormone (the enzyme secreted by the pituitary gland to stimulate the testes to secrete testosterone) levels. These findings suggest that chronic stress causes premature aging and decreased male testicular function.[31] These data also suggest an increased risk of diabetes.

While cigarette ads show virile men on horses conquering the world (and women), the reality is the exact opposite: Smoking demasculinizes men! Nicotine and conitine (a breakdown product of nicotine) increase the activity of androgen-degrading enzymes, resulting in decreased levels of testosterone.[32] A similar effect is seen in women; nicotine increases the activity of estrogen-degradation enzymes, resulting in lower serum estrogen levels.[33] In other words, not only does cigarette smoking not make you sexier, it actually makes you less sexually functional! The lowering of serum estrogen levels might also explain why smoking women have more menopausal symptoms and an increased incidence of osteoporosis.

The final lifestyle problem is alcohol. Alcoholic men have smaller testes, decreased libido, loss of sexual potency, signs of feminization (such as enlarged breasts and body hair converting from male to female pattern), loss of body hair, decreased testosterone levels, and elevated estrogen levels. The challenge, of course, is determining what level of alcohol consumption causes problems. When young males (ages 13 to 22) who abused alcohol (for an average of 3.7 years) were tested, their serum testosterone levels were less than half that of matched controls.[34] The researchers also found that the alcohol abusers' blood levels of luteinizing hormone were 20% lower, suggesting that alcohol inhibits the pituitary. At this time, modest consumption of alcohol (two drinks or less per day) does not appear to impact testosterone levels, although alcohol does have a direct toxic effect on the testes.

Estrogens and anti-androgens in the environment

One of the unfortunate side effects of the many man-made chemicals that have entered our environment (over 5,000 by some estimates) is the damage some of them do to male gonadal function. These toxins produce problems in two ways: by blocking androgen receptor sites, so testosterone can't bind to their target cells to activate the appropriate enzyme systems, and by functioning as estrogens and thus counteracting the effects of testosterone.

For several animal species, this pollution has become so severe they are becoming extinct because they are no longer able to reproduce. For example, vinclozolin, a widely used fungicide, blocks the activity of androgen hormones in the body by binding to the androgen receptor sites. This inhibits the development of male characteristics. In male rodents exposed to anti-androgen pollutants before birth, this results in failure of the testes to descend, malformed penises, and even rudimentary vaginas. As might be expected, these rodents are quite infertile when they mature. Another more prevalent example is DDE, the long-lasting breakdown product of the pesticide DDT. Roughly 60 parts per billion (ppb) of DDE effectively blocks the androgen receptor sites. Eggs of alligators from Lake Apopka (a lake so contaminated its alligators are facing extinction) have been found to contain as much as 5,800 ppb.[35] This level results in feminized infertile males.

What relevance does this have to humans? The blood of South Americans whose homes were treated with DDT to control malaria carries as much as 140 ppb of DDE. Tissues from stillborn infants in Atlanta shortly before the banning of DDT in the U.S. contained DDE levels as high as 650 ppb in the brain and 3,570 ppb in the kidneys!

Although the U.S. has banned use of DDT for over 20 years, much of the rest of the world has not. For example, Brazil and our neighbor, Mexico, both use over 1,000 tons of DDT a year—more than we ever used in the United States. Unfortunately, DDT and DDE do not respect national borders; they have spread throughout the world through animal movement and air and water currents.

Phthalates, compounds commonly used to make plastics flexible, are the most common industrial contaminants in the environment. Several of them have been found to be estrogenic. In particular, two of them, butyl benzyl phthalate (BBP) and di-n-butyl phytate (DBP) cause problems for male gonadal function. They also stimulate the growth of breast cells in culture, which may be of special significance in breast cancer. According to British studies, the average diet contains 0.5 mg DBP per kilogram of food wrapped in plastic. Far worse, however, are fatty foods such as butter and margarine, which have been found to have BBP levels as high as 45 mg per kilogram. These foods pick up the BBP from their wrappers.[36] Another very common estrogenic chemical in our environment is BHA, which is added to foods to prevent spoilage.

Other toxins also cause trouble. For example, the dioxin residues that are found in the fat of fish, meat, and dairy products reduce testosterone levels in men who eat these foods. Lead exposure reduces sperm counts and inhibits testosterone synthesis.[37]

Not enough research has been done to determine the exact level of exposure required for the various toxins to exert a clinical impact. However, considering that 15% of couples are infertile and that male infertility is the problem 30 to 50% of the time, the wise man will assiduously avoid these toxins!

Poor nutrition

The trace minerals zinc, copper, and selenium are crucial for male gonadal function. Even a mild zinc deficiency (such as found in 25 to 30% of normal people between the ages of 65 and 85) will result in decreased testosterone production and low sperm counts.[38] A severe zinc deficiency will cause shrinkage of the testes. Even short-term deficiencies have an immediate impact on male gonadal function.

One study compared the effects of varying zinc intake from 1.4 to 10.4 mg per day. The researchers found substantially lower levels of testosterone and semen in the low zinc group, despite the fact that serum zinc levels did not change. It is interesting to note that a significant amount of zinc is lost with ejaculation—semen is very high in zinc. Those with the lowest level of zinc intake lost 9% of their zinc by ejaculation.[39] Fortunately, even modest levels of supplementation help reestablish normal function.

Selenium is especially important for male gonadal function. It is needed for testosterone synthesis and also protects the sperm and testes from free radicals and heavy metals. Selenium is a crucial cofactor for the enzyme glutathione peroxidase, which protects sex cells from free radicals. Selenium may be a metabolic antidote to heavy metals and other toxic elements because it blocks their binding to important enzymes. Selenium deficiency results in reduced testosterone secretion, decreased sperm motility, and increased incidence of abnormal sperm.[40] One study measured selenium status in 41 semen donors, 23 of whom had normal sperm levels and 18 of whom had a low sperm count. Those with low sperm counts had significantly lower selenium levels.[41]

As documented in Chapter Seven, deficiencies of these trace mineral nutrients are very common, especially as we age.

Nutritional deficiencies are not the only problem. Nutritional excesses can also decrease testosterone levels. For example, one study evaluated the impact on testosterone levels of a high-fat meal in eight healthy men between 23 and 35 years of age. Drinking an 800-calorie milkshake containing 54.4 gm of fat dropped their testosterone levels by 30% compared to a shake containing only 1 gm of fat. This research suggests that the high-fat Western diet may result in chronic depletion of male testosterone levels.[42]

How to Determine If Your Male Hormone Levels Are Low

While the only accurate way to determine male hormone function is by measuring testosterone levels in the blood or urine, signs and symptoms can be suggestive. The common signs of testosterone deficiency are listed in Table 8-7.

How to Increase Male Hormone Levels

The first step in increasing male hormone levels is to control those factors that lower testosterone levels or decrease the biological activity of testosterone by blocking its binding to its target cells. This means decreasing stress, quitting smoking, and decreasing exposure to toxins, especially those that are estrogenic. Optimizing nutritional status is extremely important.

- *Dosage:* 25 mg of zinc picolinate and 150 µg of selenium each day

Although *Panax ginseng* has been asserted to be a sexual rejuvenator, few human studies support this belief. There are, however, some promising results

Table 8-7 Signs and Symptoms of Low Levels of Male Hormones[43]

Abdominal obesity	Insomnia
Atherosclerosis	Loss of aggressiveness
Depression	Loss of libido
Fatigue	Loss of male hair pattern
Impotence	Loss of muscle mass
Infertility	Osteoporosis

in animal research. Ginseng has been shown to promote the growth of the testes and increase spermatogenesis in rabbits, increase testicular nucleic acid content in rats, and increase sexual activity and mating behavior in male rats.[44] In other experimental animal studies, ginseng has been shown to increase testosterone levels.[45]

- *Dosage:* 4 to 6 gm of high quality ginseng root per day or 10 mg of ginsenosides three times a day

The Female Hormones

Hormonal function and balance are far more complex in women than men. As in the male, hormone secretion in females is controlled by the pituitary. However, while men maintain a high degree of hormonal consistency throughout their life, women's hormonal levels cycle every month and then change dramatically at about age 50.

The woman's cycle is composed of three phases: the follicular, luteal, and menstrual. During the follicular phase, the pituitary secretes primarily follicle stimulating hormone (FSH), which stimulates the follicles in the ovary to grow in size and number, to secrete estrogen, and, for one of them, to ripen into an ovum. At the end of the follicular phase, a burst of luteinizing hormone (LH) from the pituitary causes the ripe ovum to be released from the cell surrounding it, while the other follicles degenerate, with a resultant decline in estrogen production. This begins the luteal phase. During this phase, the cells that surrounded the ovum mature into the corpus luteum. The corpus luteum, in response to continued LH stimulation, secretes large amounts of progesterone.

If fertilization does not occur, the corpus luteum degenerates after about seven days. During the menstrual phase, the lining of the uterus degenerates and is excreted. The levels of various female hormones during the menstrual cycle are graphed in Figure 8-2. If fertilization does occur, the pituitary secretes another hormone, prolactin, which stimulates the breasts to prepare for lactation (milk production).

The estrogens secreted by the ovaries (β-estradiol, estrone, and estriol) are responsible for the development of the female characteristics: enlarged breasts,

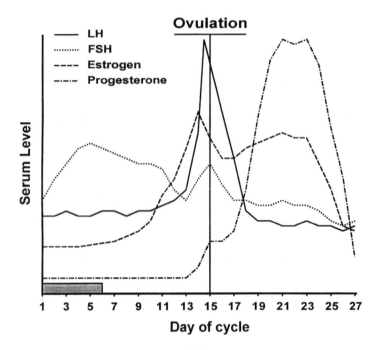

Figure 8-2 *Hormone Levels During the Menstrual Cycle*

widened hips, smooth skin, and mature female hair pattern. In addition, the estrogens play an important role in calcium deposition in the bones, growth during adolescence, muscle buildup, and also a modest amount of sodium and water retention.

The primary function of the progestins (progesterone and 17-α-hydroxy-progesterone), secreted by the corpus luteum of the ovaries, is to prepare the uterus for a fertilized ovum. Progesterone also blocks the action of aldosterone, resulting in a modest loss of sodium and water.

Anything that causes an imbalance in either the total amount or ratio of any of these pituitary or ovarian hormones can cause a wide range of health problems. The most common problems include premenstrual tension, excessive menstrual bleeding, menstrual irregularity, and menopausal problems as the normal cycling stops. In general, most hormonal problems in women are the result of low levels of estrogen or progesterone or high levels of pituitary hormones or toxic estrogen metabolites.

Low Estrogen Levels

Estrogen levels get out of balance for a number of reasons, such as cigarette smoking, nutritional deficiencies, and stress. Low estrogen levels also commonly

Table 8-8 Signs and Symptoms of Low Estrogen Levels

Amenorrhea (missing periods)
Breast atrophy
Loss of sexual desire
Menstrual irregularities (irregular periods, spotting, heavy bleeding)
Osteoporosis
Vaginal dryness

occur due to pituitary suppression after years of using birth control pills. The typical signs and symptoms of low estrogen levels are listed in Table 8-8.

How to Reestablish Estrogen Balance

While the common conventional way to restore normal female hormonal function is to provide synthetic estrogens, this approach has many problems. A substantial amount of research has documented the side effects (such as fluid retention, weight gain, and irritability) and possible increased risk of breast and uterine cancer. Fortunately, nutrition and herbs can be very useful in reestablishing normal estrogen metabolism. Plant source sex hormones are a welcome alternative to animal or synthetic estrogens because they are far safer than the synthetic estrogens or estrogens extracted from the urine of pregnant mares.

Phytoestrogens

Phytoestrogens ("phyto" means plant) are chemicals found in some foods and herbs that bind to cell estrogen receptor sites and activate estrogen-dependent activities. However, although they bind to estrogen receptor sites, they are far less active than true estrogen—about 2% as active. This turns out to have several beneficial effects: when estrogen levels are excessively high, phytoestrogens reduce overall estrogen activity, but when estrogen levels are low, phytoestrogens increase estrogen activity. The end result is normalization, which is especially useful for women at any time of estrogen imbalance, such as PMS or menopause.

Foods high in phytoestrogens include members of the umbelliferous plant family (fennel, celery, and parsley), brassica family (cabbage, broccoli, brussels sprouts), soy beans, nuts, whole grains, apples, and alfalfa. Fennel and anise are particularly high in phytoestrogens and possess confirmed estrogenic action.[46] In addition to estrogenic compounds, soy beans and the brassica family contain the anti-cancer chemicals indole-3-carbinol and sulforaphane.[47]

Soy foods are an especially rich dietary source of phytoestrogens because they contain the isoflavones genistein and daidzein.[48] One cup of cooked soy beans provides approximately 300 mg—the equivalent effect of about 0.45 mg of conjugated estrogens or one tablet of Premarin, the estrogen drug most commonly prescribed by medical doctors.[49] In addition, while estrogen replacement therapy may increase the risk for some cancers, the consumption of soy foods is associated with a significant reduction in cancer risk.

Cultivate friendly bacteria
Simply adding phytoestrogen-rich foods to your diet, however, may not be adequate. Isoflavones must first be converted to biologically active estrogenic compounds by friendly intestinal bacteria. Since the presence of friendly bacteria is, in turn, dependent upon a healthy gastrointestinal climate, all the dietary and lifestyle factors that affect a woman's digestive tract can significantly impact her hormonal health as well. One critical factor is soluble fiber (beans, oat bran, and bananas)—a primary food source for the friendly intestinal bacteria, *Lactobacillus acidophilus* and *Bifidobacterium bifidus* (see Chapter Five). Without a good supply of the food, these friendly bacteria cannot thrive.

Antibiotics frequently contribute to health problems for women. Since antibiotics decimate not only the bacterial infection for which they are prescribed, but a woman's friendly intestinal flora as well, other unfriendly flora can proliferate. As a result, a woman taking tetracycline for acne may find herself dealing with vaginal yeast infections and PMS. An imbalance in bowel flora can lead to an increase in circulating estrogen.

Balancing herbs
Several herbs have been used for centuries for the treatment of women's problems, including: dong quai (*Angelica sinensis*), alfalfa (*Medicago sativum*), red clover (*Trifolium praetens*), licorice root (*Glycyrrhiza glabra*), black cohosh (*Cimicifuga racemosa*), fennel (*Foeniculum vulgare*), and anise (*Pippinella anisum*). Some 250 plant species have been found to contain phytoestrogens.[50] Because of the balancing action of phytoestrogens on estrogen effects, it is common to find the same plant recommended for conditions of estrogen excess (such as premenstrual syndrome) as well as conditions of estrogen deficiency (such as menopause and menstrual abnormalities). Many of these herbs have been termed "uterine tonics." Several of these are discussed below.

Excessive Levels of Estrogen and Estrogen Metabolites

Excessive levels of estrogen and estrogen metabolites can be a serious problem; they lead not only to menstrual difficulties but also substantially increase the risk of endometriosis (an abnormal proliferation of the uterine lining), cervical dysplasia (precancerous cells in the cervix), and breast cancer. Unfortunately, this estrogen excess may occur with few symptoms to give warning, although some women will experience symptoms such as those found when progesterone levels are too low (see the next section). High estrogen levels are due in large part to inappropriate diet and problems with the liver's metabolism of estrogen.

A diet high in protein and fat and low in grains and fiber results in elevated levels of estrogens and toxic estrogen metabolites and an increased risk of breast and other cancers. In contrast, a vegetarian diet, especially one high in soy foods and low in fats, balances estrogen levels and helps to prevent cancer.[51] This occurs because vegetarian diets are high in phytoestrogens, which limit the body's production of estrogen, and fiber, which binds to estrogen metabolites after they are secreted into the bowels.

If a woman's diet contains inadequate fiber to bind to the estrogen metabolites, bacteria in the intestines convert them into carcinogens, which are reabsorbed into the circulation where they increase the risk of cancer. This explains why women in China and Japan, who eat a lowfat high-fiber diet, have much lower rates of breast cancer compared to women in the U.S. and Britain. However, when women of these ethnic backgrounds move to the U.S. and adopt a Western diet, their breast cancer rates elevate to the same high level.

Recent studies add further support for the importance of high-fiber, lowfat diets in women's health. In these studies, diets high in soluble and insoluble fiber and low in fat (less than 25% of daily calories) resulted in a significant increase in levels of hormonally activated phytoestrogens.[52]

In 1990, one of the principal investigators in endocrine research (and a member of one of the first research teams to show a connection between dietary fat, fiber, and breast cancer), Dr. Herman Aldercreutz published a comprehensive review paper summarizing ten years of research findings.[53] He concluded that vegetarian women have been found to have a lower risk of hormone-related diseases, such as breast cancer, for a number of reasons, including their consumption of more plant foods rich in isoflavones and many other phytochemicals, their lower intake of fat (and much lower intake of the saturated fats found in animal foods), and higher intake of fiber and essential fatty acids (abundant in flax seed oil and soy beans).

Another excellent way of protecting from the effects of excessive estrogen is exercise, which has been shown to result in a significant reduction in the risk of breast cancer. One research study compared 545 women who developed breast cancer by the age of 40 to an equal number of healthy controls. The risk of breast cancer in women who exercise at least four hours per week, or 35 minutes per day, was found to be a remarkable 60% less than sedentary women.[54]

Lowering levels of estrogen and progesterone is one of the mechanisms by which exercise is thought to exert its protective effects, so it's not surprising that physical activity has also been linked to a better frame of mind throughout the menstrual cycle. Physically active women are found to experience much less impaired concentration, bad moods, behavioral change, and pain.[55]

Low Levels of Progesterone (Corpus Luteum Insufficiency)

European physicians believe that many menstrual problems are due to inadequate function of the corpus luteum. This occurs when the corpus luteum cells in the ovary do not mature enough during the first half of the cycle, resulting in inadequate secretion of progesterone during the second half of the

Table 8-9 Signs and Symptoms of Low Progesterone Levels [56]

Cycles without ovulation	Ovarian cysts
Dysmenorrhea (painful periods)	Persistent bleeding between periods
Endometriosis	Polymenorrhea (abnormally frequent
Fibrocystic breast disease	periods)
Fluid retention	Premenstrual tension
Hypermenorrhea (heavy periods)	Secondary amenorrhea (loss of periods
Infertility	after having regular periods)

cycle. An excessive ratio of estrogen to progesterone causes many menstrual difficulties. Low progesterone levels are suspected when symptoms such as those listed in Table 8-9 occur. Progesterone levels can also be easily measured by a physician.

Corpus luteum deficiency can occur because the pituitary does not secrete enough luteinizing hormone to stimulate maturation or because of excessive secretion of prolactin from the pituitary. This latter cause appears quite common, occurring in 70% of women with low progesterone levels. As can be seen in Table 8-10, many common causes exist for progesterone deficiency. Another problem is adrenaline, the fight-or-flight hormone released during stress, which blocks the binding of progesterone to receptor sites.

Reestablishing Normal Progesterone Levels

As usual, the first step is to control all the known causes of progesterone deficiency as listed above. The next step is to use the nutrients and herbs that help reestablish the normal function of the ovaries and corpus luteum. The most important nutrients are discussed below; effective herbs are discussed in the next section, under Menopause and Menstrual Disorders.

Zinc

Zinc is an especially important mineral for progesterone production. A deficiency can also result in excessive production of prolactin. Interestingly, zinc also increases the binding of growth hormone to prolactin receptor sites, thus blocking the effects of prolactin.[63]

■ *Dosage:* 20 mg of zinc picolinate a day

Vitamin A

Another important nutrient is vitamin A. Supplementation with as little as 6,000 iu per day substantially increases progesterone levels.[64]

■ *Dosage:* 5,000 iu vitamin A per day

Table 8-10 Causes of Low Progesterone/High Prolactin

Lifestyle	Stress[57]
Toxins and Drugs	Alcohol, antidepressants, toluene[58,59,60]
Nutritional Deficiencies	Vitamin B$_6$, vitamin C, zinc[61]
Nutritional Excesses	Arginine (an amino acid high in meat), saturated fat in diet, sugar[62]

Vitamin C

Vitamin C is required for progesterone secretion. Also, the concentration of vitamin C in the corpus luteum is very high, far in excess of that which is required to facilitate hormone production. This high level may be required by the ovary's high rate of tissue remodeling and collagen synthesis during the follicular-luteal cycle. Vitamin C also is essential for collagen synthesis, which in turn is required for follicular-luteal growth, for repair of the ovulated follicle, and for corpus luteum development.[65]

Licorice root (*Glycyrrhiza glabra*)

Glycyrrhiza glabra (licorice root) has been used for a variety of female disorders for several thousand years in both Western and Eastern cultures. It is particularly useful in treating premenstrual syndrome, which is attributed to an increase in the estrogen to progesterone ratio. Licorice is believed to lower estrogen while simultaneously elevating progesterone levels.[66]

- *Dosage:* ½ tsp fluid extract of licorice root or 1 gram dried root three times a day

How to Treat Common Endocrine Disorders

Menopause

Menopause is a normal part of a woman's maturation. However, many women experience significant discomfort both during and after the transition. In addition, many women develop osteoporosis due to low estrogen levels late in life. The problems are essentially due to excessive secretion of the pituitary hormones and inadequate secretion of hormones by the ovaries. This is further aggravated by lifestyle and nutritional problems. Fortunately, the common discomforts of menopause—hot flashes, night sweats, cold hands and feet, depression, vaginal dryness and irritation, and loss of libido—all respond well to natural medicine.

Lifestyle

Research clearly demonstrates that regular physical exercise lowers the frequency and severity of hot flashes. The frequency of moderate and severe hot

Table 8-11 Health Benefits of Regular Exercise in Menopause

Relief from hot flashes	Improved ability to deal with stress
Decreased bone loss	Improved oxygen and nutrient utilization
Decreased risk of breast cancer	in all tissues
Improved heart function	Increased self esteem, mood, and frame
Improved circulation	of mind
Reduced blood pressure	Increased endurance and energy levels
Decreased blood cholesterol levels	

flashes in postmenopausal women was studied in 79 women who took part in physical exercise on a regular basis compared to a control group of 866 non-exercising women. The researchers found that the women in the group who spent 3.5 hours or more per week exercising had no hot flashes and passed through a natural menopause without needing hormone replacement therapy.[67] As can be seen in Table 8-11, regular exercise not only helps to alleviate hot flashes, but it also has many beneficial effects on mood and the health of bone and the cardiovascular system.

In contrast, cigarette smoking aggravates menopausal symptoms and can result in earlier menopause. Smokers have approximately double the rate of menopause at an earlier age. Those who stopped smoking partially reversed this effect.[68]

Nutritional support

Several nutrients have been shown to be effective in relieving hot flashes and atrophic vaginitis (the loss of vaginal elasticity and mucus secretion associated with menopause). Those with the best clinical results include vitamin E, hesperidin in combination with vitamin C, and gamma-oryzanol.

Vitamin E

In the late 1940s, several clinical studies found vitamin E to be effective in relieving hot flashes and menopausal vaginal complaints when compared to a placebo.[69] In one study, vitamin E supplementation was shown to not only improve the symptoms, but also improve the blood supply to the vaginal wall when taken for at least four weeks.[70] A follow-up study published in 1949 demonstrated that vitamin E (400 iu daily) was effective in about 50% of postmenopausal women with atrophic vaginitis.[71]

Vitamin E oil, creams, ointments, or suppositories can be used topically to provide symptomatic relief of atrophic vaginitis. Vitamin E is usually quite effective in relieving the dryness and irritation of atrophic vaginitis as well as other forms of vaginitis.

- *Dosage:* 600 iu of vitamin E (mixed tocopherols); for atrophic vaginitis, simply break open a vitamin E capsule and apply the oil directly

Hesperidin   Like many other flavonoids, hesperidin is known to improve blood vessel integrity and reestablish normal integrity of the capillary membranes, so that they won't be excessively permeable. In one clinical study, 94 women suffering from hot flashes were given a formula containing 900 mg of hesperidin, 300 mg of hesperidin methyl chalcone (another citrus flavonoid), and 1,200 mg of vitamin C daily.[72] At the end of one month, symptoms of hot flashes were relieved in 53% of the patients and reduced in 34%. Improvements were also noted in nocturnal leg cramps, nose bleeds, and easy bruising.

- *Dosage:* 500 mg of hesperidin a day

Gamma-oryzanol (ferulic acid)   A growth-promoting substance found in grains and isolated from rice bran oil, this nutrient aids in the treatment of hot flashes. Its primary action is to normalize pituitary function and promote endorphin release by the hypothalamus. Gamma-oryzanol was first shown to be effective in menopausal symptoms, including hot flashes, in the early 1960s.[73] Subsequent studies have further documented its effectiveness.

In one of the earlier studies, 8 menopausal women and 13 women who had had their ovaries surgically removed were given 300 mg of gamma-oryzanol daily. At the end of the 38-day trial, over 67% of the women had a 50% or greater reduction in their menopausal symptoms. In a more recent study, the benefits of a 300 mg per day dose of gamma-oryzanol was even more effective; 85% of the women reported improvement in their symptoms.[74]

Gamma-oryzanol is an extremely safe natural substance. No significant side effects have been produced in experimental and clinical studies. In addition to being helpful in improving the symptoms of menopause, gamma-oryzanol has also been shown to be quite effective in lowering blood cholesterol triglyceride levels.[75]

- *Dosage:* 300 mg per day of gamma-oryzanol

Herbal support
The four most useful herbs in the treatment of hot flashes are *Angelica sinensis*, *Glycyrrhiza glabra* (discussed above), *Vitex agnus-castus* (discussed below), and *Cimicifuga racemosa*. These herbs have been used historically to lessen a variety of female complaints including hot flashes. While these herbs are effective individually, combining them may produce an even greater benefit.

Angelica sinensis   In Asia, *Angelica sinensis* (also known as angelica and dong quai) has a reputation second only to ginseng. Predominantly regarded as a "female" remedy, angelica has been used in treating menopausal symptoms (especially hot flashes), as well as in such conditions as dysmenorrhea (painful periods), amenorrhea (lack of periods), metrorrhagia (heavy bleeding), and to assure a healthy pregnancy and easy delivery. Its effectiveness in relieving hot flashes appears to be due to a combination of angelica's mild estrogenic effects coupled with other components that act to stabilize blood vessels.[76]

- *Typical Dosage:* 1 to 2 gm of powdered root or 1 ml of the fluid extract of *Angelica sinensis* three times a day

Cimicifuga racemosa (black cohosh)   This herb was widely used by the American Indians and later by American colonists for the relief of menstrual cramps and menopausal symptoms. Recent scientific investigation has upheld the use of black cohosh in both dysmenorrhea and menopause. Clinical studies have shown that extracts of black cohosh relieve not only hot flashes, but also depression and vaginal atrophy.[77] In addition to exerting vascular effects, black cohosh has been shown to reduce LH levels, thus implying a significant estrogenic effect.

- *Typical Dosage:* 1 to 2 gm of powdered *Cimicifuga racemosa* berries three times a day

Ginkgo biloba   Although not traditionally considered an herb for treating symptoms of menopause, *Ginkgo biloba* extract is very useful for women during this time due to its beneficial effects on the vascular system. It appears to be especially useful in improving the cold hands and feet as well as the forgetfulness that often accompanies menopause. *Ginkgo biloba* extract has been shown to improve blood flow to the hands and feet in human clinical trials and to be effective in the treatment of peripheral vascular diseases of the extremities, including Raynaud's syndrome, a disease characterized by extremely cold fingers or toes.[78,79,80]

- *Typical Dosage:* 40 mg of standardized extract (24% flavonoids) of *Ginkgo biloba* three times a day

Menstrual Disorders and Premenstrual Syndrome (PMS)

Nutrition

As with all other health problems, poor nutrition underlies many menstrual disorders. Compared to normal women, those with premenstrual syndrome consume 62% more refined carbohydrates, 275% more refined sugar, 79% more dairy products, 78% more sodium, 53% less iron, 77% less manganese, and 52% less zinc.[81] Putting women who were on a high-fat diet on a lowfat diet results in substantial reduction of fluid and other symptoms of PMS.[82] PMS patients given a multivitamin and mineral supplement containing high doses of magnesium and pyridoxine in an uncontrolled study showed a 70% reduction in both pre- and post-menstrual symptoms.[83]

Especially useful is pyridoxine (vitamin B_6). Although not deficient according to serum and other measures, several studies have demonstrated the clinical efficacy of vitamin B_6 supplementation in treating PMS.[84] In one double-blind cross-over trial, 84% of the subjects had a lower symptomatology score during the B_6 treatment period.[85]

- *Typical Dosage:* 100 mg per day

Another important nutrient is magnesium. Deficiency is strongly implicated as a causative factor in PMS. Although serum levels are normal, red blood cell magnesium levels, a much better measure of cellular magnesium status, are significantly lower in women with PMS than in those without.[86] One clinical trial of magnesium in PMS showed a reduction of nervousness in 89%, breast pain in 96%, and weight gain in 95%.[87]

- *Typical Dosage:* 250 mg magnesium citrate

Vitex

The berries of *Vitex agnus-castus* (chaste tree), which is native to the Mediterranean, have long been used for female complaints. As the name suggests, chaste berries were used in suppressing the libido. Scientific investigation has shown that chaste berry has profound effects on pituitary function, increasing LH secretion and decreasing the secretion of FSH.[88] *Vitex* also decreases the secretion of prolactin from the pituitary gland.[89] The net result is increased activity of the corpus luteum (which is why it is used by European gynecologists for corpus luteum insufficiency) and increased synthesis of progesterone.

The most frequent indications for therapy with *Vitex agnus-castus* are menstrual disorders and premenstrual syndrome. A large study in Europe of 153 gynecologists working with 551 patients found it to be quite effective. Improvement in symptoms were found in 31.9% of patients within the first four weeks and 83.5% within 12 weeks, with 29% becoming symptom free by the end of the study. Only 11% showed no response to the treatment. About 5% reported side effects, all of them mild, with the exception of one individual who experienced heavy headaches that required cessation of therapy.[90]

- *Dosage:* 40 drops of a 1 to 5 tincture of *Vitex agnus-castus* per day

Female Infertility

Infertility in women is a common and, for many, deeply distressing problem. It's also very expensive, with the cost of artificial insemination and delivery ranging from $44,000 to $211,940.[91] Fortunately, much can be done to restore fertility once the causes are understood.

Relax

The first step is to stop worrying about it. Easy to say and hard to do, but this simple concept works for a surprising number of women. A study of 54 women who had a mean time of unexplained fertility of 3.3 years entered a behavioral treatment program designed to elicit their relaxation response. After completing the mind/body program, the women showed statistically significant decreases in anxiety, depression, and fatigue. Within six months, 34% of the women became pregnant.[92]

Avoid drugs and other toxins

The female reproductive process is a complex balance of many factors. Many toxins disrupt this process, including prescription drugs, recreational drugs, and environmental poisons. For example, in one study, approximately 1,000 women between the ages of 20 and 39 years who had been trying to conceive for at least 12 months were evaluated for recreational drug use of marijuana, LSD, speed, cocaine, or other drugs for their effects on fertility. When matched with controls, the women who used drugs, especially cocaine, had a higher incidence of reproductive abnormalities.[93]

It is not just the illegal recreational drugs that need to be avoided. The legal ones (smoking, alcohol, and caffeine) are just as much of a problem, probably because they are used more frequently. As might be expected, smoking is associated with infertility. This appears to be due to some, as yet undetermined, directly toxic affect of conitine (a break down product of nicotine) on the ovum. Research has shown that eggs taken from smoking women are more difficult for sperm to fertilize (one-third less likely) than eggs from women who do not smoke.[94]

Equally unsurprising is the affect of alcohol consumption on fertility. One study of almost 5,000 fertile and infertile women found that those who averaged one alcoholic beverage a day had a 30% increased risk of infertility, while those who drank two or more had a 60% increased risk of fertility. In addition, women who drank one or more alcoholic beverages every day had a 50% increased risk of endometriosis. This is not to say that women should never drink alcohol, but rather to exercise restraint.[95]

Even drinking caffeinated beverages has an impact on fertility. The researchers found that tea had very minimal effects on fertility, while caffeine-containing coffee and soft drinks were strongly related to decreased fertility. They found that as little as one caffeinated drink per day resulted in a remarkable 50% reduction in the monthly chance of conception.[96]

Environmental chemicals, some of which women frequently encounter (such as those found in beauty salons), are also a problem. For example, one study examined cosmetologists who worked full time in cosmetology or in other jobs during the first trimester of pregnancy. The study involved 96 cosmetologists who had had a spontaneous abortion and compared them with 547 cosmetologists who had had a single live birth. The authors found associations between spontaneous abortion and the number of hours worked per day in cosmetology, the number of chemical services performed per week, the use of formaldehyde-based disinfectants, and work in salons where nail sculpturing was performed. The problem is that many of the chemicals used in cosmetology are known to affect fertility: Many products contain solvents that have been linked to spontaneous abortion; hair dyes can be absorbed through the skin and have been associated with mutagenic and carcinogenic effects and female infertility; and fumigants commonly used in cosmetology contain formaldehyde, a well-known toxin.[97]

Maintain optimal nutritional status

As with virtually every other bodily process, the trace minerals (especially zinc, copper, and selenium) are crucial for maintaining reproductive health. Zinc deficiency leads to impaired synthesis and secretion of follicle stimulating and luteinizing hormones, abnormal ovarian development, disruption of the menstrual cycle, frequent abortion, prolonged gestation, teratogenicity (fetal abnormalities), stillbirths, difficulty in parturition, pre-eclampsia, toxemia, and low-birth-weight infants. Copper is critical for the enzymes that produce the elastin and connective tissue that make up the arteries and other structural tissues of the body. Deficiency results in spontaneous abortions. Selenium is critical for protecting the fragile ova from free radical damage. Deficiency results in infertility, abortion, and retained placenta. Selenium deficiency in a mother may also lead to muscle weakness in the child. Selenium requirements increase in pregnant and in lactating women as a result of selenium transport to the fetus.[98]

Herbs

For Marilyn, mentioned at the beginning of the chapter, I recommended a combination of three herbs [squaw vine (*Mitchella repens*), heloniasis (*Chamaelirium luteum*), and black haw (*Viburnum opulus*)]. Although they have historically been used to help women reestablish their hormonal balance, supposedly by stimulating the pituitary, I could find no clinical studies evaluating their efficacy. Nonetheless, they've been so useful for my infertile patients, I continue to recommend them.

- *Dosage:* 1 tbl of tincture of squaw vine, heloniasis, and black haw three times a day

Male Infertility

About 15% of couples in the U. S. have difficulty conceiving a child. In about one-third of the cases of infertility, it is the male who is infertile; in another one-third, both the male and the female are responsible. Current estimates suggest about 6% of men between the ages of 15 and 50 are infertile.

In about 90% of the cases of male infertility, deficient sperm production is the problem. Although it only takes one sperm to fertilize an egg, in an average ejaculate, a healthy man will eject nearly 200 million sperm. However, because of the natural barriers in the female reproductive tract only about 40 sperm will ever reach the vicinity of an egg. A strong correlation exists between the number of sperm in an ejaculate and fertility.

Total sperm count as well as sperm quality of the general male population has been deteriorating over the last few decades. Since 1940, the average sperm count has dropped from 113 million per ml to 66 million in 1990. Adding to this problem, the average amount of semen fell almost 20%, from 3.4 ml to 2.75 ml. Combined, these changes mean that men are now

Table 8-12 Common Causes of Falling Sperm Counts

Increased scrotal temperature	Tight-fitting clothing and briefs
	Varicose veins in the scrotum
Environmental	Environmental pollution
	Environmental estrogens
	Heavy metals (lead, mercury, arsenic, etc.)
	Organic solvents
	Pesticides (DDT, PCBs, DBCP, etc.)
	Overuse of alcohol, tobacco, or marijuana
Dietary	Increased intake of saturated fats
	Reduced intake of fruits, vegetables, and whole grains
	Reduced intake of dietary fiber
	Nutritional deficiencies

supplying only about 40% of the number of sperm per ejaculate compared to 1940 levels.

Why some males are infertile

The downward trend in sperm counts appears to be due to environmental, dietary, and lifestyle changes in recent decades. Table 8-12 lists the most common causes of low sperm counts. As can be seen, most of these are controllable through improvements in lifestyle.

Reestablishing male fertility

Because sperm formation is closely linked to nutritional status, it is critical that men with low sperm counts have optimal nutritional intake. This means consuming a healthful diet and taking nutritional and herbal supplements that support sperm formation. In addition, it appears to be important for men with low sperm count to keep their scrotum cool, quickly treat any genitourinary infections, and avoid dietary and environmental sources of estrogens.

Maintain a cool scrotum

The scrotal sac normally keeps the testes at a temperature of between 94 and 96°F. At temperatures above 96°F, sperm production is greatly inhibited or stopped completely. Typically, the mean scrotal temperature of infertile men is significantly higher than that of fertile men, and reducing scrotal temperature in infertile men will often restore fertility. This temperature reduction is best done by wearing loose underwear and pants, avoiding hot tubs, and periodically taking a cold shower, especially after exercising.

Genitourinary tract infections

A wide number of bacteria, viruses, and other organisms can infect the male genitourinary system. *Chlamydia trachomati*, a sexually transmitted disease, is the most common as well as the most serious of infections in the male genitourinary tract. Typically, the symptoms will be pain or burning sensations upon urination or ejaculation. During an acute chlamydia infection, antibiotics are essential. Chlamydia is sensitive to tetracyclines and erythromycin. Unfortunately, because chlamydia lives within human cells, it may be difficult to totally eradicate the organism with antibiotics alone, which is why support for the immune system is essential (see Chapter Four).

While acute chlamydial infections are usually associated with severe pain, chronic infections of the penis, testes, or prostate can exist with little or no symptoms. Some research shows that 28 to 71% of infertile men have evidence of a chlamydial infection.

Estrogens and other environmental toxins

As discussed above, we are now exposed to many estrogens in our food and environment that damage male gonadal function.[99] Although many synthetic estrogens, such as DES, are now outlawed, many livestock and poultry are still hormonally manipulated, especially dairy cows. Cow's milk contains substantial amounts of estrogen due to modern farming techniques.

The rise in dairy consumption since the 1940s inversely parallels the drop in sperm counts. Avoidance of hormone-fed animal products and milk products may be important for men with low sperm counts or testosterone levels. Organic dairy products may be safer because the animals are not treated with hormones or antibiotics. There are reports that estrogens have even been detected in drinking water.[100] Purified or bottled water may be a suitable option to prevent exposure.

Many of the chemicals with which we have contaminated our environment in the past 50 years are weakly estrogenic. Most of these chemicals—including PCBs, dioxin, and DDT—are resistant to biodegradation and eventually make their way into our bodies. For example, even though DDT has been banned for nearly 20 years, it is still often found in the soil and in root vegetables such as carrots and potatoes. These toxic chemicals are known to interfere with spermatogenesis. Again, as discussed in Chapter Seven, organic vegetables tend to have significantly lower levels of toxins.

Yet another toxin especially damaging to male fertility is aflatoxin, which is produced when foods become contaminated with fungi. Peanuts are especially susceptible. For example, a study evaluated 100 males giving semen samples who were attending an infertility clinic and compared them to 50 normal men in the same community. The mean aflatoxin concentrations in the infertile men was 60% higher than that found in the fertile men. Especially disconcerting was the finding that 50% of the sperm in the infertile men with elevated aflatoxin levels was abnormal compared to fertile men (10 to 15%). Feeding rats a diet contaminated with aflatoxin produces the same negative effects on the sperm and fertility.[101]

Fortunately, other research suggests a simple way of protecting sperm from such toxins. Garlic has been shown to neutralize many toxins, including aflatoxin. In a dose-dependent manner, meaning the more you eat the better the results, garlic blocks the binding of aflatoxin to DNA (the way it causes damage).[102] The message is clear: If you want healthy sperm, then avoid toxins and eat garlic.

Nutritional support

Sperm are especially susceptible to free radical damage since they contain a high concentration of polyunsaturated fatty acids in their membrane, actively produce free radicals from their metabolism, and lack defensive enzymes. Free radical or oxidative damage to sperm is thought to be responsible for many cases of low sperm count since high levels of free radicals are found in the semen of 40% of infertile men.[103,104] Men exposed to increased levels of environmental free radicals are much more likely to have abnormal sperm and sperm counts.[105] Cigarette smoking is also associated with decreased sperm counts as well as an increased frequency of abnormal sperm, presumably due to the high levels of free radicals and other toxins in the smoke.[106] All of these factors combine to make the health of the sperm critically dependent upon antioxidants. Antioxidants such as vitamin C, beta-carotene, selenium, and vitamin E have been shown to be very important in protecting the sperm against damage.

Vitamin C   Vitamin C is especially important in protecting the sperm's genetic material (DNA) from damage. Ascorbic acid levels are much higher in seminal fluid compared to other body fluids, including the blood. In one research study, when dietary vitamin C was reduced from 250 mg to 5 mg per day in healthy human subjects, the seminal fluid ascorbic acid decreased by 50% and the number of sperm with damage to their DNA increased by 91%.[107] Providing supplemental vitamin C appears to be especially helpful for infertile men.

In one study, 30 infertile but otherwise healthy men received either 200 mg or 1,000 mg of vitamin C or placebo daily. After one week, the 1,000 mg group demonstrated a 140% increase in sperm count, the 200 mg group a 112% increase, and the placebo group no change. After three weeks, both vitamin-C groups continued to improve, with the 200 mg group catching up to the improvement of the 1,000 mg group. The most impressive result of the study was that at the end of 60 days, all of the vitamin-C group had impregnated their wives, compared to none for the placebo group. [108]

- *Dosage:* 1,000 mg of vitamin C a day, best in divided doses

Zinc   Perhaps the most critical trace mineral for male sexual function, zinc is involved in virtually every aspect of male reproduction, including hormone metabolism, sperm formation, and sperm motility. Zinc deficiency is characterized by decreased testosterone levels and sperm counts. Zinc levels are typically much lower in infertile men, with low sperm counts indicating that a low zinc status may be the contributing factor to the infertility. Supplementing with zinc appears to be very helpful for infertile men. One study of men with infertility of greater than five-years duration found that some of them had sperm counts of less than 25 million per ml.[109] The men were provided a supplement of zinc sulfate (60 mg elemental zinc daily) for 45 to 50 days. In the 22 patients with initially low testosterone levels, mean sperm count increased by a remarkable 250%! Their testosterone levels also increased, and 9 out of the 22 wives became pregnant during the study. In contrast, in the 15 men with normal testosterone levels, although sperm count increased slightly, there was no change in testosterone level, and no pregnancies occurred. In other words, the zinc worked for the men who were deficient in this mineral.

- *Dosage:* 25 mg of zinc picolinate a day

Vitamin B$_{12}$ Another nutrient of great value for infertile men is vitamin B$_{12}$, a deficiency of which leads to reduced sperm counts and sperm motility. Even in the absence of a deficiency, supplementation appears to be worthwhile in men with sperm counts of less than 20 million per ml. In one study, providing 1,000 mcg per day of vitamin B$_{12}$ to men with sperm counts of less than 20 million per ml resulted in 27% of them increasing their sperm production to over 100 million.[110]

- *Dosage:* 1,000 µg of vitamin B$_{12}$ a day

Summary

Endocrine dysfunction is surprisingly common. Between low thyroid function (25%), low levels of DHEA (most people over age 50), low levels of testosterone in men (25%), and imbalances of estrogen and/or progesterone in women (about 50%), most of us suffer from some level of endocrine dysfunction.

The most common causes of dysfunction are alcohol and other toxins, stress, smoking, and nutritional deficiencies, especially of zinc and selenium. Reestablishing normal hormonal balance has a remarkably positive impact on our heath and sense of well-being. Total wellness can be usually be achieved by optimizing endocrine function through the use of specific nutrients and herbs. Sometimes, however, supplying synthetic hormones is necessary when the body can't be stimulated to produce adequate amounts of needed hormones.

Chapter Nine

Enhancing Rejuvenation

You need to study this chapter if you suffer from any of the following:
- *Symptoms:*
  Loss of distance focus
  Loss of memory
  Loss of strength and/or agility
  Loss of sexual interest and ability

  Out-of-control blood sugar
  Pigmentation spots on the skin
  Premature aging
  Receding gums

- *Diseases:*
  Alzheimer's disease
  Cancer
  Congestive heart failure
  Depression
  Diabetes

  Macular degeneration
  Osteoarthritis
  Osteoporosis
  Parkinson's disease

Behaviors that increase risk:
- A high-meat diet
- Eating foods containing additives
- Excessive alcohol consumption
- High level of exposure to toxins
- High level of exposure to oxidants, such as ultraviolet light from the sun
- Inadequate amounts of fruits and vegetables in the diet
- Inadequate sleep
- Inadequate physical activity
- Smoking

Thumbnail: Quick Help for Stimulating Regeneration

- *General:*

  Avoid all toxins, especially organic solvents (e.g., paint thinner) and aluminum

  Aerobic exercise: one-half hour of aerobic exercise three times a week

  Strength training: weight training once or twice a week

- *Diet:*

  Avoid simple sugars

  Eat onions or garlic at least once a day

  Eat five or more servings of fruits and vegetables a day

  Eat at least 3 oz of soy products a day

  Eat at least 4 oz of blueberries (or other blue/black berries) a day

  Replace coffee with green tea

- *Supplements:*

  (in addition to a daily multivitamin and mineral supplement)

  Vitamin C: 1,000 mg per day

  Vitamin E (mixed tocopherols): 400 iu per day

  Vitamin B_{12}: 1 mg per week

  Coenzyme Q_{10}: 20 mg per day

  Glucosamine sulfate: 1,000 mg per day

  Glutathione: 100 mg per day

  Chromium: 125 mcg a day

  Magnesium: 400 mg per day

  Selenium: 125 mcg per day

  Flax seed oil: 1 tbl per day

- *Herbs:*

  Panax ginseng: 100 mg of standardized extract three times a day

  Ginkgo biloba extract: 40 mg three times a day

  Crataegus oxyacantha: 600 mg standardized extract a day

To most of us, progressive degeneration with age seems an unavoidable fact of life. Yet, while aging is inevitable, degeneration isn't. Our unhealthful lifestyles and toxic modern environment greatly accelerate the process, and much can be done to improve the situation. The basic concept is that the body normally repairs most damage in a timely and effective manner. It is only when damage becomes excessive or repair deficient that degeneration occurs. The greater the imbalance between damage and repair, the faster our rate of aging and degeneration. In this chapter we look at each of the major degenerative processes we suffer as we age. We'll explore the ways we can prevent the degeneration and actually stimulate regeneration.

Real-Life Messages About Regeneration

Osteoarthritis

Leaning heavily on a cane, Janet a 50-year-old university professor, limped into our teaching clinic at Bastyr University. She had such a bad case of osteoarthritis that she was scheduled for a hip replacement in three weeks. Before going through the pain and expense of this highly invasive procedure, she decided to see if we had some magic herb to cure her condition. I vividly remember the look of disappointment on the students' faces as Janet came in—they were eager for cases they could learn from, but this woman's condition seemed to have progressed far beyond our ability to help her.

Fortunately, I was aware of several ways to stimulate regeneration of her joint cartilage, but first, we had to decrease the rate of damage. Possibly nowhere else is the impact of an imbalance between wear-and-tear and repair-and-regeneration so graphically demonstrated as in the cartilage of the joints. Since the cartilage has a very poor blood supply, if the trauma to the joints is excessive, even a healthy repair process can't regenerate the cartilage rapidly enough. The problem is significantly aggravated by the most common medical therapy: aspirin. Aspirin, while it decreases the pain, also blocks the cartilage repair process, actually increasing the rate of degeneration! (I'll describe this surprising result in more detail below.)

Our first step in helping Janet was to determine the ways in which she was overly stressing her joints. We immediately determined that muscle tension and joint misalignment were causing far too much trauma to her hips. Added to that was her history of running on hard surfaces with poor shoes. As an avid jogger, she had run 50+ miles a week for over 20 years, and it had all caught up to her. The x-rays of her hips showed that not only was there virtually no cartilage left in her hip joint but also a considerable amount of calcification around the joint. The combination of the two easily explained her pain and limited range of motion.

Our treatment program was of necessity intense: (1) Massage to loosen her muscles, spinal and joint manipulation to reestablish normal alignment, and corrective exercises to establish proper posture and joint motion. (2) Half an hour a day of diathermy (a way of applying deep heat) to the joint to increase blood supply. (3) Strict avoidance of aspirin and other NSAIDs (non-steroidal anti-inflammatory drugs, e.g., acetaminophen, ibuprofen, etc.), and all members of the nightshade family (i.e., potatoes, tomatoes, peppers, and eggplant) since in some susceptible individuals eating these foods damages the joints. And (4) supplementation with several nutrients to stimulate joint regeneration: niacinamide (although the mechanism is unknown, Dr. William Kaufman 30 years ago demonstrated joint regeneration, as proven by x-rays, in hundreds of osteoarthritis patients using niacinamide[1]), glucosamine sulfate, vitamin C, and flavonoids.

Within a month, Janet no longer needed her cane. Within two months, her x-rays showed a small amount of improvement. Within three months, she took a walking tour of Europe. Then disaster struck. Against my adamant admonitions that it was too soon, she entered and ran in a 10-km marathon. Her joint pain immediately returned. At this point, she decided to get the hip replacement.

In retrospect, I realize that while we were very successful in the physical realm, we had missed dealing with the psychological—Janet's fanatical desire to run regardless of her pain and disability. Don't misunderstand me, I am not against running or intense exercise at any age. I personally understand the fanaticism—at 49 I am still an avid basketball player, despite damaged cartilage in both my knees. However, I do so with appropriate attention to strengthening my joints and limiting my playing to my rate of regeneration, i.e., I only play full-court basketball twice a week. (It is possible my wife, Lara, disagrees with this personal assessment of my ability to maintain an appropriate balance.)

- *The message:* Our bodies have a tremendous ability to regenerate, if given the right help. But there are limits. Niacinamide and glucosamine sulfate will help cartilage regenerate, but it takes time and care.

Receding Gums

Jennifer was only 45, but had already had two operations for receding gums. Her periodontist had just advised her that she was going to need yet another operation. She knew there had to be a better way and so came to see me. The causes of her problem were quickly evident. She admitted to being a heavy smoker and eating a very poor diet. I advised her on how to improve her diet, directed her to a smoking cessation program, provided some herbs to help break the addiction, and prescribed large dosages of vitamins A and C and folic acid.

She took the supplements and did little else. When I asked why she didn't even take the herb to help stop smoking, she replied she wasn't ready to quit! Needless to say, her gums continued to recede. Then her husband, only five years her senior, had a heart attack, which he survived. Suddenly they both became extremely health conscious. Both stopped smoking and adopted a healthful lowfat, almost vegetarian diet. Over the ensuing months, not only did Jennifer's gums start to grow back, but her husband's atherosclerosis improved.

- *The message:* Simple nutrients and stopping damaging habits such as smoking will help the gums regenerate, but there has to be a will before there is a way.

Use It or Lose It

I had the good fortune of knowing both my grandfather and great-grandfather. Coming from hearty Italian stock, they lived simple lives, ate well, and were always physically active. They lived long into their 90s and suffered virtually no degenerative disease (except my grandfather, who developed cataracts at age 80).

I vividly remember one summer in college when my father was building a cabana for the family swimming pool. He hired some of my college buddies to help with the foundation. Specifically, he wanted them to help me and my grandfather push wheelbarrows full of concrete up a steep incline to dump into the forms. This was a challenging task. The wheelbarrows were very heavy and a misstep would result in disaster, so significant strength, endurance, agility, and coordination were required. My grandfather, at age 75, nonchalantly pushed more than a dozen loads of concrete up the slope into the foundation, while my college friends, who were larger than he was and less than a quarter his age, couldn't even manage one. I remember being so proud that day of my tough old grandfather. In retrospect, I realize I should have been appalled at the poor physical conditioning of the supposed prime of U.S. youth.

- *The message:* Use it or lose it. Age is no deterrent to strength, endurance, coordination, or agility.

Physiological Function and Age

If we look at how the physiological function of animals in the wild changes with age, we find that they maintain a high level of function until the very end of their full life-span, at which point they deteriorate very quickly. Humans, in contrast, start to degenerate shortly after they reach adulthood and suffer a relentlessly progressive loss of physiological function as they grow older (see Figure 9-1). With decreasing function comes increasing debility and decreasing ability to maintain health in the face of environmental challenges.

An extremely important concept, one promulgated by Dr. Jeffrey Bland and others, is the difference between life-span and health-span. Health-span is actually more important than lifespan because it is the portion of life in which good health is experienced. After all, why would we want to live longer if the additional time is spent in a hospital bed suffering from a painful disease?[2]

Some Causes of Excessive Degeneration

Degeneration occurs when the rate of damage exceeds the rate of repair. As graphically demonstrated by Janet's problems with osteoarthritis, this occurs for essentially two reasons: excessive damage and/or inadequate repair. Tables 9-1 and 9-2 list the typical causes of these. For most of us, the most common and important causes are overuse, environmental toxins (especially oxidants), and inadequate nutritional resources to ensure optimal functioning of the repair systems. Each of these is discussed in context in the subsections below.

How Free Radicals Cause Aging and Degeneration

According to the free radical theory of aging, which was first proposed in the 1950s, the rate of aging is proportional to the level of oxidative damage from free radicals.[3] Uncontrolled free radicals cause progressive damage to cell membranes,

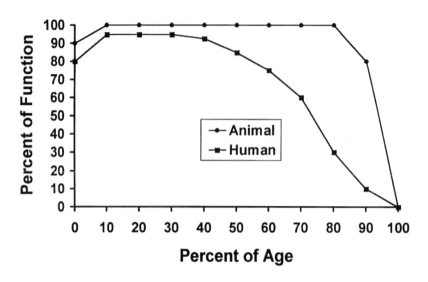

Figure 9-1 *The Deterioration of Physiological Function with Age*

enzyme systems, and DNA, resulting in problems ranging from cellular dysfunction to enzyme inactivation to cellular death to cancer. Dr. B. N. Ames,
who has researched cancer and mutagens for several decades, has estimated
that the average human cell sustains 10,000 DNA free radical "hits" per day.[4]
Although most of these are repaired, unrepaired damage accumulates with age.
As the damage accumulates, first cellular and then organ dysfunction occur,
ultimately leading to degeneration of the nervous system, the endocrine system, and the immune system.

A considerable amount of research shows a direct correlation within and
among species between health, longevity, and antioxidant defenses. For example,

Table 9-1 Causes of Excessive Damage

Cause	*Effect*
Overuse	Excessive damage
Exposure to environmental pollutants	Toxins both directly damage tissues and poison the enzyme systems needed for repair and regeneration. Several tissues, such as the nerves and immune system, are especially sensitive to toxins.
Excessive free radicals	Directly damage cell walls, DNA, enzyme systems, etc.
Poor metabolic function	Poor metabolic function results in the production of non-end product metabolites, which build up over time until cellular processes are strangled and the cell becomes dysfunctional or dies.

Table 9-2 Causes of Inadequate Repair

Cause	Effect
Inadequate rest	Most of the body's regenerative processes take place during sleep. Insufficient rest results in inadequate opportunity for repair and regeneration.
Excessive stress	By activating the fight-or-flight systems, stress turns off the regenerative systems.
Poor blood supply	Inadequate blood supply results in needed nutrients not being available and regeneration-blocking wastes not being removed.
Neurological defect	Organ function and regeneration requires neurological stimulation.
Inadequate nutrition	Repair and regeneration enzymes cannot function without their required vitamins and minerals.
Loss of DNA repair accuracy	When our DNA is damaged, special cellular enzymes clip out the damaged pieces and replace them with correct pieces. Over time and when adequate nutrients are not available, this process becomes inaccurate.

fruit flies that produce above-normal levels of the enzymes (superoxide dismutase and catalase) that neutralize free radicals live one-third longer and have a delayed loss of physical performance.[5]

Not only longevity but also long-term health and functional ability are greatly influenced by our ability to control free radicals. For example, free radical attack and cumulative oxidative damage have been shown in humans to be associated with most degenerative conditions, including cancer, atherosclerosis, cataracts, macular degeneration, inflammatory bowel disease, autoimmune diseases, arthritis, chronic lung disease, neurologic disorders, premature aging, and inappropriate cell death.[6] Without a doubt, free radical damage is a major cause of premature aging and debility. The role of free radicals in chronic disease is so significant that a large section of Chapter Five is devoted to describing how free radicals cause damage and the nutrients and herbs that can be used to neutralize them.

Fortunately, studies indicate that the use of supplemental antioxidants and avoiding chemical toxins in the environment will significantly improve our health and longevity.[7]

How to Recognize Excessive Degeneration

When examining a new patient, one of my first actions is to look in his or her mouth, because nowhere else is a person's balance between regeneration and

Table 9-3 Signs and Symptoms of Excessive Degeneration

Chronic unexplained fatigue	Out-of-control blood sugar
High blood pressure	Pigmentation spots on the skin
Loss of distance focus	Premature aging
Loss of memory	Premature wrinkling
Loss of strength and/or agility	Premature graying of hair
Loss of sexual interest and ability	Receding gums
Mental impairment, e.g., short-term memory loss	Varicose veins

degeneration so easily viewed. In the mouth, bacteria, chewing, and breathing all cause constant damage to the cells lining the mucous membranes and gums. The healthy body quickly repairs damaged cells, with the average surface cell being replaced every two to three days. However, when trauma becomes excessive, for example due to gum infections or smoking, or repair is deficient (for example due to a deficiency in folic acid or vitamin C), the lining cells are not replaced as rapidly as they are damaged, and the gums slowly recede.

Table 9-3 lists common signs and symptoms of excessive degeneration and Table 9-4 the common diseases associated with aging and degeneration. However, most of us know premature aging when we see it. People rapidly growing old and suffering progressive loss of function and increasing dependency are all too common in the U.S. So much of it is unnecessary, as we'll see in the next section.

The Keys to Rejuvenation

The basic key to health and longevity is to eliminate unnecessary damage and promote tissue regeneration. Without question, much of what we recognize as aging is simply the accumulation over time of unrepaired damage, much of it from free radicals. The general keys to stimulating rejuvenation are pretty obvious: avoid toxins; eat a whole-foods, relatively vegetarian diet; optimize repair and protective enzymes through nutritional and herbal supplements; get adequate rest; and exercise regularly.

These principles are well-demonstrated by the study of the natural course of osteoarthritis. This disease is well-known as a common, progressive loss of cartilage in the major joints, which is accompanied by progressively worsening joint pain and dysfunction. Rheumatologists will tell you that cartilage cannot regenerate and that all that can be done is to control the pain and inflammation. However, some very interesting research contradicts this common belief.

When osteoarthritis patients were followed over several years, x-ray evaluation of their joints found that those who were treated conventionally, i.e., with aspirin and other nonsteroidal anti-inflammatory agents (NSAIDs), continued to lose cartilage in their joints, and their disease worsened as expected.

Table 9-4 Diseases Commonly Associated with Aging and Degeneration

Alzheimer's disease	Huntington's disease
Amyotrophic lateral sclerosis	Macular degeneration
Angina pectoris	Mitral valve prolapse
Cancer	Osteoarthritis
Cardiomyopathy	Osteoporosis
Cervical dysplasia	Parkinson's disease
Congestive heart failure	Retinitis pigmentosa
Depression	Scleroderma
Diabetes	

In contrast, osteoarthritis patients who did not use aspirin actually had an increase in the thickness of the cartilage in their joints.

By decreasing the pain, aspirin allows the joints to continue to be misused (for example, due to muscle imbalance or misalignment of the joints). Equally important, aspirin and other NSAIDs actually block the collagen synthesis required for cartilage repair.[8] Damage to the joints is actually aggravated by pain relievers, which allow the damage to continue, because the body's warnings (pain) can now be ignored, and because they also contain a toxin that blocks the repair mechanisms.

Considering how poorly we take care of ourselves and the cavalier way we take drugs to block the body's cries for help, is it any surprise that the incidence of chronic degenerative diseases continues to increase? The appalling statistics are that more than 80% of Americans aged 60 and over suffer from at least one serious chronic degenerative disease, such as cancer, atherosclerosis, osteoporosis, macular degeneration, or diabetes. While some degree of degeneration is inevitable as we grow older, we suffer far too much and at too early an age.

The bottom line: Listen to your body. If something hurts, don't just cover up the pain with anti-inflammatory drugs and analgesics. Ignoring your body's messages just continues the damaging activities and inhibits your body's effort toward repair. Doesn't it make more sense to simply find out what is wrong and then to help your body fix it? Natural medicine has known for centuries many excellent ways of preventing and treating the common degenerative diseases that plague our society. Provided below are strategies for maintaining total wellness and preventing degeneration.

Eat Lots of Organically Grown Fruits and Vegetables

The "wear-and-tear" theories of aging have long assumed that sub-optimal nutrient status during the last decades of life was the natural, unavoidable consequence of aging. However, recent research shows that the nutritional deficiencies of aging are simply the results of poor diets and poor digestion—both of which are reversible.[9]

Tissue regeneration is highly dependent on the availability of the essential nutrients, which are needed by the enzymes that repair damage and regenerate cells. These essential nutrients are best provided by a diet of whole, organically grown foods, especially fruits, vegetables, nuts, seeds, beans, and fish. The data continue to accumulate that a diet high in fruits and vegetables can help prevent cancer and many other chronic degenerative diseases.[10] Unfortunately, Americans, as a whole, are still not eating enough fruits and vegetables. A recent survey of 23,699 adults in 16 states found that only one in five was eating five or more servings a day. The worst dietary offenders were men, the young, and the less educated.[11]

This lack of fruits and vegetables in the diet probably helps explain the appalling nutritional status of older Americans. A survey of 474 Americans 65 to 98 years of age found that virtually all were deficient in at least one nutrient and a whopping 40% of the men and 35% of the women had an intake of less than two-thirds of the RDAs (Recommended Dietary Allowances) for at least five essential nutrients.[12]

The situation is even worse when one considers that, at least in the opinion of nutritionally oriented physicians, the RDAs seriously underestimate our real nutritional needs. This concern about the adequacy of the RDAs, which at one time was considered controversial, is now being substantiated by hard data. One group of researchers, after studying nine vitamins, found that the RDAs of at least four (B_2, B_6, B_{12}, and D) needed to be increased. In the interest of accuracy, it must be noted that they recommended a decrease for one nutrient, vitamin A.[13] Better than the RDAs, however, are what might be called the SONAs, or Suggested Optimal Daily Nutrient Allowances, which are discussed in Chapter Seven.

Eating organically grown foods is also important. Organically grown foods contain micronutrients such as the essential trace minerals and less pesticides and other toxic contaminants. A pretty dramatic example of the importance of eating whole foods and decreasing exposure to toxins can be found in one of the most rapidly growing tissues in the body, sperm. Rather than perform a dry laboratory measurement of nutrient and toxin content of organic foods, some clever researchers decided to do a real-world experiment: They compared the sperm count of men who were members of an organic farmers association with three groups of blue-collar workers (printers, metal workers, and electricians). The men who ate the food they grew without the use of pesticides or chemical fertilizers were found to have much higher sperm counts.[14]

If you are wondering about your nutritional status, don't ask your family doctor to perform blood levels to determine adequacy. Research has shown that while blood tests may show normalcy, cellular tests can show serious deficiency. Cellular tests detect deficiencies 30 to 60% more often than serum tests.

Supplement Your Diet with Key Nutrients

While a whole-foods diet is necessary for optimal health, more and more research is showing that supplementing with key nutrients and several herbs helps prevent and reverse many of the problems of aging. These are dosages of nutrients that are substantially in excess of the RDAs, which are simply not a good enough guide to determining our optimal nutrient needs. See Table 7-3 in Chapter 7 for a listing of what a good multi-vitamin and mineral supplement should contain.

Use a Multivitamin and Mineral Supplement

Start with a high quality multivitamin and mineral supplement. Even in supposedly healthy older adults, researchers found that supplementation with a modest potency multivitamin and mineral preparation had a significant positive impact on their health. I say supposedly healthy, because the definition of health that the researchers used was absence of overt diagnosable disease—a very poor definition. In this double-blind study, a total of 96 Canadians aged 66 to 88 were provided either a multivitamin or a placebo. The only evaluation of the health impact of the supplement they used was incidence of infection. Over a period of one year, the researchers found a whopping 52% decrease in the frequency and length of infection (23 days of infection-related illness in the treated versus 48 in the placebo group).[15]

The supplement contained very modest levels of a handful of nutrients. At 100% of the RDA or less: vitamin A (400 mg retinol), vitamin D (400 mcg), selenium (20 mcg), and copper (1.4 mg); at 100 to 200% of the RDA: vitamin B$_6$ (3 mg), vitamin B$_{12}$ (4 mcg), vitamin C (80 mg), iron (16 mg), and zinc (14 mg); and significantly above the RDAs: folate (400 mcg), vitamin E (44 mg) and beta-carotene (16 mg). Very modest levels with remarkable results.

It is interesting to note that, with the exception of vitamin E, the levels of nutrients listed above can be supplied by a whole-foods diet that uses generous amounts of brewer's yeast, blackstrap molasses, sea vegetables, pumpkin and squash seeds, and whole-grain products.[16]

Vitamins E and C and selenium

In addition to a good multivitamin and mineral supplement, some nutrients need to be supplied in higher dosages. For example, as discussed in several sections below, antioxidants are extremely important in preventing many of the pathological processes of aging. Each day, I recommend consuming 400 iu of vitamin E (mixed tocopherols), 1,000 mg of vitamin C, and 125 mcg of selenium.

Magnesium

Magnesium is one of the more common mineral deficiencies in older adults. Even in apparently healthy senior citizens, it is usually deficient.[17] Magnesium is especially important for men, because a deficiency can cause the arteries of the heart to spasm, resulting in a heart attack. Epidemiological studies have shown that areas with low magnesium in the water supply have a higher incidence of heart disease. Deficiency can occur from decreased intake of foods rich in magnesium, eating foods depleted of magnesium due to poor farming techniques, decreased absorption, and disorders and medications that impair magnesium absorption. For all men over 40, I recommend supplementing their diet with 400 mg of magnesium citrate a day. Good dietary sources of magnesium include green foods (magnesium is the mineral ion of chlorophyll), beans, and whole grains.

Essential Fatty Acids

Essential fatty acids should be consumed liberally. Aging is associated with a dramatic decrease of essential fatty acids (EFAs) in the membranes of the cells. Because EFAs are critical for cell membrane structure and many physiological processes, this decline probably plays a significant role in many degenerative conditions. Many culinary plants and medicinal herbs owe their culinary and physiological effects to their volatile oils. This recognition lead to an experiment to determine the effect of volatile oils from almonds, nutmeg, pepper, and thyme on fatty acid metabolism in the liver of old mice. They found that thyme oil exerted the greatest protection against age-associated declines in essential fatty acid content. The authors speculated this was due to its antioxidant activity.[18] I recommend 1 tbl of flax seed oil a day. But make sure it is produced under nitrogen (rather than air) and refrigerated in a dark bottle. As a rich source of fatty acids, it becomes rancid very easily (which gives the normally sweet oil a bitter flavor).

Supplement Your Diet with Rejuvenating Herbs

Several herbs have been found to be remarkably helpful in both preventing and reversing several of the more severe degenerative processes, while the use of others has been associated with greater health and longevity. They exert these beneficial effects through a wide variety of mechanisms, ranging from organ-specific protection from free radicals and environmental toxins, to improvement in blood supply to areas where it is in short supply, to enhancement of wound healing. While I generally recommend that herbs only be used when needed, the following herbs seem to be of even more value when used regularly.

Camellia sinensis (Green tea)

Drink green tea. In a very large epidemiological study of 2,254 women in Japan, it was found that as green tea intake increased from less than three, to four to nine, to greater that ten cups per day, serum HDL cholesterol (the good cholesterol) increased, LDL cholesterol (the bad cholesterol) decreased, and

Table 9-5 Abnormalities Normalized by *Eleutherococcus senticosus*[20]

Function	Normalization Action
Adrenal	Impedes hypertrophy induced by stress Impedes atrophy induced by cortisone
Thyroid	Impedes hypertrophy induced by hormones Impedes atrophy induced by toxic chemicals
Kidney	Increases renal capacity in pyelonephritis (a serious inflammatory condition of the kidneys)
Blood pressure	Decreases high blood pressure by helping reverse atherosclerosis Increases blood pressure when too low
Blood glucose	Reduces blood sugar when too high Increases blood sugar when too low
Leukocyte	Reduces high white cell count induced by the injection of milk under the skin Increases low white cell count induced by toxins from the intestines
Erythrocyte	Reduces high red cell count induced by toxins (such as cobaltous nitrate) Reduces low red cell count induced by drugs (such as phenylhydrazine)
Stress	Reduces overactivation of the adrenal cortex in response to stress Prevents stress-induced thymic and lymphatic atrophy
Radiation	Protects against radiation exposure
Cancer	Inhibits carcinogenesis (from such toxins as urethane, 6-methylthiouracil)
Cholesterol	Reduces liver biosynthesis
DNA	Stimulates DNA synthesis

liver function improved.[19] As discussed below, drinking green tea also decreases the risk of cancer. These effects are apparently due to green tea's substantial concentrations of phytochemicals called catechins. These and other polyphenols constitute as much as 30% of the dried weight of green tea leaves and may result in as much as 1,500 mg per cup of brewed tea.

The Ginsengs
The herbs with the most research as general rejuvenators are the ginsengs: *Panax ginseng* and *Eleutherococcus senticosus*.

Eleutherococcus senticosus (Siberian ginseng)   Used in Russia for centuries, it functions as an "adaptogen," which means it normalizes human physiology regardless of the direction of pathology. Table 9-5 summarizes its remarkable ability to stimulate a function when it is low or tune it down when high.

All these beneficial effects provide real-world health promotion. *Eleutherococcus* appears to be effective in treating immune depression (especially chronic infections), fatigue, atherosclerosis, angina, high blood pressure, kidney disease (such as acute pyelonephritis), stress, and various neuroses.[21] It is not surprising that it contributes to an overall sense of well-being.

Eleutherosides are the constituents that exert Siberian ginseng's many beneficial effects, which is why I recommend a standardized extract containing 1% eleutherosides.

- *Dosage:* 100 mg three times a day of standardized extract (1% eleutherosides)

Panax ginseng (Korean ginseng)   Used for several thousand years in Asia, it functions as a tonic, prophylactic agent, and restorative. Modern research has shown that this adaptogen is effective in improving physical and mental performance in a wide variety of stressful situations. It even helps those who are healthy. For example, in a double-blind, cross-over study on university students in Italy, administration of a ginseng extract was found to improve performance on attention (cancellation test), mental arithmetic, logical deduction, integrated sensory-motor function (choice reaction time), and auditory reaction time. The students taking ginseng also reported a greater sensation of well-being.[22] Korean ginseng also helps relieve many of the problems of aging and chronic disease, including chronic fatigue, diabetes, male sexual debility, cancer, immune depression, high blood pressure, high cholesterol levels, wound healing, liver detoxification of poisons, and radiation exposure.[23]

Ginseng has also been used for decades by athletes to improve their performance, although there has been an absence of compelling human research to support such use. However, animal research has shown that it substantially increases resistance to physical or chemical stress.[24] In a particularly impressive study, the time to exhaustion was increased up to 183% in the mice that were given ginseng 30 minutes prior to exercising, compared with controls.[25]

- *Dosage:* 500 mg a day of ginseng root powder containing 5% ginsenosides

Speed Wound Healing and Prevent Scarring

Once a tissue has been damaged, several steps are needed for repair: inflammation to stop further damage and remove the damaged tissues, deposition of collagen (but not too much), and regrowth of tissue—all of which are critically dependent on the availability of required nutrients. In addition, throughout the entire process, the damaged area needs to be protected from infection because the normal mechanical protective surface has been penetrated.

As noted before, our white cell response is critically dependent on vitamin C. Five hundred to a thousand mg per day of vitamin C has been shown to increase the mobility of white cells and increase their entry into damaged or infected areas. Zinc is necessary for several of the enzymes involved in bactericidal activity.

Next, fibroblasts enter to begin the deposition of collagen. Vitamin C, iron, and alpha-ketoglutarate are required for the enzymes that form collagen out of the amino acids proline and lysine. Vitamins A and B_6 and the minerals copper and zinc play key roles in the crosslinking necessary for collagen to develop the necessary strength.

Finally, the body produces new cells to replace the damaged ones. Zinc and copper are crucial for the enzymes involved in protein synthesis.[26]

This whole process of healing seems to be greatly aided by the herb *Centella asiatica.*

Centella asiatica (Centella or Gotu kola)

One of the herbs with the best documented wound-healing and tissue-repair activity is centella.[27] Although the exact mechanism of action has not yet been fully determined, its terpenoids, including asiatic acid, madecassic acid, and asiaticoside, have been shown to stimulate the synthesis of collagen, the first step in tissue repair.[28] As might be expected, adding vitamin C further increases the rate of collagen synthesis.

Experimental studies on centella's wound-healing mechanisms have shown that asiaticoside, given orally, not only increases the rate of collagen synthesis but also stimulates hair and nail growth, increases blood supply to connective tissue, increases the formation of mucin and structural molecules such as hyaluronic acid and chondroitin sulfate (needed for cartilage repair), and increases the strength of skin.[29]

Clinically, centella has been shown to increase the rate of healing of a wide variety of tissue disruptions, including anal fissures, bladder ulcers, burns, dermatitis, hemorrhoids, keloids, leprosy, lupus erythematosus, stomach ulcers, perineal lesions, periodontal disease, retinal detachment, scleroderma, skin ulcers, surgical wounds, and varicose veins.

Most widely studied has been the use of *Centella asiatica* in the treatment of wounds.[30] It has been shown to decrease healing time and reduce scar tissue formation in: surgical wounds such as episiotomies and ENT (ear, nose, and throat) surgeries, skin ulcers due to arterial or venous insufficiency, traumatic injuries to the skin, gangrene, skin grafts, schistosomiasis lesions, and perineal lesions produced during childbirth.

Just as important as its ability to increase the rate of wound healing has been centella's efficacy in preventing scarring and even reversing keloids and hypertrophic scars. Keloids and hypertrophic scars are formed when the healing process gets stuck in the late inflammatory phase for too long, resulting in excessive deposition of collagen. In some people, this can go on for months or even years without progressing to the final healing phase. Centella helps by reducing the inflammatory phase of scar formation while enhancing the final healing phase.[31]

In one study, a total of 227 patients with keloids or hypertrophic scars were treated by oral administration with a standardized centella extract (effective dosage 60 to 90 mg). The centella extract was used alone in 139 patients (the curative group) and 88 used the extract along with surgical scar revision (preventive group). In the curative group, 116 patients (82%) were found to have benefited from the extract, either by relief of their symptoms or by disappearance of the inflammatory phase. In a double-blind substudy of 46 of the 139 patients, 22 out of 27 receiving the extract improved while only 9 of 19 given a placebo improved.[32] Similar clinical improvement was observed in 72 of the 88 patients (79%) in the preventive group.

Centella's inhibition of out-of-control scarring may explain why it is so effective in treating scleroderma, a disease characterized by excessive and inappropriate collagen synthesis. Several clinical trials have shown that centella helps reverse the disease, decreases skin induration and joint pain, and improves finger motility.[33]

The standardized extract from Centella asiatica has also been effectively used in the treatment of patients with second- and third-degree burns. Daily local application and/or intramuscular injections of the extract gave excellent results if the treatment was begun immediately after the accident. The extract prevents or limits the shrinking and swelling of the skin caused by skin infections (a common problem in burns), inhibits scar formation, increases the rate of healing, and decreases fibrosis.[34]

Several studies have demonstrated that standardized extracts of Centella asiatica are effective in the treatment of varicose veins and venous insufficiency. This appears to be due to centella's ability to enhance the connective tissue structure of the veins, reduce inflammation and scarring in the veins, and improve blood flow through the affected limbs.[35] Significant improvement in symptomatology (such as feelings of heaviness in the lower legs, numbness, and night cramps), physical findings (a lessening of edema, spider veins, leg ulcers, and vein swelling), and functional capacity (improved venous flow) was observed in approximately 80% of patients in the clinical trials.

Centella asiatica and its extracts are very well-tolerated, especially orally. However, the topical application of a salve containing centella has been reported to cause contact dermatitis in a few people. The majority of clinical studies on Centella asiatica have used proprietary formulas available in Europe (e.g., Madecassol, TECA, and Centelase).

- *Dosage:* 60 to 120 mg per day of standardized extract (containing asiaticoside [40%], asiatic acid [30%], madecassic acid [30%], or madecassoside [1 to 2%]) when needed to assist in wound healing or tissue repair

Maintain Optimal Weight

In just the past decade, the weight of the average American adult has increased 10 pounds, resulting in a very serious increase in health risk. We went from 26% of adult Americans being overweight in 1981 to 34% in 1991. This increase is largely due to a decrease in exercise. The prevalence of sedentary adults increases with age from 54.6% among those aged 18 to 34 years old, to 58.9% of those aged 35 to 54, to 61.9% of those aged 55 or older.[36]

Increasing Strength by Using Super Slow

At 49 years of age, I am quite physically active, playing full-court basketball twice a week with guys 10 to 20 years younger and using a Stairmaster once a week. In addition, for several years, I've used weights once a week, at times with an exercise trainer, to improve my strength. I followed the typical program of three sets of 10 to 12 repetitions. The end result was that I was able to jump 16 inches off court when going after a rebound.

I then learned of Super Slow, a different way of increasing strength. Instead of a large number of repetitions, this method emphasizes very slow movement (a count of ten up and five down) while holding a weight heavy enough to cause total muscle exhaustion by six repetitions. It is the most difficult physical activity I have ever subjected myself to, but the dramatic results were worth the effort. After only six sessions, my vertical leap increased two inches; after 12 sessions my leap increased another two inches for a total improvement of 25%. My shoulder size increased so much that my suit jackets became tight, and I had to purchase larger shirts! Even better, the procedure takes only half as much time as the older, far less effective, multiple repetition method.

- *The message:* A smart exercise program can result in improvement in strength regardless of age or physical fitness.

Research shows that thinner people live longer and suffer from less degenerative disease. These findings come from a huge prospective study of over 19,000 middle-aged men followed for 27 years. Researchers found that those who are lean live significantly longer than those who are either extremely under- or overweight.[37] The message is clear: Eat less, weigh less, and live longer—but don't overdo it.

Excess weight is also a serious problem for our children. According to one study, 75% of children now consume more total fat and saturated fat than the recommended amounts—which many physicians think are still too high.[38]

Keep Physically Strong

The research is clear, older people are physically weaker because they are more sedentary. The old adage "use it or lose it" couldn't be truer or more appropriate—rest is *not* what people need as they age. William J. Evans, M.D., of Tufts University, who has researched this area for several decades, describes aging as nothing more than the accumulated results of a lifetime of inactivity.

After the age of 40, the average person loses 6.6 pounds of muscle each decade. At age 20, 90% of the volume of the thigh is muscle, but by age 90 it is only 30% muscle, with the rest being fat and bone. With the elderly having

Table 9-6 Unhealthful Results of Inactivity

Slower metabolic rate resulting in low energy
Fatigue
Less strength
Lower aerobic capacity
Poorer regulation of blood sugar levels, resulting in increased risk of adult-onset diabetes
A worse ratio of LDL cholesterol to HDL cholesterol, resulting in an increased risk of atherosclerosis
Increased risk of high blood pressure
Decreased bone density, resulting in increased risk of osteoporosis
Decreased ability to maintain a constant internal body temperature

only one-third the muscle of the young, it is not surprising that they feel weak and even feeble.[39] The good news is that even a modest strengthening program can double or triple an elderly person's strength in only a few months. Even at the age of 96, men and women can substantially increase the strength and size of their muscles.[40]

The research shows that slowly moving weights heavy enough to cause complete muscle fatigue after six repetitions (if you can lift the weight eight times or more, it is too light) is the most efficient. The best results are obtained when every muscle group is exercised twice a week. As listed in Table 9-6, inactivity is a serious health problem.

Get Adequate Rest

Adequate sleep is absolutely necessary for long-term health and regeneration. While many different physiological processes occur during sleep, perhaps the most important for rejuvenation are the increased secretion of growth hormone and the scavenging of free radicals in the brain.

Many of the benefits of sleep are probably mediated through growth hormone. It has been called the "anti-aging" hormone. Several research projects are now studying the rejuvenating effects of injections of growth hormone. The reason for the excitement is that it stimulates tissue regeneration, liver regeneration, muscle building, breakdown of fat stores, normalization of blood sugar regulation, and a whole host of other beneficial processes in the body. In other words, it helps convert fat to muscle! While small amounts are secreted at various times during the day, most of its secretion occurs during sleep.

Some preliminary research suggests that growth hormone secretion can be increased by nutrition. One research project found that 2 gm of glutamine ingested over a 20-minute period 45 minutes after a light breakfast increased serum growth hormone levels in eight of nine healthy male volunteers between 30 and 64 years of age. The long-term effects of this supplementation are unknown, so it's premature to recommend.[41]

Sleep functions as an antioxidant for the brain because free radicals are removed during this time. In fact, sleep is required to ensure that there is minimal neuronal damage due to free radical accumulation during waking. Most people can tolerate a few days without sleep and fully recover. However, chronic sleep deprivation appears to accelerate aging of the brain. Animal research shows that prolonged periods of sleep deprivation cause neuronal damage.[42]

As people age, they tend to sleep less, with the average person 50 years of age or older sleeping almost two hours less than they did as a teenager. This diminished opportunity to secrete growth hormone and scavenge free radicals in the brain probably plays a significant role in the degeneration of aging. Several nutrients and herbs can help reestablish an adequate level of rest.

Melatonin

One of the best sleep aids is melatonin. Supplementation with melatonin has been shown in several studies to be very effective in helping induce sleep, in both children and adults, and in those with normal sleep patterns as well as those suffering from insomnia. Providing melatonin to those with sleep disorders shows that it decreases the amount of time it takes to fall asleep and helps make the sleep deeper. Interestingly, melatonin levels fall from adulthood to old age, at which time virtually no melatonin rhythm can be observed. Melatonin appears to be safe, even at high dosages. However, only low dosages are needed with as little as 0.1 mg resulting in a significant drop in sleep latency (the time required to go to sleep). Melatonin has even been observed to be a potent inhibitor of cancer growth, possibly due to its stimulation of natural killer T lymphocytes.[43]

- *Dosage:* Between 3 and 6 mg an hour before sleep.

Valerian (*Valeriana officinalis*)

Valerian is one of our best herbal sleep aids. Its centuries of traditional use is now being documented with clinical research. For example, in a double-blind study involving 128 subjects, an aqueous extract of valerian root improved subjective ratings for sleep quality, decreased sleep latency and left no "hangover" the next morning.[44] It works well for insomniacs, with a double-blind clinical trial showing 44% reporting perfect sleep and an additional 45% reporting improved sleep. No side effects were reported.[45]

Keep Your Mitochondria Strong

Every cell of the body requires metabolic energy to function. Energy production takes place primarily in special organs in the cells called mitochondria. Within the mitochondria, enzymes of the Krebs cycle metabolize carbohydrates and fatty acids to produce ATP, the energy currency of the body. Without ATP, most of our enzymes fail. One reason that people who exercise regularly have more energy is that a side effect of exercise is the proliferation of mitochondria in their cells. Just as our muscles grow when we stress them through exercise, so do our mitochondria. This means more energy not only for exercising but for all the other important activities in our lives.

A growing body of evidence suggests that the number and energy production efficiency of mitochondria may be the most accurate measure of biological age. Aging can be seen as the cumulative result of accumulated damage to the mitochondria.[46] After 70% of the mitochondria are damaged, they can't regenerate, and the cells become dysfunctional. Most of the damage to the mitochondria is the result of oxidative damage from free radicals, nitrous oxide and several toxins, some of which come from unhealthful bacteria in the gut. While some free radicals come from environmental toxins, most are created as a side effect of the production of energy in the mitochondria from oxygen and fuel.

Glutathione is the main antioxidant protecting the mitochondria. Glutathione is available through two routes: diet and synthesis. Dietary glutathione (found in fresh fruits and vegetables, cooked fish and meat) does not appear to be affected by the digestive processes and is well absorbed from the intestines into the bloodstream.[47] Unfortunately, glutathione does not cross the mitochondrial membrane very well. Fortunately, the mitochondria can synthesize glutathione internally, although people with liver disorders, such as cirrhosis, make less.[48]

Certain nutrients, such as N-acetyl cysteine (NAC), glycine, and methionine, help increase the synthesis of glutathione, and these substances do cross the mitochondrial membrane. N-acetyl cysteine is a precursor for glutathione and NAC supplementation raises intracellular levels of glutathione. This is one of the reasons that supplementation with large oral and intravenous dosages of NAC has been used to help decrease the toxicity of chemotherapy drugs used to treat cancer.[49]

- *Dosage:* 100 mg of glutathione per day

Keeping Your Cardiovascular System Healthy

We produce energy in two basic ways: aerobic and anaerobic metabolism. Aerobic metabolism (which occurs in the mitochondria) is far more efficient, with the cells able to produce 18 times as much energy per unit of fuel metabolized. In addition, far fewer toxins are produced in the process. The only way to ensure aerobic metabolism is to maintain optimal blood supply, which means regular exercise, a strong heart, and open blood vessels. Regular exercise is especially important, because it not only keeps the heart strong and the mitochondria pumping out ATP, but also improves mental health and neurological, hormonal, and immune functions.

However, when engaging in a vigorous exercise program, remember that the body's requirement for antioxidants increases. Supplemental vitamin E has been shown to be especially effective in lowering the oxidative stress reactions of exercise.[50] Dietary supplementation with antioxidants is a very important part of a healthful exercise regime, especially for those exercising in polluted cities, at high intensity, or at high elevations.

In addition to regular exercise, we need to prevent (or if it has already developed, reverse) atherosclerotic blockage of our arteries. There is now no doubt that diet can both prevent and reverse cardiovascular disease. Although aspirin is the current medical fad for prevention of heart attacks, several studies have shown that dietary modifications are more effective. The research that has received the most media attention has been the work of Dr. Dean Ornish. His research was so well-done and the results of his program so impressive compared to both a control group and conventional bypass surgery, that several insurance companies now cover his treatment as an alternative to bypass surgery.

Ornish's basic approach is to combine a lowfat vegetarian diet with an exercise, visual imagery, and stress-reduction program. After one year, objective tests and subjective reports documented significant regression of atherosclerosis of the heart blood vessels.[51] Of particular significance is the fact that, unlike those receiving bypass surgery, these people's arteries don't re-clog since they are now living a heart-healthy lifestyle.

Although most of the popular media coverage has focused on total cholesterol as a measure of risk, a far more accurate measure is the amount of oxidized LDL cholesterol (this is partly offset if the HDL cholesterol is high). It is oxidized LDL cholesterol that is so damaging to our arteries. Oxidized LDL cholesterol increases with our total cholesterol level and when the cholesterol in the food we eat is oxidized. It also increases when our level of antioxidants is inadequate. Fortunately, there is much we can do to decrease oxidized LDL cholesterol and increase HDL cholesterol.

Relying on conventional medical cholesterol-lowering drugs is not a good idea. For example, a worldwide research project found that although clofibrate decreased cholesterol levels, it actually increased the mortality rate 36%! While it may decrease mortality from heart disease, the drug's side effects increase other causes far more.[52] Treatment with the nutrients and herbs discussed below, on the other hand, results in lower cholesterol without side effects.

Keeping Your Arteries Open

The first step to keeping your arteries open is to reduce the total amount of cholesterol since, if properly done, this will reduce the amount of LDL cholesterol (the kind that builds up and clogs the arteries). We get cholesterol in two ways: externally from the food we eat and internally from our own normal metabolic processes. It does little good to eat a low cholesterol diet (although that will help us to avoid oxidized cholesterol) if we are over-producing cholesterol internally or not removing it from the blood at the normal rate. Trans-fatty acids (in margarine, shortening, and many processed foods) and elevated levels of blood sugar interfere with normal cholesterol metabolism. Several nutrients and herbs have been shown by both laboratory and clinical research to help the body eliminate excessive cholesterol.

Garlic

One of the best and cheapest nutrients is garlic, which has been shown to decrease the rate of cholesterol synthesis. Both raw and processed garlic contain several compounds (ajoene, 2-vinyl-4H-1,3-dithiin, and diallythiosulfinate allicin) that inhibit an enzyme (HMG-CoA reductase), which is necessary for the synthesis of cholesterol.[53] Supplementation of peripheral arterial occlusive disease patients (a form of atherosclerosis so severe those afflicted have trouble even walking) with encapsulated garlic powder (800 mg per day) improved walking distance, reduced blood pressure, reduced spontaneous platelet aggregation (blood clotting), and decreased total and LDL cholesterol levels in the blood.[54,55] The improvement in walking distance was noted after five weeks and correlated with the decrease in platelet aggregation.

The problem with coffee

While garlic helps, some types of coffee pose a problem for those with elevated cholesterol levels. Some coffee bean oils (Arabica) contain a high proportion of a compound called *kahweol*, which raises triglyceride and cholesterol levels. However, some types of coffee (Robusta) have no kahweol and do not elevate cholesterol.[56] Coffee brewed with paper filters has lower levels of kahweol, whereas percolated coffee has the highest, since the filter paper absorbs the kahweol.

Niacin

In the widely publicized Coronary Drug Project, the vitamin niacin was the only lipid-lowering agent found to not only prevent heart disease but to also increase longevity. In contrast to those using placebo, the patients who were supplemented with niacin reduced their mortality 11%.[57]

The problem with niacin is that it causes uncomfortable flushing 20 to 30 minutes after ingestion. To avoid the unpleasant flushing, timed-release formulations have been produced. Unfortunately, these formulations cause liver damage in 52% of those using the time-release product over a long period of time. A better solution is a form of niacin called inositol hexaniacinate. This form has been used extensively in Europe and has been shown to lower cholesterol levels and improve peripheral blood flow in intermittent claudication (blockage of the blood supply to the periphery). It has far fewer unpleasant side effects and is even slightly more effective than niacin alone.[58]

Useful herbs

Glucomannan, a polysaccharide derived from konjac root (*Amorphophallus konjac*), is an effective aid in the treatment of high cholesterol. Even in healthy men, administration of 3.9 gm per day over four weeks resulted in a

10% decrease in total cholesterol, a 7.2% drop in LDL cholesterol, a 23% decrease in triglycerides, and a 2.5% drop in blood pressure with no change in diet.[59] No side effects were noted. Obviously, the results would be improved by also incorporating a healthier diet.

In rats fed a high-fat diet, an extract from the leaves of *Gymnema sylvestre* has been shown to decrease serum total cholesterol, LDL cholesterol, triglycerides, and very low density lipoprotein, while elevating HDL cholesterol—all very important in preventing and reversing atherosclerosis.[60]

In patients with severe atherosclerosis who have had plaques surgically removed from their arteries, adding 15 gm of guar gum daily decreased their total cholesterol by 17% and their LDL cholesterol by 26%.[61]

Ways to Decrease Oxidized Cholesterol

The second step is to avoid foods with high levels of oxidized cholesterol. Basically, this means any cholesterol-containing food that is cooked at high temperatures in the presence of air, e.g., scrambled eggs, fried bacon, grilled beef, etc. We can also protect our LDL cholesterol from oxidization by taking antioxidants.

One of the best antioxidants is vitamin E. The minimum dose of alpha-tocopherol needed to significantly decrease the susceptibility of LDL cholesterol to oxidation is 400 iu per day.[62] However, vitamin E supplementation is far more effective when used in conjunction with a cholesterol-lowering diet, which has been shown by angiography to actually reverse atherosclerosis.[63] Those with elevated serum lipids should also consume a diet rich in carotenoids, which provide additional protection, especially for non-smokers.[64]

The evidence for the beneficial effects of antioxidants in the treatment of atherosclerosis and heart disease is very strong. Vitamins C and E, selenium, acetyl-cysteine, coenzyme Q_{10}, carotenes, and catechins have all shown beneficial results in clinical trials.[65,66,67]

Not only does garlic reduce cholesterol levels (as we discussed above), but it has also been shown to be an effective antioxidant, protecting the heart and arteries from oxidized lipids.[68]

Ways to Increase HDL Cholesterol

Finally, we need to increase the proportion of HDL cholesterol in our bodies. Changes in lifestyle, nutritional supplements, and several herbs have been shown to increase levels of HDL cholesterol.

Exercise

The best way to increase HDL cholesterol is to exercise regularly. Research has shown a direct correlation between the amount of exercise and the amount of HDL elevation. For example, one study evaluated 2,906 healthy, non-smoking males and found a gradual increase in high density lipoprotein with increased miles run. Most of the improvement occurred between distances of 7 to 14 miles per week, with little additional improvement above 14 miles a week.[69]

- *Typical dosage:* One-half hour three times a week of any exercise that increases your pulse rate by 50%

The role of alcoholic beverages

Moderate alcohol consumption (one drink a day) appears to decrease the risk of heart disease, probably because alcohol increases HDL cholesterol and plasminogen activator (which helps decrease clots in the blood vessels). However, this is not a prescription for alcohol abuse; higher levels of alcohol consumption have the opposite effect, increasing the risk of a heart attack.[70]

I must admit to considerable trepidation about recommending the consumption of alcohol. We are all aware of the serious personal and social damage that alcoholism and drunkenness cause—$110 billion annually in medical expenses and lost productivity, at least 50% of all fatalities from motor vehicle accidents, and immeasurable personal and family grief. Yet the media regularly carries articles about how drinking alcohol decreases the risk of heart attacks, the leading cause of death in men. Some very interesting research gives us some guidance in making the decision.

Several epidemiological studies over the last decade have demonstrated that light-to-moderate alcohol consumption modestly lowers the risk of heart attacks in both men and women. However, the results have been variable, and there has been considerable controversy about whether the benefits outweigh the risks, which forms of alcohol are most effective, and why alcohol consumption elevates serum HDL cholesterol.

Some excellent work appears to have found a key criterion for determining which men are most likely to decrease their risk of a heart attack by consuming alcohol. First, a bit of background. Most of us are aware of our blood type—A, B, AB, and O. However, few are aware that there are several other blood group subtypes. Of special importance here is a blood group subtype called Lewis. According to research, men with the Lewis phenotype Le(a-b-) have a significantly increased risk of heart attacks, which the researchers suggest is due to a close genetic relation with insulin resistance.

The researchers studied 3,383 men aged 53 to 75 years and recorded the diseases that the men developed and their mortality during a four-year period. At the start, they excluded 343 men with any history of heart disease. They then measured the remaining men's blood subtypes, alcohol consumption, physical activity, tobacco smoking, serum lipids, body-mass index, blood pressure, prevalence of high blood pressure and non-insulin-dependent diabetes mellitus, and social class. After four years, they found that in the 280 men with Le(a-b-) blood subtype, alcohol was a significant factor in their risk of heart disease. That is, the men in this group who consumed the equivalent of three drinks a day (of any type of alcohol) decreased their incidence of heart attack by a remarkable 75%! However, it should be noted that in the other 2,649 (90.4%) men with other phenotypes, there was a only limited negative association with alcohol consumption. The researchers concluded, "In Le(a-b-) men, a group genetically at high risk of heart disease, alcohol consumption seems to be especially protective."[71]

Obviously, drinking alcohol is a personal decision that is affected by social, religious, and other factors. Those who are unable to control their drinking should not drink, and drinking before driving, boating, or operating any major machinery is always a very bad idea. However, if you have blood group Le(a-b-), moderate alcohol consumption may be a good idea, at least until further research finds less controversial and risky ways of decreasing your risk of heart attacks. Your doctor can order this blood test for you.

While ethanol may be the beneficial factor in drinks for some people, it may be other constituents of alcoholic beverages that are the real champions. In animal research, the consumption of red wine and dark grape juice, but not white wine, is associated with reduced incidence of experimental atherosclerosis. These beverages contain a wide variety of naturally occurring compounds, especially several flavonoids such as anthocyanidins, flavanols, and flavones. These compounds are potent antioxidants and have demonstrated significant platelet inhibition (which reduces blood clots) in vitro.[72] The biological activity of these compounds explains at least some of the heart protective properties of red wine and purple grape juice.

Other Ways to Help Keep Your Blood Vessels Open

Gingko

The herb Ginkgo biloba also appears to help inhibit the development of, and even reverse, atherosclerosis. In rabbits given a high-fat diet, Ginkgo biloba extract (GBE) decreased lipid disturbances, inhibited plaque formation, and increased HDL cholesterol.[73] It works in humans as well; ginkgo has been found to be effective reversing the atherosclerosis found in intermittent claudication (a disease characterized by severe pain in the legs due to insufficient blood supply). In one double-blind study, 20 patients, aged 44 to 73 with serious blockage of the arteries, were given either 320 mg of GBE daily or placebo. After four weeks, the treated patients were found to have a 38% improvement in blood supply. Ginkgo also helps by decreasing platelet and red blood cell clotting and improving oxygen and glucose uptake by the peripheral tissues.[74]

Omega-3 fatty acids

Several population studies have shown an inverse relationship between fish consumption and heart disease, with one showing an effect with as little as one serving of salmon a week.[75] These results appear to be due to the omega-3 fatty acids in fish. Interestingly, autopsy studies have shown that the highest degree of coronary heart disease is found in those with the lowest concentration of omega-3 oils in their fat tissues. And, as might be expected, those with the highest concentration of omega-3 fatty acids had the least degree of development of atherosclerosis.[76]

If you don't like fish, omega-3 fatty acids from plant foods, such as walnuts and flax seeds, appear to be just as effective. The Mediterranean diet, which is high in these fatty acids, has been shown to decrease mortality 60%.[77] For example, the inhabitants of Crete get their increased levels of these important fatty acids through their consumption of walnuts and purslane; they also consume large amounts of olive oil. Supplementation with omega-3 oils in the form of flax seed oil or EPA- and DHA-rich fish oils also appears to be effective.[78]

Glycosaminoglycans

Glycosaminoglycans (GAGs), which are derived from the aorta of animals, are also valuable in the prevention of heart disease. They are made up of several compounds, including dermatan sulfate, chondroitin sulfate, and related hexosaminoglycans. Apparently, these nutrients help the blood vessels by preventing oxidative damage to their inner lining, inhibiting blood clot migration into the middle part of the blood vessel walls, and inhibiting the formation of fat and cholesterol deposits in the arteries.[79] In addition, GAGs lower LDL cholesterol and raise HDL cholesterol. Research has even shown that GAGs increase blood supply to the brain and help relieve poor blood supply to the peripheral tissues.[80]

Strengthen Your Heart

Clearly, the most important way to protect and strengthen your heart is to exercise regularly and maintain open blood vessels. Unfortunately, as we age, most people develop various forms of cardiovascular disease, ranging from atherosclerosis to cardiac failure (congestive heart failure). Several nutrients and herbs are especially helpful in keeping our heart strong, or if cardiovascular disease has developed, restoring health to our heart.

Promoting better functioning of heart tissue is an important, though frequently overlooked, component of the overall treatment of many types of cardiovascular disease. Degenerative lesions of the heart muscle impair pump function and can be found in most types of cardiovascular disease, including high blood pressure, atherosclerosis, and cardiac failure. These lesions apparently result from repeated insults, such as ischemic events (meaning periods of inadequate blood supply to the heart that are not bad enough to cause a heart attack, but bad enough to damage the heart muscle), inflammation, severe stress (the flight-or-fight syndrome releases catecholamines from the adrenals that, while they help us run faster, can damage the heart), and nutritional deficiencies.

Fortunately, the mechanical function of a failing heart can be reversed by providing optimal nutrition to regenerate the damaged heart muscle. One

Curing a Weak Heart

Anna came to see us in the teaching clinic, complaining of trouble sleeping at night. Questioning revealed that shortly after lying down she would awaken, having trouble breathing and needing to urinate. It all added up to a diagnosis of congestive heart failure—a condition in which the heart is too weak to adequately pump blood through the body. This results in dizziness and fainting due to inadequate blood to the brain and the build-up of fluids in the tissues throughout the body, especially the legs.

When the person lies down to sleep, gravity causes the fluids to move from the legs into the lungs, resulting in breathing problems at night. Due to the severity of her symptoms, I referred her to an internist friend of mine, who confirmed the diagnosis. She, of course, recommended the cardiac drug digoxin. I didn't want to start Anna on this drug since, while it would have helped her in the short run, over time her heart would continue to weaken.

Instead, we began her on a program of nutrients to rebuild her heart (coenzyme Q_{10}, vitamin B complex, and antioxidants), plus *Crataegus oxyacantha* (hawthorn berry) to improve the blood supply to her heart and gently increase the strength of contraction of the heart muscle. I've used this protocol (taught to me by Dr. Bastyr) quite successfully for several patients, and, as expected, within a few weeks Anna's heart strengthened. Six months later, I had Anna re-evaluated by my internist friend again, who could now find no problems with her heart!

- *The message:* Just like any other tissue of the body, the heart will regenerate given proper nutritional and herbal care.

of the best nutrients for strengthening and regenerating the heart muscle is coenzyme Q_{10}.

Coenzyme Q_{10} (CoQ_{10})

The therapeutic use of CoQ_{10} in preventing and reversing cardiovascular disease has been well-documented in both animal studies and human trials. In animals, supplementation with CoQ_{10} reduced the amount of heart muscle that died or became inflamed when the blood supply to the animals' hearts was blocked, and when chemicals and viruses were used to try to damage the heart.[81,82]

Research has shown that CoQ_{10} deficiency is common in cardiac patients. Heart muscle biopsies of patients with cardiac diseases showed a CoQ_{10} deficiency in 50 to 75% of cases.[83] As one of the most metabolically active tissues in the body, the heart may be unusually susceptible to the effects of CoQ_{10} deficiency.

A particularly common heart problem is angina pectoris, the heart pain that comes when there is an inadequate supply of blood to meet the needs of the heart. It's the last step in atherosclerotic progression before a heart attack. But don't wait for angina pains to indicate your heart is in trouble—the grim data is that in more than 50% of people, the first sign of serious problems with the heart's blood supply is a heart attack, and half of those having an attack die immediately. Fortunately, CoQ_{10} can help.

In a double-blind, placebo-controlled, crossover trial of 12 patients with stable angina pectoris, supplementation with 150 mg per day of CoQ_{10} resulted in a 53% reduction in the frequency of anginal attacks.[84] In another study, 17 patients with mild congestive heart failure received 30 mg of CoQ_{10} per day. All patients improved and nine (53%) actually became asymptomatic after four weeks.[85]

In another study, 20 patients with congestive heart failure due either to ischemic or hypertensive heart disease were treated with 30 mg per day of CoQ_{10}. After two months, 55% percent of the patients reported subjective improvement and 30% showed a "remarkable" decrease in chest congestion. Patients with mild disease tended to improve more often than those with more severe disease. Subjective improvements in congestive heart failure were confirmed by various objective tests, including increased cardiac output, stroke volume, cardiac index, and ejection fraction.[86] Some research indicates that CoQ_{10} might be useful in severe cardiac failure, where it could be used to reduce the dosage of digitalis and the risk of digitalis toxicity.

The most severe form of degeneration of the heart muscle is cardiomyopathy. While theories abound to explain it (viral infection, autoimmune reaction, etc.), the cause is essentially unknown. I believe that, for most people, cardiomyopathy is simply the end result of life-long abuse of the heart (i.e., chronic nutritional deficiencies, poor blood supply, excessive hormonal stress, inadequate aerobic exercise, etc.).

A significant deficiency of CoQ_{10} has been found in the blood and heart tissue of patients with severe cardiomyopathy, and supplementation with oral CoQ_{10} for two to eight months increases myocardial CoQ_{10} levels by 20 to 85% and substantially improves heart function.[87] In one double-blind trial, daily administration of 100 mg of CoQ_{10} for 12 weeks significantly increased the volume of blood pumped by the heart, reduced shortness of breath, and increased muscle strength. These improvements lasted as long as the patients were continuously treated (three years in this study). However, cardiac function deteriorated again when CoQ_{10} was discontinued. Of 80 patients treated, 89% improved while on CoQ_{10}.[88]

Another heart problem benefiting from CoQ_{10} supplementation is mitral valve prolapse. It affects both children and up to 10% of women. While most suffering the condition have no symptoms, some suffer palpitations and, in severe cases, heart failure. In a double-blind, placebo-controlled study of children with mitral valve prolapse, supplementation with 2 mg per kilogram of body weight for eight weeks resulted in improvement in seven out of eight children, with no improvement in the placebo group.[89] Relapse frequently occurred in patients who stopped the medication within 12 to 17 months, but rarely occurred in those who took CoQ_{10} for 18 months or more. Apparently this useful nutrient was able to stimulate regeneration of the heart weakness that allowed the mitral valve to collapse.

Finally, CoQ_{10} is of great value in treating hypertension. In animals, experimental induction of hypertension leads to a CoQ_{10} deficiency, which can the be corrected by CoQ_{10} supplements. In humans, a deficiency of CoQ_{10} was found in 39% of patients with high blood pressure compared to 6% of those with normal blood pressure.[90] Providing these patients with 60 mg of CoQ_{10} for eight weeks resulted in a highly significant decrease in blood pressure, with 54% of patients experiencing a mean blood pressure fall of greater than 10%.[91] This beneficial effect on blood pressure was usually not seen until after at least 4, and in some cases 12, weeks of therapy, so be patient!

Although the way CoQ_{10} helps decrease high blood pressure is not fully known, animal research suggests that it works by decreasing the secretion of hormones and biological chemicals that cause fluid retention and an elevation of blood pressure.[92]

- *Dosage:* 25 mg of coenzyme Q_{10} per day

Crataegus oxyacantha (Hawthorn berry)

One of the best herbs for helping to strengthen the heart is the hawthorn plant. While traditionally the berry has been the part most used, recent research has shown that other parts of the tree are also of value. A considerable amount of clinical research demonstrates just how effective the procyanidines and other flavonoids (a group of plant pigments that offer significant protection against free radical damage) in the hawthorn plant are in helping to improve the heart. *Crataegus* has been shown to improve the blood supply to all parts of the heart and the peripheral vascular system, modestly increase the strength of contraction of heart muscle, increase the tolerance of the heart muscle to low levels of oxygen, and improve exercise tolerance.[93]

Hawthorn's ability to strengthen the heart results in significant clinical improvement in conditions such as congestive heart failure, a common problem as people age. For example, using 600 mg a day of hawthorn extract resulted in significant improvement in patients with early-stage congestive heart failure. These patients' symptoms (such as shortness of breath when lying down) improved, they were able to ride bicycles for longer distances, and their blood pressure improved.[94] In another study, 132 patients with more advanced heart failure were treated with 900 mg of hawthorn extract. After eight weeks, they had a 50% decrease in symptoms and improved ability to cycle.[95]

- *Dosage:* 120 mg standardized extract three times a day

Maintain Neurological and Mental Function

While I don't want to get into a theological or philosophical debate on the subject, I believe most of us would agree that our experiences of life are virtually all mediated through our brain and nervous system. We need to keep them in top shape! A common misunderstanding is that we are born with a fixed number of neurons, which then degenerate and become fewer with age; in essence, our brain function peaks in young adulthood, and it's all downhill from there and nothing can be done about it. Happily, this turns out to be inaccurate.

If we are healthy and not exposed to brain toxins, there is actually no decrease in the number of nerve cells after the age of 30. While we can't increase the number of neurons in our brain, we *can* increase the number of connections to the neurons, with fully engaged neurons making as many as 20,000 connections, which makes our brains work better.

Marian Cleeves Diamond, Ph.D., has been studying the brains of rats and humans for several decades, resulting in the publication of 150 research studies and three books. The results of her work are clear: Rat brain size and function can be substantially affected regardless of age, with old rats (equivalent to a 90-year-old human) showing as much change as young rats. Providing rats with an enriched environment (the more diverse the better) that changes constantly (yes, even rats get bored with the same toys) results in several very significant effects: increased size of the cortex (the higher function part of the brain) and increased blood supply to the brain, neuron cell size, number of neuron connections, and size of synapses. Amazingly, Cleeves Diamond could demonstrate increases in brain size after just four hours of stimulation! These changes add up to rats better able to perform progressively more complex functions.

In contrast, stress causes just the opposite effects, with the brain of stressed animals actually getting smaller. In other words, the more we use our brain, the better it works, unless we damage it by stress and toxins.

Considering the high incidence of dementia and other degenerative diseases of the brain, we apparently need to do a much better job of stimulating and protecting our brains and nervous system. This is especially the case as we get older since the risk of developing diseases of an aging brain (dementia, Alzheimer's disease, Parkinson's disease, and amyotrophic lateral sclerosis) increases 15-fold between 65 and 85 years of age.

Once these diseases develop, they may not be reversible, at which point we are limited to improving function as best we can and limiting further degeneration. Obviously, prevention is the best approach. A considerable amount of research shows that this degeneration is caused primarily by three factors: poor blood supply to the brain, nutritional deficiencies, and brain-specific toxins—all of which are controllable.

Improve Blood Supply to the Brain

Unlike most other tissues, the brain has very little energy reserves and therefore is extremely susceptible to hypoxia, i.e., poor blood supply. As one of the most metabolically active tissues of our body, the brain uses large amounts of energy, which must be provided by a constant supply of glucose and oxygen. When cerebral circulation is inadequate, even if for only a few minutes, a chain reaction occurs that quickly results in brain dysfunction, then damage to the cell membranes of the neurons, and finally, irreversible cellular death. Cerebral vascular insufficiency is an extremely common condition in the elderly of developed countries due to the high prevalence of atherosclerosis.

Obviously, getting regular exercise and keeping the blood vessels open and the heart strong are absolutely essential to keeping our brain and nervous system healthy. In addition, several nutrients and herbs are especially helpful.

Ginkgo biloba

Without question, Ginkgo biloba is the oldest, most effective, and most researched herb for helping the brain. Its medicinal use can be traced back to the oldest Chinese materia medica (books explaining the medicinal use of herbs). At least as far back as 2,800 B.C., ginkgo leaves were used in Chinese medicine for their ability to benefit the brain. Gingko's effects on the brain are truly remarkable, ranging from increasing blood supply to improving neuronal function to protecting the brain from neurotoxins and the damaging effects of poor blood supply. Ginkgo has been shown to be quite effective in not only reversing many of the neurological diseases of aging, but even improving the mental function of supposedly healthy young adults. The most researched form is the standardized extract called Ginkgo biloba extract (GBE).

In a large number of studies, GBE has been shown to substantially increase blood supply to the brain, resulting in regression of the cerebral vascular insufficiency often seen in the elderly. It appears that by increasing cerebral blood flow, and therefore oxygen and glucose utilization, Ginkgo biloba extract offers relief from the commonly expected "side effects" of aging and may even offer significant protection against their development. Furthermore, GBE's anti-clumping effect on platelets offers additional protection against blood clots in the brain, a major cause of strokes. Particularly interesting is GBE's ability to normalize the circulation in the hippocampus and striatum, the areas of the brain most affected by blood clots.[96]

GBE also is remarkable in its ability to prevent the metabolic and neuronal disturbances that occur during cerebral ischemia (low blood supply) and hypoxia (low oxygen supply). It accomplishes this by enhancing oxygen utilization and increasing cellular uptake of glucose, thus restoring normal energy production. More specifically, GBE improves mitochondrial respiration, diminishes cerebral edema, improves cell membrane function, stabilizes lysosomal membranes so they don't release their cell-destructive digestive enzymes during hypoxia, and inhibits the action of enzymes that might have been released by the lysosomes.[97]

Another problem with aging is the loss of receptor sites in the brain for neurochemicals. For example, in rats aging results in a 22% drop in receptor sites. Fortunately, GBE reverses this trend.[98] However, long-term use is probably necessary to achieve this effect.

These improvements in brain blood supply and neuron function add up to considerable benefit for those suffering from diseases of the brain and neurological degeneration. In the elderly, ginkgo has been shown to increase mental performance and improve the sense of balance, short-term memory, vertigo, headaches, ringing in the ears, lack of attention, and depression. It has even been shown to be beneficial in treating Alzheimer's disease (discussed below). These beneficial effects undoubtedly account for GBE currently being the most widely prescribed drug in Europe.[99]

Ginkgo also appears to be of value in supposedly healthy young adults. In a double-blind study of healthy young women, reaction time and tests of memory improved significantly after the administration of GBE.[100]

- *Typical dosage:* 40 mg three times a day of the standardized extract (24% ginkgo heterosides)

Brain-Damaging Nutritional Deficiencies

Because the brain is so metabolically active, it has tremendous need for a regular supply of micronutrients. It's not surprising then that a deficiency of almost any nutrient can cause brain dysfunction. However, several nutrients are particularly important and commonly deficient, especially in the elderly (see Table 9-7).

Deficiencies of vitamins B_6, B_{12}, and folic acid cause neurological abnormalities and mental deterioration of older adults as well as an increased incidence of cardiovascular disease. Studies indicate that metabolic insufficiency or frank deficiency of these vitamins is common in older people, and that B_{12} deficiency is a common cause of dementia in the elderly. [102,103]

Most physicians rely on the development of a certain type of anemia before they begin to suspect vitamin B_{12} or folate deficiency. Unfortunately, research shows that the neurological and mental defects show up at least six months before blood changes.[104] Simple blood measurement of these vitamins is also unreliable because the body tries to maintain normal levels in the blood even long after a serious cellular deficiency has occurred. A far better method is to ensure that adequate amounts of these nutrients are in your diet and supplements. If a deficiency is suspected and not responding to supplementation, see a nutritionally oriented physician (such as a holistic medical doctor or

Table 9-7 Nutrients That Impact the Brain and Nervous System[101]

Nutrient	Impact	Effect of Deficiency
Thiamin (B$_1$)	Energy production	Brain fatigue
Riboflavin (B$_2$)	Neurotransmitter control	Neuropathy
Niacin	Neurotransmitter control	Dementia
Pyridoxine (B$_6$)	Neurotransmitter control	Neurological problems
Cobalamin (B$_{12}$)	Nerve function	Dementia
Folic acid	Nerve function	Dementia
Choline	Acetylcholine synthesis	Memory problems
Pantothenic acid (B$_5$)	Energy production	Brain fatigue
Inositol	Nerve function	Peripheral neuropathy
Tocopherol (E)	Protection from free radicals	Nerve degeneration
Iron	Energy production	Neurological problems
Zinc	Smell and taste	Loss of smell and taste
Copper	Neurotransmitter control	Neurological problems
Chromium	Blood sugar regulation	Diabetic neuropathy
Taurine	Neurotransmitter control	Seizures
Carnitine	Cognition	Dementia
Magnesium	Neurotransmitter control	Sleep disturbances, nervous exhaustion
Tetrahydrobiopterin	Neuronal excitation	Dementia
Tryptophan	Neurotransmitter production	Depression
Phenylalanine/tyrosine	Neurotransmitter production	Depression

naturopathic doctor) for the sophisticated functional tests that are better measures of the adequacy of these vitamins.

Vitamin B$_{12}$ deficiency can be caused by low uptake (such as in strict vegetarians), malabsorption, gastritis, lack of acid in the stomach, or lack of intrinsic factor (a special compound that ensures absorption of vitamin B$_{12}$). A very common condition of the elderly is a condition called gastric atrophy. In this condition, the cells and glands of the stomach have degenerated, and the stomach is no longer able to produce adequate amounts of stomach acid or of intrinsic factor. In one study, low stomach acidity was found in over half of those over the age of 60.[105] (For more discussion of digestive disorders such as this, see Chapter Seven.)

Elsewhere in this book, we've talked about the importance of the essential fatty acids for appropriate inflammatory balance, optimal immune function, and protection from atherosclerosis. In the elderly, dietary fatty acid supplementation has been shown to improve mental function as measured by task performance.[106] In adult dyslexics, DHA supplementation improved reading ability and behavior. It also improved night vision, again supporting its importance for the retina.[107]

Avoiding Brain and Nerve Toxins

The high levels of essential fatty acids in the brain its high level of metabolic activity and make the brain especially susceptible to toxins and damage. The need to protect this delicate organ is undoubtedly one of the reasons the blood/brain barrier developed.

Microglia in the brain monitor the health of surrounding cells and become highly phagocytic (meaning they eat and destroy) if they detect injured cells. In this state, they resemble the macrophages (see the description in Chapter Four) found in the blood. Like the macrophages, they migrate to the site of injury and ingest pathogens; they also secrete digestive enzymes to digest pathogens, dying cells, and other debris.

Normally, the microglia secrete growth factors important for the formation and maintenance of the central nervous system. Like other white cells, they tend to overreact to damage to ensure that all the pathogens are destroyed and cellular debris is removed. The microglia are activated by anything that injures the brain, such as trauma from a concussion (which may explain the progressive brain dysfunction seen in boxers), infection (such as AIDS, meningitis, and encephalitis), lack of blood supply (such as from atherosclerosis and strokes—interestingly, microglia are activated within minutes of a stroke, long before the neurons actually die), and many chemical toxins, several of which are unfortunately common.

As might be expected, uncontrolled or excessive activation of the microglial cells appears to play a significant role in common degenerative brain disorders, such as multiple sclerosis, Parkinson's disease, amyotrophic lateral sclerosis, Alzheimer's disease, and the dementia of AIDS.[108] It appears that, in some situations, a vicious cycle is initiated after some trigger pushes the microglia into a hyperactive state, especially when the inflammatory processes of the body are out of control (see Chapter Six).

For example, a low blood supply event (such as a micro-stroke) damages a group of brain cells, resulting in activation of the microglial cells. But instead of stopping after the damaged cells are removed, the microglia overreact and release too many proteases (which chew holes in the membranes of surrounding healthy cells), initiate the production of amyloid precursor protein (a degenerative form of protein that is secreted to wall off damaged tissues), and secrete the cytokine interleukin 1 (which increases inflammation and induces other cells to produce amyloid as well). To make matters worse, the microglia also produce free radicals, which further damage membranes, proteins, and the DNA, and, perhaps most importantly, cause the amyloid proteins to clump together, finalizing damage to the cells in the area. The end result is the formation of plaques such as those found in Alzheimer's disease, which are extremely damaging to the brain.

Obviously, if we want to keep our brains functioning well as we age, we must protect our neurons from damage. Some of the ways to protect the brain are obvious, i.e., keep the blood supply to the head wide open and don't box! Others, however, are less obvious, especially the chemical toxins.

Organic solvents

One class of common chemical toxins of particular significance to the health of the brain are the organic solvents, i.e., the chemicals found in paint, paint thinner, cleaning fluids, gasoline, kerosene, and lighter fluid, among others. Recent studies have shown the development of neurological disorders in patients following prolonged exposure to n-hexane (petroleum distillate), ingestion of petroleum products, and the abuse of solvents. Whether these damaging effects are due to microglial cell activation or direct toxicity to the neurons is unclear at this time.

Mental function in patients exposed to organic solvents improves as toxicity lowers. Brain recovery from solvent exposure can be accelerated through the use of phospholipids, such as found in those lecithin and egg yolks.[109]

There is a compelling body of evidence that suggests that exposure to organic solvents, such as paint thinner and n-hexane, appears to induce such degenerative brain disorders as Parkinson's disease in susceptible individuals.[110,111] This may be partly due to a genetic weakness in the afflicted individuals' cytochrome P450 (see Chapter Five for a full discussion of this important detoxifying enzyme), which results in an increased toxic reaction to environmental poisons.[112]

Free radicals

Brain cell membranes contain the highest percentage of unsaturated phospholipids of any cells in the body, making them extremely susceptible to lipid peroxidation (the damaging of lipids by free radicals). Free oxygen radicals damage membrane lipids and cellular organelles, resulting in neuronal death. Signs of oxidative damage to the brain are seen in amyotrophic lateral sclerosis, Huntington's disease, Parkinson's disease, and Alzheimer's disease patients.[113,114]

To limit this type of damage, we need to decrease our exposure to oxidants, e.g., ozone in the atmosphere, rancid foods, and toxic chemicals, and increase our consumption of antioxidants both in foods and supplements, i.e., carotenoids, flavonoids, vitamins C and E, beta-carotene, selenium, and antioxidant herbs.

Vitamin E, in particular, has been shown to directly protect the nerves from oxidative damage and result in improved neurological function after supplementation.[115] The bioflavonoids found in *Ginkgo biloba* appear to be especially protective of nervous tissue since they stabilize membranes and scavenge free radicals.

Food allergy

Although the concept of food reactions remains controversial to the traditional medical establishment (even though these observations have been made

A Mysterious Depression

Ed earned his living as a psychological counselor. He was so good at it that I often referred patients to him. One of the reasons he was so good was his own personal history of episodes of depression, one of which had been so bad he was hospitalized. Several days of intensive psychotherapy were required before he was functional enough to leave the hospital. Through constant counseling, he was able to live a normal life but continued to suffer from bouts of depression.

Ed consulted me to see if I could find a nutritional reason for his problem. Careful history taking and physical examination revealed a relatively good diet (he was also taking an excellent multivitamin and mineral supplement) and no apparent physical problems. I was mystified, but for some reason I suspected that he might be allergic to wheat. I instructed him in how to perform a food challenge test, and had him avoid wheat and all other grains for four days. On the morning of the fifth day, he ate one piece of bread, with stunning results.

About a half hour after eating the bread, Ed described his reaction as similar to an experience he had had as a youth when smoking very strong marijuana. For a period of over an hour, he became so "high" that he started hallucinating and became so hyperactive he described it as "clinical mania." After two hours of this, he "crashed" and became so depressed he couldn't get out of bed until the next day. This extreme reaction was such a surprise to him that he repeated the challenge test a week later with the same, though less intense results. As might be expected, he religiously avoided wheat thereafter!

■ *The message:* Food reactions can powerfully influence our mental and emotional function.

since the turn of the century), those of us involved in nutritional medicine are confident in our belief in the significant role that food intolerance and food allergy play in attention deficit hyperactive disorders (ADHD) in children. This belief has been further reinforced by a study of 26 children with significant ADHD. The researchers began with an open trial where they eliminated multiple allergens from the children's diet. Then, they enrolled the 19 (73%) who appeared to respond favorably in a double-blind, placebo-controlled food challenge. They found that these children responded to reactive foods and artificial colors with ADHA and improved when all the offending items were removed. Children with eczema were most responsive to this approach.[116] This research reaffirms the work of Dr. Joseph Egger, who has published several studies in this area that consistently show that foods, especially food additives, can seriously damage a child's mental and emotional health.[117]

Is there any reason to believe that the mental and emotional functioning of susceptible adults doesn't suffer from the same sensitivity to foods and food additives? This problem has been recognized by clinical ecologists (physicians who specialize in the effects of environmental toxins and food allergies on health) for several decades.[118] The typical signs of brain dysfunction seen after a person eats a food to which he or she is allergic include headache, lethargy, drowsiness, irritability, hyperactivity, confusion, depression, and difficulty concentrating.

Maintaining a Strong Musculoskeletal System

Osteoporosis

Osteoporosis, which literally means "porous bone," is a significant problem for the elderly, especially women. Over her lifetime, the average women loses 35 to 50% of her bone, while men lose about a third less. This heavy bone loss results in collapse of the spinal column and, in the U.S., over 1.5 million spontaneous fractures every year of such bones as the hips. Most of this can be avoided through exercise, nutritional supplements, and special foods.

Exercise
Physical fitness is the major determinant of bone density.[119] One hour of moderate physical exercise three times a week has been shown to prevent bone loss. In fact, this level of exercise has actually been shown to increase the bone mass in postmenopausal women.[120] In contrast to exercise, immobilization doubles the rate of urinary and fecal calcium excretion, resulting in a significant negative calcium balance.[121]

Nutrition
Supplementation with calcium has been shown to be effective in reducing age-related bone loss.[122] Many experts recommend a daily calcium intake of 1,500 mg, which, considering the typical American diet (meat-eating Americans typically consume excessive amounts of protein that when metabolized cause the excretion of calcium), requires supplementation in the range of 1,000 to 1,200 mg. However, the most widely used form of supplement, insoluble calcium carbonate, requires a good digestive system, especially adequate hydrochloric acid in the stomach, for absorption. Since most older women are deficient in gastric acid, most of the supplemented calcium is unabsorbed.

A far better choice are the soluble, ionized forms of calcium, such as calcium citrate, calcium lactate, calcium aspartate, or calcium gluconate. Research has shown that while about 45% of the calcium in calcium citrate is absorbed in patients with reduced stomach acid, only 4% of the calcium in calcium carbonate is absorbed.[123] It has also been demonstrated that calcium is more bioavailable from calcium citrate than from calcium carbonate in normal subjects.[124]

However, many other nutrients are needed as well as calcium. For example, boron supplementation (3 mg per day) improves bone mineral status,[125] as does magnesium supplementation (400 mg per day),[126] and vitamin K.

Vitamin K works by a different mechanism than the minerals; it is necessary to ensure the quality of the protein matrix on which the calcium is deposited. A deficiency of vitamin K can lead to impaired mineralization of the bone, and markedly depressed serum vitamin K levels have been found in patients with fractures due to osteoporosis, with the severity of fracture strongly correlated to the level of circulating vitamin K.[127] Vitamin K deficiency is common in individuals with chronic gastrointestinal disorders or poor fat absorption and in some who have used large amounts of antibiotics.

Calcium, boron, magnesium, and vitamin K are found in green leafy vegetables and may be one of the reasons that vegetarians have less osteoporosis. (Another is that vegetarians usually do not consume excessive amounts of protein.)

- *Daily dosages:* 800–1,000 mg of calcium citrate; 500 mg magnesium citrate; 3 mg of boron–3 mg/d; 1 mg of vitamin K

Some Habits to Avoid
Coffee, alcohol, and smoking all induce a negative calcium balance and are associated with an increased risk of developing osteoporosis.[128] Because smokers tend to drink more coffee and alcohol and consume a diet high in refined carbohydrates, it is very difficult to control for these other variables when trying to determine why smokers have a 15 to 30% lower bone mineral content compared to non-smokers. In its relationship to osteoporosis, smoking may be more an indicator of lifestyle rather than a direct cause.

Maintain Good Joint Function

Arthritis
Arthritis is the most prevalent chronic condition in both men and women aged 45 to 69 years of age in the U.S. Osteoarthritis is the most common form of arthritis and a serious cause of dysfunction and reduced quality of life in older adults. As discussed at the beginning of this chapter, it results primarily from progressive degeneration of the cartilage due to an imbalance between the wear and tear on a joint and the ability of the body to regenerate the joint, and it is aggravated in the long run by standard drug therapy (i.e., nonsteroidal anti-inflammatory drugs). Much can be done nutritionally to stimulated regeneration of the joint cartilage to help restore normal function. This is thoroughly discussed below under "How to Prevent and Reverse Common Problems of Aging." The other common type of arthritis, rheumatoid arthritis, is discussed in Chapter Six.

Chronic Back Pain

Another common joint problem of the elderly is chronic low back pain. The best way to prevent and reverse this condition is through appropriate corrective exercises, plus expert massage and spinal manipulation to reestablish proper musculoskeletal alignment.

The most common medical approach to back pain, i.e., bed rest, is probably the worst treatment, just as is ignoring the pain and overusing the back. Among patients with acute low back pain, continuing ordinary activities within the limits permitted by the pain led to a more rapid recovery than either bed rest or back-mobilizing exercises.[129] In a large research study, patients with acute, nonspecific low back pain were randomly given three treatments: bed rest for two days (67 patients), back-mobilizing exercises (52 patients), or the continuation of ordinary activities as tolerated (67 patients). After 3 and 12 weeks, the patients in the normal activity group had better recovery than those who were prescribed either bed rest or exercises. They experienced a shorter duration of pain, lower pain intensity, improved lumbar flexion, and fewer days absent from work. Recovery was slowest among the patients assigned to bed rest.

Expert mobilization and manipulation are particularly useful in speeding up the recovery and returning to activity. However, don't overdo them—pain means stop! Appropriate strengthening exercises, after the acute episode is over, speed recovery and improve lumbar function. In one study, 90% of patients subjected to vigorous exercise regimes had a good or excellent outcome based on several measurement criteria.[130]

Maintaining Visual Function

Age-related macular degeneration is the leading cause of blindness in elderly Americans. A quarter of those 65 years of age and a third of those over 75 show signs of macular degeneration. Susceptibility of the retina to oxidative damage appears to be a key factor in the development of macular degeneration. Ultraviolet light from the sun creates free radicals that damage the fatty acids within the retina. Since the lens focuses most of the light entering the eye precisely on the macula, it's not surprising that most of the damage occurs there.

It has been known since 1982 that antioxidant supplementation decreases the production of free radicals in the retina of animals.[131] Human research has shown that the higher the levels of antioxidants found in the blood, the lower the incidence of age-related macular degeneration.[132] A recent study of 421 people found that those in the top quintile of "antioxidant index"—a composite of serum levels for carotenoids, vitamins C and E, and selenium—had only 30% the incidence of age-related macular degeneration as those in the lowest quintile.[133]

As might be expected, research has shown an inverse correlation between dietary intake of fruits and vegetables high in carotenes and macular degeneration.[134] The carotenoids that appear to confer the greatest protection are lutein and zeaxanthin, which are found in tomatoes and dark green, leafy vegetables, especially spinach and kale. Supplementation (5 mg per day) with these carotenoids dramatically elevates macular lutein and zeaxanthin levels and the safety appears to be very high.[135] Interestingly, beta-carotene itself, found in red-orange vegetables, appears to have little value for the prevention of macular degeneration.[136]

Zinc also appears to be quite useful for protecting the eye. Two enzymes important for retinal function, retinol dehydrogenase and superoxide dismutase, are zinc dependent. To see if zinc would help patients with existing macular degeneration, researchers provided a group of 151 patients either 80 mg of zinc per day or placebo. After two years, they found the zinc group retained their visual acuity 42% better than the untreated group.[137]

Ginkgo biloba has been shown to be of special value in the prevention of macular degeneration because its antioxidant flavonoids protect the retina of the eye from free radical damage. These effects also appear to be of benefit in preventing diabetic retinopathy, another common cause of blindness in the elderly.[138]

Preventing Cancer

Without a doubt, one of the greatest concerns people have about aging is cancer, since so many of us develop some form of cancer as we grow older. Fortunately, there is much we can do to decrease our risk. For example, a considerable amount of research has shown that a vegetarian diet reduces the rate of cancer while also increasing longevity.[139] Much of the benefit appears to be due to its high content of fruits, vegetables, essential fatty acids, and soy products.

Eat a Diet Rich in Fruits and Vegetables

A review of 13 epidemiological studies, 9 cohort studies (a way of gathering data that looks at subgroups of people for trends), and 115 case-control studies concluded that the consumption of higher levels of fruit and vegetables is consistently associated with a reduced risk of cancer at most sites. The protection is strongest for skin and mucous membrane (called epithelial) cancers, particularly of the intestinal and respiratory tracts. The association exists for a wide variety of vegetables and fruits, and there was some suggestion that raw forms are more effective in lowering risk.[140] Another review of over 200 studies found that low fruit and vegetable intake resulted in twice the risk of most cancers (esophagus, oral cavity, larynx, pancreas, stomach, colon, rectum, lung, breast, cervix, ovary, uterus, and bladder) compared to those who had a high intake.[141]

The protective effects of fruits and vegetables have been attributed to several constituents, including carotenoids, vitamins C and E, selenium, dietary fiber, dithiolthiones, glucosinolates, indoles, isothiocyanates, flavonoids, phenols, protease inhibitors, plant sterols, allium compounds, and limonene. These constituents may complement and overlap in mechanisms of action, including (1) induction of detoxification enzymes, (2) inhibition of carcinogens (such as nitrosamine) formation, (3) enhancement of the formation of anti-cancer agents, (4) dilution and binding of carcinogens in the gastrointestinal tract, (5) altered hormone metabolism, and (6) antioxidant effects, among others.

Some researchers suggest that cancer may be a disease of maladaption due to reduced intake of certain foods that are metabolically necessary. They believe that vegetables and fruits contain the anticarcinogenic "cocktail" to which our bodies have adapted, and if we abandon this plant-oriented diet, we may suffer the consequences.[142]

Eat more soy products

We have known for a long time that women in the Far East have a much lower incidence of breast cancer than women in the West. For example, women in Japan suffer only one-quarter the incidence of breast cancer of women in Great Britain. A considerable amount of research shows that one of the main reasons for this remarkable difference is the much greater consumption of soy products by Japanese women, which results in a much higher consumption of isoflavones (150 to 200 mg) each day.

A similar, but different effect is seen in rates of prostate cancer. Whereas both Japanese and Western men experience the same incidence of prostate cancer, the mortality in Japanese men is much lower because their prostate cancers grow much more slowly. Again, the difference has been attributed to the consumption of soy products.[143]

Soy beans and some grains (especially rye) and seeds (especially flax) contain compounds identified as lignans (such as matairesinol and enterodiol from rye) and isoflavonoids (such as genistein and daidzein from soy). These are converted by health-promoting bacteria in the intestines to phytoestrogens, which help lower the risk of cancers, especially those mediated by the sex hormones.

These compounds have several valuable properties: They bind to estrogen receptors thus blocking the cancer-promoting effects of estrogen, they function as antioxidants neutralizing free radicals, they block enzymes that activate carcinogens, and they inhibit the growth of cancerous tissue.[144] A mere 3 oz a day of soy products is sufficient to provide protection.

Herbs to Help Prevent Cancer

Several herbs have been shown to be especially helpful in lowering the risk of cancer and, if it develops, in supporting the body's efforts to eliminate the cancer.

Shiitake mushroom (Lentinus edodes)   The shiitake mushroom is a mainstay of the Japanese diet and may be another reason for their much lower incidence of cancer. If you've had cancer or have a strong family history of cancer, then *Lentinus edodes* may be a very important herb for you. Its active constituent is a polysaccharide, lentinan, which powerfully stimulates the immune system, suppresses chemical and viral carcinogens, directly attacks cancers, and prevents cancer recurrence or metastasis after surgery. It has been shown to prolong the life-span of patients with advanced and recurrent stomach, colorectal, and breast cancer. Side effects are virtually unknown.[145]

- *Dosage:* 3 gm of the dried mushroom or 100 mg of lentinan daily

Garlic (Allium sativum)   Consumption of garlic is associated with a decreased risk of colon cancer, with those consuming the most, enjoying the greatest benefit.[146] Breast, oral, and skin cancer cells have all been shown to be inhibited by garlic.[147] Several constituents of garlic, including ajoene, diallyl sulfide and disulfide, S-allylcysteine, and allicin, have shown anticarcinogenic potential.[148]

- *Dosage:* ½ clove (or equivalent in processed) garlic twice a day

Green tea (Camellia sinensis)   World-wide, 2.5 millions tons of dried tea are consumed each year, 20% of which is green tea. Consumption of green tea is associated with a lower risk of cancers of the skin, esophagus, and stomach.[149] Green tea appears to work through several mechanisms, possibly the most important being its ability to stimulate detoxification enzymes, including free-radical scavenging catalase and glutathione peroxidase. The benefits from green tea appear to be due to one of its components, the epicatechins, which have been found to be especially effective in preventing both chemical and radiation-induced skin cancers.[150] In an experimental study, skin cancer was induced in mice using a combination of the chemical carcinogen DMBA and ultraviolet light (UVB). Providing the mice with green tea decreased their incidence of skin cancers.[151]

The role of the gut in cancer

The health of the gut also plays an important role in determining the risk of cancer. For example, a considerable amount of recent research has shown a connection between toxins in the bowel and breast cancer.[152] Bile acids, including the known carcinogen lithocholic acid, are found in the bowel in concentrations 100 times those of the blood. Normally, bile acids are eliminated from the bowel by being absorbed by fiber. However, a low-fiber diet, combined with unhealthful bacteria in the gut (which increase production of pathogenic bile acids), results in increased levels of these carcinogens. Supplementation with health-promoting lactobacilli helps to inhibit the toxic bacteria and decrease production of toxic bile acids.[153] And eating a high-fiber diet is essential.

How to Prevent and Reverse Common Problems of Aging

Alzheimer's Disease

In the U.S., 5% of those over the age of 65 suffer severe dementia while 10% suffer mild to moderate dementia. Over the age of 80, the incidence of mild to severe dementia is 20 to 25%. Postmortem studies have shown that 50 to 60% of all cases of dementia are the result of Alzheimer's disease (AD). The tremendous increase (ten-fold) of AD in this century in the U.S. population over the age of 65 is one reason why AD is referred to as "the disease of the 20th century."

AD is a classic example of brain atrophy and degeneration, with pockets of neurons being replaced by plaques containing amyloid proteins. While the etiology of AD has been extensively researched, the cause is still not fully understood. However, it appears to be some combination of toxin exposure, free radical damage, excessive glial cell activity, and poor blood supply.

The role of aluminum in Alzheimer's disease

One of the toxins receiving the most attention as a possible causal factor is aluminum because biopsies of the degenerative neurotangles seen in the brains of Alzheimer's patients show high levels of this toxic mineral. Whether the aluminum concentration develops in response to AD or initiates the lesions has not yet been determined, but significant evidence shows that it contributes, possibly very significantly, to the disease.

A study of 356 healthy people has shown that serum aluminum concentration increases as people age. Those with Alzheimer's disease have significantly higher aluminum levels than both normal people and patients with other types of dementias, such as from alcohol, atherosclerosis, and stroke.[154] Trying to remove the aluminum appears to help some, but it's probably too late after the disease is well-established. For example, intramuscular injections of desferrioxamine (a chelating agent for the removal of iron and aluminum) over a two-year period showed a significant slowing of the rate of decline in 48 Alzheimer's disease patients.[155]

Even in those without mental disease, elevated aluminum levels are associated with poorer mental function. For example, in a study of dialysis patients, the 13 patients who had a positive aluminum deferoxamine test (a measure of the amount of aluminum in the body) were compared to 13 who had a negative test. Subjecting the entire group to four attention tests and two memory tests revealed that those with higher levels of aluminum had a moderate to considerable disturbance of mental function.[156]

Where does the aluminum come from? Unfortunately, it is in our water supply, food, antacids, and deodorants. The aluminum in water is in a more bioavailable and thus potentially toxic form. Researchers measured the aluminum absorption of tap water by adding a small amount of soluble aluminum in a radioactive form to the stomach of animals. They discovered that the trace amounts of aluminum from this single exposure immediately entered the animal's brain tissue. The frightening news is that aluminum in water not only occurs naturally, it is also added (in the form of alum) to treat some water supplies.[157] In addition, calcium citrate supplements appear to increase the efficiency of absorption of aluminum (but not lead) from water and food.[158]

Now that I've scared you, what can you do? Scrupulously, maybe even fanatically, avoid all known sources of aluminum. Although I couldn't find any research that looked at this obvious possibility, don't used aluminum-containing antacids. Millions of Americans regularly self-medicate with antacids for the relief of heartburn, stomach pain, and ulcers. Since many of these (read the labels) use aluminum salts to neutralize the stomach acid, taking such antacids may be a very serious mistake. While the average person consumes a bit less than 10 mg of aluminum a day from food and water (much more in areas with an aluminum-contaminated water supply), consuming aluminum-containing antacids increases that by a factor of 10 to 100![159]

Other potential sources of aluminum include: underarm deodorants, clay (yes, that medicinal clay that is so useful for detoxification is made of aluminum salts—they are supposedly inert, but I'm not taking any chances), cooking acid foods in aluminum pots and pans, wrapping food with aluminum foil, and nondairy creamers. Aluminum is also found in baking powder and table salt; it is added to keep them from becoming lumpy. Finally, avoid food grown in areas of high acid rain, which increases the availability of aluminum for absorption by the plant.[160]

You can also decrease absorption of aluminum by making sure your diet is high in magnesium, as this useful mineral competes with aluminum for absorption, not only in the intestines but also at the blood/brain barrier.[161]

Ginkgo biloba

The efficacy of ginkgo in improving blood supply to the brain has been very well-documented. This effect has been helpful in senile dementia, including those with Alzheimer's disease. In a randomized, double-blind study, 40 Alzheimer's patients were given either 80 mg of gingko or placebo three times a day. Using a large battery of tests, the researchers found significant improvements in memory, attention, psychopathology, psychomotor performance, functional dynamics, and neurophysiology within one month. Improvement continued over the three months of the study.

These results contribute to the growing evidence that free radical damage plays an important role in the mental decline seen in senile dementia. As a potent antioxidant and brain-cell protective agent, ginkgo is a useful tool for slowing mental decline. It is important to note that this study used an unusually high dose. Most past research and clinicians have used a 40 mg dose three times a day. The higher dose of 80 mg may cause transient headaches or dizziness initially.[162] Although long-term studies with Alzheimer's patients to determine the maximum effect of ginkgo still need to be done, we know from other long-term use that it is very safe.

- *Dosage:* 40 mg *Ginkgo biloba* extract three times daily

Cancer

If cancer does develop, adding antioxidants to a conventional cancer treatment regime may significantly improve survival. In one study of patients with small-cell lung carcinoma, providing antioxidant nutrients resulted in better tolerance for radiation and chemotherapy and significantly prolonged survival time.[163] According to nutrient need, the researchers used vitamin A (15,000 to 40,000 iu per day), beta-carotene (10,000 to 20,000 iu per day), vitamin E (300 to 800 iu per day), vitamin C (2,000 to 5,000 mg per day), manganese (97 to 194 mg per day), and sodium selenate (856 to 3,424 mcg per day).

Cataracts

Many elderly people develop cataracts. Cataracts are caused by carbohydrate disorders such as diabetes (see below), nutritional deficiencies (such as vitamin B_2 and tryptophan), chemical toxin exposure (such as dinitrophenol and naphthalene), drugs (ergot, corticosteroids, and phenothiazines), and exposure to oxidants (such as ultraviolet light). Most of these damage the lens of the eye through the creation of free radicals. Antioxidant nutrients, both as supplements and in foods, help to prevent the development of cataracts.

It is well-known that the function of vitamin C in the fluid of the eye is to act as an antioxidant and protect the lens. Vitamin C has been shown to be modestly effective in protecting the fatty acids of the lens against lipid peroxidation. Vitamin E has also been shown to provide modest protection of the lens from lipid oxidation. Recent work suggests that supplementing the diet with vitamins C and E decreases the risk of cataract formation by 50 to 70%.[164]

Glutathione, a nutrient that is present in high concentrations in the lens, may be even more important than these vitamins in the prevention of cataracts. Glutathione is important because it is involved in a number of reactions that help to detoxify hydrogen peroxide and free radicals, and it can reduce protein disulfides (a damaged form of protein in the lens). Concentrations of glutathione drop sharply with the development of cataracts.

Rats on a diet deficient in selenium (the trace mineral required for the enzyme) have shown cataracts in the second generation. In addition to free radicals, high sugar levels can induce cataracts by binding with lens proteins to form opaque protein disulfides. Glutathione appears to help prevent the binding of sugar to proteins and thus the formation of the opaque proteins. Glutathione levels are reduced when we are exposed to high levels of toxins since it is also a key nutrient in several detoxification processes in the liver.[165]

Diet is important too. Researchers conducting the Nurses Health Study found that eating spinach correlated with better protection from cataracts than any other food, including foods high in other antioxidants. Those who ate spinach five or more times per week had only half the risk of developing cataracts compared to those who rarely ate this food.[166]

Especially helpful for protecting the lens of the eye are the anthocyanidins found in blueberries (*Vaccinium myrtillus*). Supplementation with 80 mg three times a day in conjunction with vitamin E was found to prevent progression of cataracts in 97% of 50 patients.[167] (This is the equivalent of eight ounces of blueberries a day.)

- *Daily dosages:* 1,000 mg of vitamin C, 400 iu of vitamin E, 100 mg of glutathione, 80 mg of anthocyanidins

Diabetes

Out-of-control blood sugar is especially damaging to many tissues of the body. Unfortunately, diabetes mellitus is very common in the United States, affecting approximately 4.5% of the population. The prevalence of diabetes is rising (at 6% per year), and it is now the seventh leading cause of death in the U.S. In 1992, while diabetics accounted for only 4.5% of the U.S. population, their care required roughly 14.6% of the total U.S. health care dollar. This is obviously a common and costly problem.

Epidemiologically, diabetes has been linked to the Western lifestyle and is uncommon in cultures that consume a primitive (unrefined foods) diet. However, as cultures switch from their native diets to the foods of commerce, their rate of diabetes increases, eventually reaching the same proportions seen in Western societies. The problem appears to be due to toxic or viral damage to the pancreas, the consumption of simple carbohydrates (i.e., sugar and refined carbohydrates), and nutritional deficiencies. While juvenile-onset diabetes (which accounts for 10% and is called insulin dependent diabetes mellitus) is due to lack of insulin because of a damaged pancreas, the much more common adult-onset diabetes (call non-insulin dependent diabetes mellitus) is due to lack of tissue sensitivity to insulin, the levels of which are often above normal. Diet, specific nutrients, and some herbs help prevent and reverse this resistance of the cells to insulin.

Diet and Nutrition

The place to start is diet—all refined carbohydrates (i.e., sugar, refined flour, fruit juice, honey, etc.) must be removed from the diet and replaced with whole foods. Research has shown that a whole-foods diet (i.e., fruits, vegetables, beans, nuts, seeds, and whole foods) is effective in reversing the insulin resistance seen in adult-onset diabetes. It contains starches (which require less insulin than simple sugars), high levels of fiber, a diverse array of natural antioxidants, and an increased proportion of omega-3 fatty acids, and the essential trace mineral chromium. Plus, it is devoid of agricultural chemicals and growth-promoting substances.[168]

Considerable experimental and epidemiological evidence indicates that chromium levels are a major determinant of insulin sensitivity.[169] Chromium, an essential micronutrient, functions as a cofactor in the glucose tolerance factor, which is required for insulin to activate cellular uptake of sugar. Chromium deficiency is widespread in the U.S. due to modern agricultural techniques and the consumption of refined foods. Supplemental chromium has been shown to significantly improve glucose tolerance; decrease fasting glucose, cholesterol, and triglyceride levels; and increase HDL cholesterol by increasing insulin sensitivity.[170] Chromium is available in yeast (1 tbl twice a day) or as a supplement (200 to 400 mcg a day). Chromium is not, however, by itself a panacea for diabetes.

Disturbances in the metabolism of the essential omega-6 fatty acids is a key factor for many of the damaging effects of diabetes.[171] Examination of the blood of diabetics has shown that they are deficient in DGLA (di-homogammalinolenic acid). (See Chapter Six for more discussion of the metabolism of essential fatty acids.) This deficiency makes the tissues less responsive to insulin, decreases the levels of the anti-inflammatory prostaglandins PGE1, and increases the inflammatory thromboxanes. This results in spontaneous blood clots and arterial contractions, which cause a local decrease in blood supply. This in turn decreases availability of oxygen and other nutrients for the nerves and other tissues. Over time, the result is death of the nerves and local tissue damage.

Fortunately, supplementing with essential fatty acids helps. In rats with chemically induced diabetes, nerve function could be returned to normal after ten days of supplementation with evening primrose oil that contained 9% GLA.[172] This research has now been reproduced in humans.

In one double-blind trial, 22 patients with confirmed diabetic neuropathy received 4 gm of evening primrose oil (containing 360 mg of GLA) or placebo daily. After six months, the group taking evening primrose oil showed a significant improvement in nerve function, as well as normalization of heat and cold sensitivity, numbness, pain, weakness, and paresthesias (loss of sensitivity).[173] Interestingly, there was no improvement in blood sugar regulation; the benefits were due to local effects on the nerves.

Daily vitamin C supplementation has also been found useful for treating adult-onset diabetes. This important nutrient improved protection against oxidative stress and decreased fasting plasma insulin (remember those with this type of diabetes have too much insulin since their tissues don't respond to insulin like they should), glycosylated hemoglobin (a measure of the average blood sugar levels), total cholesterol, and LDL cholesterol.[174] The dosage was a modest 500 mg twice a day.

Herbal help for diabetes

Many herbs have been used through the centuries to improve blood sugar regulation and alleviate the side effects of diabetes. Fenugreek seeds, *Aloe vera*, and onions and garlic are especially helpful in normalizing blood sugar and insulin levels.

Fenugreek seeds (Trigonella foenum graecum)   Shown to reduce fasting and postprandial (after a meal) blood sugar levels in both juvenile and adult-onset diabetic patients, this herb appears to work by improving cell sensitivity to insulin.[175] Twenty five grams of fenugreek seed a day does the job, decreasing the spilling of sugar in the urine by 53% in juvenile diabetics. Apparently both natural and defatted and debitterized forms work, and although the natural form may be more effective, the processed forms are easier to eat.

Aloe vera   Adding ½ tsp daily of dried *Aloe vera* sap to the diet of adult-onset diabetics in one study dramatically reduced their mean blood glucose levels from 273 to 151 mg/dl.[176] Animal research suggests that *Aloe vera* works by stimulating increased synthesis of insulin.

Onions and garlic   These foods help to normalize blood sugar regulation. The sulfur-containing compounds in onions (*Allium cepa*) and garlic (*Allium sativum*) appear to work by decreasing the rate of elimination of insulin by the liver.[177] One to seven ounces of onions (either raw or boiled) resulted in a substantial drop in blood sugar levels.[178]

■ *Dosages:* ½ oz of fenugreek seeds and ½ clove of garlic twice a day

Osteoarthritis

Osteoarthritis develops because of an imbalance between damage and regeneration. As mentioned above, the conventional medical treatment actually increases the rate of progression of the disease in the name of relieving the symptoms. Naturopathic treatment, on the other hand, uses several nutrients to help stimulate regeneration of the joint cartilage.

Glucosamine sulfate is an especially effective therapy for osteoarthritis; it significantly enhances cartilage regeneration. It is very effectively absorbed by the body; in one study, 90% of a radio-labeled dose entered the blood supply as glucosamine. It reaches a peak after eight to ten hours and has a half life of 70 hours, meaning it stays in the body a long time, becoming part of normal tissue. It diffuses from the blood into the bones and articular tissue.[179] Glucosamine's most important role in treating osteoarthritis is in increasing the ability of cartilage to synthesize both sulfated mucopolysaccharides and protein. This helps restore the balance between cartilage erosion and regeneration.

These metabolic effects show up clinically in good results. In a typical example of several clinical trials, 40 patients with osteoarthritis of the knee compared the efficacy of 1.5 gm of glucosamine sulfate with 1.2 grams of ibuprofen daily, using a double-blind protocol. Pain scores decreased faster during the first two weeks in the ibuprofen group than the glucosamine-treated group. However, by week eight, the glucosamine-treated patients reported a lower pain score.[180] Other studies have shown that the pain relief continues for weeks after the supplementation with glucosamine sulfate is discontinued. Adverse reactions are very rare.

- *Dosage:* 500 mg glucosamine sulfate three times a day

Depression

Depression is a common problem as people age. Because it is usually due to diminishing brain function, the best approach is to improve function of the brain and nervous system as discussed above. Several herbs have been shown to gently and safely elevate mood.

St. John's wort (*Hypericum perforatum*)

One of the best herbs for mood elevation is St. John's wort. It is a remarkable healing herb, which has been used to treat a variety of ailments for over 2,000 years. It has been used to treat bed wetting, wound healing, diarrhea, stomach upset, and burns, but perhaps its most important use is to alleviate depression. In one typical study, 105 patients with mild-to-moderate depression of short duration were given 300 mg of St. John's wort three times a day or a placebo over a four-week period; 67% of the St. John's wort group demonstrated improvement in their symptoms (sadness, hopelessness, helplessness, worthlessness, exhaustion, headache, and poor sleep) with no reported side effects.[181]

Twenty-eight controlled studies in Europe treated approximately 1,500 depressed patients with consistently positive results in mild-to-moderate depression. However, St. John's wort is probably not effective in severe cases, including those with psychotic symptoms and in those where the depression is associated with an increased suicide risk.

Hypericum extract, the most active constituent in St. John's wort, was compared to the synthetic antidepressant Maprotilin in 102 patients suffering from depression. The sum score on the Hamilton Depression Scale fell about 50% for both groups after four weeks. While the patients taking Maprotilin suffered side effects such as tiredness, dry mouth, and heart problems, the *Hypericum* patients reported no side effects.

Another multi-center, randomized, double-blind study compared the efficacy of *Hypericum* extract (300 mg three times a day) with the antidepressant Imipramin (25 mg three times a day). After six weeks, both showed comparable clinical efficacy.[182]

Hypericin is the pigment that gives its flowers their characteristic red color. It appears to work as a monoamine oxidase (MAO) inhibitor. MAO is an enzyme responsible for breaking down the brain chemicals serotonin and norepinephrine. Blocking the breakdown of these brain neuropeptides probably accounts for its anti-depressive effects. Although St. John's wort is not as powerful as prescription MAO inhibitors, the same types of precautions need to be followed. Those using full dosages of St. John's wort should avoid foods high in tyramine (e.g., smoked or pickled foods), and alcoholic beverages (beer and wine). Those taking tryptophan, tyrosine, cold and hay fever remedies, amphetamines, and narcotics should not use St. John's wort. Use of *Hypericum* with these might cause a rapid and dangerous elevation in blood pressure.

- *Dosage:* depression that makes you unable to live your life normally requires the attention of a physician. If you are not taking an MAO inhibitor, take 300 mg of *Hypericum* twice a day and avoid smoked or pickled food and alcoholic beverages.

Ginkgo biloba

Ginkgo's ability to increase blood supply to the brain, decrease the effects of oxidizing chemicals on the brain, and improve mental function are all useful in treating depression. A randomized, placebo-controlled, double-blind study of 40 patients aged 51 to 78 years evaluated how well gingko would work for those suffering from mild-to-moderate cerebral dysfunction combined with depressive episodes and who had not responded well to treatment with tri- and tricyclic antidepressants.

During the study, the patients continued using their antidepressant drugs. After four weeks, the Hamilton Depression Scale of the resistant patients taking ginkgo decreased from 14 to 7. After eight weeks, it declined further to 4.5. By contrast, the placebo group showed little change. These outstanding results show that drugs and herbs can work effectively together. The patients even showed a significant improvement in cognitive function. Probably the antidepressant drugs were not able to get high enough concentrations to the brain, which is why the gingko's enhancement of blood flow to the brain helped.[183]

Not only has ginkgo been found beneficial in treating the resistant depression found in patients with cerebrovascular insufficiency and early senile dementia, it even helps mental function in those with brain injuries.[184] In a comparative double-blind study, treatment with *Ginkgo biloba* extract (80 mg twice a day) was compared to placebo in elderly subjects with senile dementia of atherosclerotic origin. After six weeks, the treated patients showed less depression, apathy, irritability, hostility, and fatigue.[185]

- *Dosage:* 80 mg *Ginkgo biloba* extract three times a day

Sexual Dysfunction

As men get older, achieving an erection becomes progressively more difficult, a condition known as erectile impotence or erectile dysfunction. Fortunately, as seen in Table 9-8, most of the causes are known and controllable.

Table 9-8 Causes of Erectile Dysfunction

Physical (85%)	Drugs (e.g., alcohol, antihistamines, anti-hypertensives, anti-cholinergics, antidepressants, anti-psychotics, tobacco, tranquilizers, etc.)
	Endocrine disorders (e.g., diabetes, hypothyroidism, low testosterone levels, elevated prolactin levels, elevated estrogen levels)
	Atherosclerosis
	Neurological disorders (e.g., multiple sclerosis)
	Other (e.g., pelvic surgery or trauma, vascular abnormalities)
Psychological (10%)	Depression
	Performance anxiety
	Stress
Unknown (5%)	

Most often, erection problems are due to poor blood supply to the penis. In fact, atherosclerosis of the penile artery is the primary cause of impotence in about half of men over the age of 50 with erection problems.[186] In addition, many of the other causes noted in Table 9-8. produce impotence by inhibiting proper blood flow to the penis. Many things can be done to prevent or correct these problems, probably the most important of which is reversing the atherosclerosis and using herbs to improve the blood supply.

Just as *Ginkgo biloba* improves blood supply to the brain of the elderly, it also improves blood supply to the penis. In one study, fifty men with proven arterial erectile impotence were treated with 240 mg of *Ginkgo biloba* extract daily for nine months. They were divided into two groups: those who could achieve an erection when a drug combination (papaverine and phentolamine) was injected into their penis and those who did not respond to the injection. In the first group, all patients regained spontaneous and sufficient erections after six months. What made this study and the results so special is that both subjective and objective data was gathered. In the first group, not only did they regain normal sexual function, but they also experienced an objective increase in blood supply to the penis indicating a reversal of the underlying pathology of the diseased arteries. In the second group, erectile function was regained in two-thirds when GBE was combined with penile injection of prostaglandin PGE1 (whose formation in the body is supported by essential fatty acids). No side effects were noted during treatment.[187]

Beneficial results have also been shown in men with proven arterial erectile dysfunction who did not react to papaverine injections. In this study, 50% of 60 such men regained potency after six months of receiving 60 mg of GBE daily, with the first signs of response surfacing after six to eight weeks.[188]

While the herbs yohimbine (from the bark of *Pausinystalia johimbe*) and muria puama (*Ptychopetalum olacoides*) have received more popular press for sexual dysfunction, these herbs are not as effective clinically as gingko and can have significant side effects. For example, yohimbine can cause anxiety, panic attacks, elevated blood pressure, excessive heart rate, and headaches. It is especially contraindicated for those with kidney disease and a history of psychological disorders. Muria puama has received little research attention, so its potential negative side effects are unknown.

(Women should refer to Chapter Eight for advice on maintaining sexual function.)

Benign Prostatic Hyperplasia (BPH)

The incidence of benign prostatic hyperplasia is estimated at 50 to 60% of men between 40 and 59 years of age. The projected annual overall cost of hospital care and surgery for BPH is over $1 billion in the U.S. alone. I have successfully treated many men with chronic enlargement of their prostate with nutrition and herbs.

Zinc

Paramount to effective treatment of BPH is adequate zinc intake and absorption. Zinc deficiency becomes more prevalent with age and supplementation has been shown to reduce the size of the enlarged prostate and to reduce symptomatology in the majority of patients.[189] The clinical efficacy of zinc is probably due to its critical involvement in many aspects of androgen (male hormone) metabolism. One of the actions of zinc is to inhibit the activity of 5-alpha-reductase, the enzyme that converts testosterone to dihydrotestosterone.[190] This form of testosterone is toxic to the prostate and contributes to the chronic swelling.

Essential fatty acids

Essential fatty acids are also crucial for proper functioning of the prostate. The administration of essential fatty acids results in significant improvement for many BPH patients. All 19 subjects in an uncontrolled study showed diminution of residual urine, with 12 of the 19 having no residual urine by the end of several weeks of treatment.[191] These effects appear to be due to the correction of an underlying essential fatty acid deficiency, because these patients' prostatic and seminal lipid levels and ratios are often abnormal.[192]

Cernilton

One product I have found especially effective is an extract from flower pollen with the commercial name, Cernilton. Controlled clinical trials have documented its efficacy in treating BPH in men without such complications as urethral stricture, prostatic stones, and bladder neck sclerosis. For example, in

Correcting BPH Naturopathically

Jonathan was 50 years old and having trouble urinating and waking at night to urinate. He had a chronic feeling of fullness in his rectum and a declining interest in sex. As usual in our society, it was his wife Adrian who dragged him into my office. His diet was typically American, i.e., pretty poor. However, he was in surprisingly good physical condition although my physical exam revealed the expected enlarged prostate.

His therapy was straightforward: zinc picolinate (40 mg per day), flax seed oil (1 tbl twice a day) and the herb saw palmetto (320 mg per day of the standardized liposterolic extract). He didn't notice any change for six weeks. After that he noticed progressively less trouble urinating. After three months, he no longer had to get up at night to urinate. At his wife's next regular checkup, she thanked me for his substantial increase in "marital activities."

- *The message:* Although benign prostatic hyperplasia is very common as men age, it is usually easily correctable with good nutrition and the appropriate herb to help speed the rejuvenating process.

one such study, one tablet three times a day was found to produce complete symptomatic relief in 36%, with an additional 42% improving significantly. As usual with most herbs, there were virtually no reported side effects.[193] Apparently, the flower pollen works by decreasing the inflammatory reactions in the prostate while also inhibiting microbes.

Saw palmetto *(Serenoa repens)*

Saw palmetto has been used for centuries for the treatment of BPH, first by Native Americans and later by European herbalists and naturopathic doctors. A considerable amount of research has documented its efficacy, even when compared to the leading drug, finasteride (Proscar). For example, in a large open trial with 505 men, after 90 days, 88% of the patients and attending physicians considered the saw palmetto therapy successful. Prostate symptoms, quality of life, urine flow rates, residual urinary volume, and prostate size all improved. The daily dose was 320 mg.[194] Typically, saw palmetto increased peak urine flow from 9.5 ml per second to 13.2 ml per second.

A recent double-blind study of 200 men with BPH found that 20 mg of a standardized phytoserolic extract of saw palmetto improved virtually every symptom.[195] Especially significant was that their peak urine flow increased from 9.9 ml per second to 15.2 ml per second. β-sitosterol apparently works by inhibiting the production of inflammatory prostaglandins in the prostate.

Summary

All of us say we want to live longer. But what we really mean is that we want to live healthy longer. There's not much point in living to a ripe old age if we are, well, overripe. I don't think many of us are interested in adding years of pain and disability to our lives and becoming a burden to our families. Fortunately, we can do much to ensure good health almost to the end of our lives. This requires that we keep all our parts working the way we need them to work and do everything we can to prevent damage and support continual rejuvenation. The basic approach is simple, avoid toxins and lifestyle behaviors that damage the organs we need for health, and utilize the key nutrients and herbs that strengthen them.

Now that you've finished this chapter, refer back to Chapter Five and work to eliminate general toxins and ensure that your detoxification systems are working optimally. Next, review this chapter (Nine) again to become fully aware of and committed to carefully avoiding the organ specific toxins that have been identified here. Finally, develop a nutritional supplementation program that provides general protection for all of your organs and additional specific protection where, based on family history or any dysfunction you've already developed, you need it the most. Now that you understand more about how your body works, you should find the list of the key nutrients and behaviors at the beginning of this chapter (p. 263) useful in preventing degeneration and promote rejuvenation.

Chapter Ten

Live in Harmony with the Psychosocial/Spiritual/Life-Force

You need to study this chapter if you suffer from any of the following:

- *Symptoms*
  Frequently feel overwhelmed by everything you are expected to do
  Find yourself furious when someone cuts you off in traffic or drives a
    bit too slowly
  Find your heart and mind still racing at night when you try to go to sleep
  Sleep poorly, yet wake up early unable to go back to sleep
  Get angry frequently
  Laugh infrequently
  Feel your life has little meaning, your existence serves no purpose
  Feel you have little control over your life, health, or well-being

- *Diseases*
  Cancer
  Chronic fatigue
  Depression
  High blood pressure
  Cardiovascular disease
  Insomnia
  Irritable bowel disease

Behaviors that increase risk:

- Fit the profile of the Type A personality: driven, irritable, perfectionistic
- Are constantly late because you've over-scheduled yourself

This chapter was primarily written by my wife Lara Pizzorno, M.A. As one of the first women graduating from Yale Divinity School in the 1970s, she has studied and written about the mind/body/spirit connection for two decades. I've added stories of patients from my practice that illustrate these important principles.

- Frequently eat on the run, in your car, while doing household chores—and get an upset stomach as a result
- Rarely relax and feel guilty when you do
- Have few or shallow friendships
- Feel there is no one to whom you can turn to for support
- Give your intimate relationships what's left of your energy after you've done everything else
- Don't exercise regularly
- Don't connect with nature in some regular way, e.g., gardening, walking, outdoor sports
- Dislike your work but are afraid to leave your job
- Have a pessimistic explanatory style, i.e., when something bad happens, you assume it's all your fault, will always be this way, and will spoil everything you do
- Don't have a commitment to something you consider a higher value
- Don't have a satisfying spiritual life

Thumbnail: Quick Help for Harmonizing the Life-Force
- Prioritize—then live according to your values
- Spend more time every day with your loved ones
- Take time to meditate or pray
- Develop a hobby that puts you in contact with nature
- Join a church, synagogue, or other group that provides spiritual and social support
- Exercise daily
- Focus on what you can be thankful for and give thanks daily
- Whenever you have the opportunity to be kind or helpful—grab it!

Since Descartes separated mind from body in the 17th century, Western conventional medicine has attempted to explain disease independently of mind, in terms of germs, environmental agents, or wayward genes. Today, however, scientists have begun to challenge this fundamental assumption and, as Bill Moyers' 1993 PBS television series, "Healing and the Mind," documented, we are in the midst of a medical revolution that puts mind firmly back into the health-or-disease equation. Jon Kabat-Zinn, Ph.D., director of the Stress Reduction Clinic and associate professor of Medicine at the University of Massachusetts Medical Center, sums up the shift in perspective:

> Over the past several hundred years, we've tended to look at disease as being more or less a function of the physical body, and to look at thoughts, feelings,

emotions, and social interactions as being in the domain of the mind . . . But as we begin looking at chronic illnesses like cancer and heart disease, which aren't infections, we see more and more evidence that how we live our lives and, in fact, how we think and feel over a lifetime can influence the kinds of illnesses that we have.[1]

Our beliefs, spiritual values, and family life have a profound impact on our physical health. Emotional imbalances, unhealthy beliefs, lack of meaning in life, and dysfunctional family life can fundamentally impair many of our body's healing processes.

The evidence is not just clinical observation, but chemical fact. An explosion of research in the new and rapidly expanding field of psychoneuroimmunology is revealing physical evidence of the mind/body connection that is changing our understanding of disease. Scientists no longer question whether our minds impact our health but are now researching the mechanisms of action through which our minds affect our bodies. The implications of the connections uncovered in just the last 20 years point toward a holistic health paradigm in which our potential for total wellness is exponentially increased.

Real-Life Messages from the Mind/Body

Mind As Slayer

Early in my practice, a 25-year-old nurse, Adrian, came to see me. She was obviously quite upset, breaking into tears as she related that her sister had just had her kidney removed, and she had the same condition. A few months before, her older sister had been found to have dangerously high blood pressure. Her medical workup revealed a rare, but serious, condition: renal artery stenosis.

A small number of women, aged 20 to 30, for no known reason (although it is more common in cigarette smokers), grow fibrous tissue around the large arteries supplying blood to their kidneys. This results in contraction of the arteries, causing a progressive decrease in blood supply to the kidneys—a serious problem because the kidneys play a major role in regulating blood pressure.

Normally, when blood pressure drops too low, the kidneys receive too little oxygen. This causes them to secrete the enzyme renin, which activates a polypeptide called angiotensin. Its activation results in constriction of the blood vessels, stimulation of the adrenals to secrete a hormone (aldosterone), which promotes the reabsorption of salt and water by the kidneys, and increased strength of contraction of the heart. The end result is an increase in the amount of blood in the body and elevation of blood pressure. More blood flows to the kidneys (as well as the rest of the body) relieving their hypoxia. Normally, this system works effectively, maintaining our blood pressure in a range that ensures proper functioning of the organs of the body. However, for these patients, the system is deranged. In order for the kidneys to have an adequate supply of blood, the rest of the body has to have too much. The result is an elevation of blood pressure, often to dangerously high levels. Unfortunately, this condition is relentlessly progressive and thought to be hereditary. The primary method of treatment is major surgery to either remove the kidney with the damaged artery or to transplant a major artery from another organ to the kidney. Adrian's sister had her kidney removed.

After her sister's operation (which was successful), Adrian went to her family doctor, who found her blood pressure to also be greatly elevated, just like her sister's. He advised her that she had the same condition and would need to be scheduled for surgery before her kidney was too badly damaged to be saved. Distraught, she decided to seek a second opinion.

Looking at her, I was surprised to hear of her problem; she appeared quite healthy and a few questions revealed a healthy lifestyle. But physical examination did indeed show a significantly elevated blood pressure.

Twenty years ago, the best way of diagnosing renal artery stenosis was by placing a stethoscope on the abdomen over the kidneys and listening for a sound described as a *bruit*, and by measuring the amount of renin in the blood and/or the amount of aldosterone in the urine. Despite careful listening over her kidneys, I could not hear a bruit. However, as only about 50% of those with renal artery stenosis have a bruit, I decided to perform the expensive test on her urine. A few days later, she brought in the urine that she had collected over a 24-hour period. I again took her blood pressure, just to be sure—it was still very high.

Her urine test came back normal.

While the urine test wasn't perfectly reliable, the probability of both the physical and the laboratory exams providing false negatives was pretty small. This caused me to consider other causes of her hypertension.

While a student, I had been quite interested in the research documenting the remarkable impact of belief and stress on many aspects of health. In particular, I had been greatly influenced by the work of Hans Selye, M.D., whose book, *Stress of Life*, I continue to recommend to students. Hypertension is one of the conditions commonly caused by fear and stress.

I invited Adrian back to my office and gave her the results and my interpretation that her fear and stress were the real causes of her high blood pressure, not renal artery stenosis. I'll never forget the sudden look of surprise and then relief that crossed her face as the meaning of my words sank in. I recommended that she read Selye's book and referred her to a counselor friend of mine for a stress reduction program. Within a week, her blood pressure was back to normal. Over the ensuing several months, I regularly checked her blood pressure, and it continued to remain normal.

- *The message:* Fear and an out-of-control imagination can seriously damage our health.

Mind As Healer

When my daughter Raven was seven years old, she started developing warts on her fingers. Over the ensuing year, her warts not only continued to grow in size and number on her hands, but also started to affect her face. I realized it was time to treat her. I had her apply thuja oil to her warts each day, an age-old naturopathic therapy that I've used successfully with many patients. Imagine my surprise when after a month not only had her warts not improved, they had actually spread! I then hit the books, asked for advice from some of my colleagues, and had her try a different herb, a thick, dark-brown extract. After a month of use, we had permanently stained several sheets and pillowcases, but my poor daughter's warts were even worse. In fact, she now had the worst case I had ever seen. With great reluctance and embarrassment, we had her see a medical doctor to have them frozen off with liquid nitrogen—a painful but effective treatment. It took several treatments to get them all. A month later, not only had they all come back, but they were worse than ever! Over the ensuing year, her warts were frozen off several times but kept returning, looking worse each time.

Finally, in desperation, we referred Raven to a hypnotist to teach her self-hypnosis and visualization. Raven, always a very determined girl, did her visualizations faithfully for ten minutes every night. After two months, all her warts were gone. Even now, ten years later, she has never again had to suffer from the unsightly condition.

In her own words, here's what she did:

> I began by staring upward and closing my eyes. I concentrated solely on my breathing, blocking everything else from my mind. I visualized numbers, starting with a "1," then putting a "2" beside it, then a "3," and so on up to as many numbers as I could see at the same time. I then imagined doing a favorite thing, to help me relax as much as possible and to be happy. I then imagined myself starting at the fifth level of an elevator and sinking deeper into my mind with every level the elevator descends. In this deep meditative state, I visualized my immune system attacking the warts. I imagined medieval weapons chopping the warts to pieces. After the visualization, I ascended in the elevator and at the top, opened my eyes.

- *The message:* The mind has a tremendous ability to heal, especially when we help it along.

How the Mind/Body Connection Works

Research has discovered that the brain and body communicate using a flood of chemical messengers that hook up to receptors on the surface membranes of our cells, and that our very thoughts, moods, and attitudes have a significant impact on which chemical messengers are sent and how they are received. Candace Pert, Ph.D., former chief of Brain Biochemistry at the NIH, whose landmark discovery of opiate receptors in the brain led to an understanding of how neuropeptide messengers link brain and body, calls them, "the biochemical correlates of emotion," because their composition and activity are directly dependent on our states of mind. These neurotransmitters translate our every fleeting thought, reaction, and emotion—conscious or unconscious—into physiological changes. They're found not just in the brain but in the immune system, endocrine system, heart, lungs, intestines—in short, everywhere. The more we know about these messenger molecules, the more evident it becomes that we are not a mind in a machine but a single integrated entity; these peptides constitute a "psychosomatic communication network" in which the mind is literally spread throughout the body.[2]

Body and Mind Are One

By causing the release of neuropeptides, which communicate directly with every cell in our bodies, our moods and attitudes become incarnate. Body and mind are two manifestations of the same process. Feelings and thoughts seem intangible but produce a cascade of changes in the body, generating messenger molecules that direct every cellular action, telling each of our cells when to divide, which genes to turn on and when, to make more of this protein or less of that one. In other words, karma has a chemical basis. We are not only what we eat, but what we think.

Mind/body medicine, however, asserts that what goes on in our heads is only a co-factor in determining our health; a person should not be blamed for "causing" his or her own illness. Recognizing that we are an integrated mind/body in which all parts constantly interact simply acknowledges that our susceptibility to disease is determined by multiple factors, not dictated by single agents beyond our control, such as genes or germs. What the mind/body model urges is that the mind's input should not be ignored, but utilized. While we are just beginning to learn what causes the brain to turn off and on our internal healing systems, the tantalizing prospect is that we can learn to use our minds to promote our physical as well as mental health.

That hopes of using the mind as healer are realistic is demonstrated by research showing that the brain and the immune system are in constant dialogue. A recent study at UCLA found that the experience of intense emotions affects immune activity. Margaret Kemeny, Ph.D., assistant professor of Psychiatry and Biobehavioral Sciences at UCLA, asked actors and actresses to think about various scenarios. The experience of intense happy or sad feelings caused an increase in natural killer cells in their bloodstream—cells produced by the immune system as a first line of defense—within 20 minutes.[3] Another study lead by Kemeny found that among 36 people with genital herpes, those who were depressed experienced more recurrences of symptoms and had significantly lower levels of suppressor cytotoxic T cells. Depression, stress, anxiety, hostility, fatigue—all were found to reliably predict poorer suppressor T cell function.[4]

David Felten, M.D., Ph.D., professor of Neurobiology and Anatomy at the University School of Rochester and his wife, Susan Felten, Ph.D., have shown that, in addition to neuropeptides, our immune systems are wired to our nervous systems via nerve fibers going into virtually every immune system organ and forming direct contacts with immune system cells. Their research provides significant evidence that the brain generates signals which influence hormonal outflow and that hormones and neurotransmitters influence activities of the immune system. They've also discovered that it's not a one-way street—products of the immune system also influence the brain. That is, the way we choose to react to the experiences of our daily lives is instantaneously registered by the autonomic nervous system and telegraphed to the brain where it affects—for good or for ill—our immune system's effectiveness.[5] Dr. Robert Ader has demonstrated the healing potential of this connection in experiments based on classic conditioning techniques, in which rats with overactive immune responses (in humans, such responses can lead to autoimmune diseases such as arthritis) learned to suppress their own immune systems.[6]

Not only have researchers discovered that neuropeptides carry messages capable of suppressing the immune system, but they have also discovered that insufficient amounts of various neuropeptides can render us more susceptible to disease. "Viruses use the same receptors as neuropeptides to enter into a cell," explains Dr. Pert, "so depending how much of the natural peptide for that receptor is around, the virus will have an easier time or a harder time getting into the cell." What this means is that our emotional state can affect our susceptibility to becoming sick from the same dose of a virus. Even the HIV virus uses a receptor normally used by a neuropeptide, and AIDS statistics graphically illustrate our wide range of susceptibility. By 1985, the blood test that screens for antibodies against the HIV virus showed that approximately 2 million people had been infected, but by 1987, only some 30,000 of these had been diagnosed as having developed AIDS. It has been estimated that for every living adult with AIDS, there are from 100 to 300 infected, antibody-positive people with no disease.[7] Are emotions and beliefs the reason some develop AIDS rapidly after infection, while others are asymptomatic for years?

To underscore the importance of cognitive and emotional factors in the onset of viral diseases, John Mason, Ph.D., an endocrinologist and stress researcher at Yale Medical School, points to the fact that, for decades, biological scientists have observed that most of the microbes that infect humans are already in our bodies and instigate a disease process only when other factors lower our immunity. Mason notes, "It is common, in fact, for many pathogenic microorganisms to be harbored within hosts without producing disease or illness. A complex assemblage of intervening 'host resistance' machinery has a major role in determining whether infection will progress into illness or not."[8] Even Louis Pasteur, father of the germ theory, recognized that "internal causes" (how people react to life and their environment) can be more decisive than a germ. On his deathbed, he remarked, "Le germe n'est rien; c'est le terrain qui est tout" (The microbe is nothing, the soil is everything).[9] In short, no microbe, germ, or virus, no pathogen is, by itself, sufficient cause for the onset of disease, but merely an agent capable of inducing specific symptoms in a susceptible host.

Our Thoughts Affect Our Health

A series of studies have shown that when groups of people are exposed to the same conditions and environments, not everyone gets sick. How resistant we are is definitely affected by how we look at problems—our "cognitive appraisal." The messenger molecules our thoughts produce orchestrate chemical changes in our central nervous system and immune defenses. For twenty years, Lawrence Hinkle, Ph.D., of Cornell Medical College in New York, directed studies of the illness patterns of more than 3,500 people divided into five groups, each of which shared the same environments and work conditions.[10] One-fourth of the individuals experienced more than half of the illnesses and over two-thirds of the total days of disability. One group was composed of 1,297 telephone operators, some of whom were frequently ill while others were seldom sick. Researchers found that the frequently ill individuals were more dissatisfied and discontented in general. Episodes of illness typically occurred in clusters when the person had conflicts with family, felt threats to status, loss of support, or excessive demands from others. Another group was composed of 139 managerial employees in a corporation. Again, although alike in age, sex, occupation, income, social and economic status, diet, and hereditary backgrounds, some managers were frequently ill and others rarely. Those often ill were usually high school graduates who had become managers without having gone to college. They habitually perceived more threats and challenges and smoked more, possibly to relieve the perceived stress in their lives, than those in the healthy group (who were generally college graduates).[11]

How We Handle Stress

Stress, like germs, has typically been thought of as a powerful external agent before which we are hapless victims, but research has shown that stress per se does not produce disease. After fifty years of researching stress, Hans Selye, the father of stress theory, concluded that it is not the stressors in our lives, but the way we react to them that counts. In his book, *Stress of Life*, Selye makes the point with a hypothetical example: What happens if you pass a helpless drunk who verbally insults you? If you ignore the abuse, you're not likely to experience any physiological ill effects, but if you let it anger you, "You will discharge adrenalines that increase blood pressure and pulse rate, while your whole nervous system becomes alarmed and tense in anticipation of combat. If you happen to be a coronary candidate, the result may be a fatal heart attack." What caused your death? The drunk? His insults? No, Selye explains, "Death was caused by choosing the wrong reaction."[12]

A team of behavioral scientists at the University of Chicago led by Suzanne Kobasa, Ph.D., and Salvatore Maddi, Ph.D., tested the popular theory that high stress equals high risk of illness from a new perspective—they tracked a group of 200 business executives at Illinois Bell Telephone Company during the AT&T divestiture to focus not on who got sick, but who didn't. Half the executives reported many symptoms, while the other 100 had few. The healthy executives were found to have a fundamentally different way of looking at and dealing with stress than those who got sick. The healthy managers saw change as inevitable and an opportunity for growth rather than a threat to security.

When confronted with problems, instead of being overwhelmed or seeing them as insurmountable, their habitual reaction was what Kobasa and Maddi dubbed "optimistic cognitive appraisal," a coping strategy that gave them a sense of inner control. In addition, they were deeply involved in their work and families, and their commitment gave them a sense of meaning, direction, and enthusiasm. Executives who had what Kobasa and Maddi described as three "resistance resources"—psychological hardiness (a sense of control, challenge, and commitment); social support; and regular exercise—had a less than one in ten chance of suffering a severe illness in the near future. In contrast, among the high-stress managers who had neither psychological hardiness nor support and didn't exercise, the probability of severe illness was higher than nine chances in ten.[13]

Richard Rahe, co-developer of the Social Readjustment Rating Scale—the checklist widely used to measure stress—conducted studies of Navy recruits at the Naval Health Research Center in San Diego, which also showed that stress does not automatically equal distress. Neither the number nor severity of stressful events could account for whether an individual became sick. The crucial factor was the meaning the person attached to the events. Cholesterol levels rose sharply only in those recruits who saw training as onerous, depressing and likely to end in failure. Those who found training challenging, even if somewhat frightening, experienced no rise in cholesterol.[14]

A study of air traffic controllers, an occupation noted for severe stress, also found that attitude, not amount of stress, was the determining factor in who got sick. C. David Jenkins, Ph.D., professor of Preventive Medicine and Community Health at the University of Texas, Galveston, headed the 27-month study. Participants were evaluated initially and every nine months thereafter. Unlike most studies, which analyze the frequency of illness after the fact, Jenkins's researchers plotted predictive data based on the assumption that Type A personalities—competitive, aggressive, easily angered, always in a hurry, and in a constant struggle against time and the environment—would be sick more often.

They were—Type As had three times the minor illnesses and injuries than the more relaxed Type Bs. Hypertension, a disease known to plague air traffic controllers, was not related to how much stress an individual experienced, but how he or she handled it. People who expressed it, let it out, and tried to do something about it, did not develop high blood pressure. Those who denied feeling stressed and claimed, "Everything is great. I'm stress-free," were the ones most likely to develop hypertension. Jenkins also discovered a protective factor: competence. Men picked by their peers as the most effective in their work did not get sick.[15]

People who are cynical or have hostile attitudes or suppressed anger have also been found to have more atherosclerosis and blockage of coronary arteries and to be more likely to have heart attacks.[16] A 25-year study of 255 physicians, who took a battery of psychological tests while at the University of

North Carolina Medical School, revealed that those with higher hostility scores had four times greater incidence of heart disease and six times the mortality than the rest of the group.[17]

Just as our cardiovascular and immune systems can be compromised by perceptions of chronic stress, another line of defense on the molecular level can also be affected. Researchers at Ohio State University College of Medicine and Comprehensive Cancer Center have reported impaired DNA repair in highly distressed people who have difficulty coping.[18] The DNA repair system is a basic line of defense against cancer. When cells are damaged by free radicals, chemicals, or radiation, the DNA repair system—if it's not compromised—keeps mutations from occurring and tumors from developing.

Our Mental States Affect the Foods We Crave

Another way in which our mental state may render us more susceptible to cancer is in its effect on our food choices. Research shows that the kind of mental or emotional state we are in, how confident or uncertain we are about coping with the problems we face, can determine which foods we seek. People who are anxious, depressed, or under chronic stress often crave sweets or high-fat junk food. Such foods increase brain levels of serotonin, a hormone that causes a temporary calming, satisfying feeling. Most antidepressant drugs work by elevating serotonin levels, so what we are doing when we turn to junk food for comfort is "self-medicating."[19] However, when junk foods are habitually eaten and crowd out cancer-protective foods such as whole grains, fresh vegetables, and fruits, our immune system's ability to prevent cancer may be compromised.

Pessimistic Thought Patterns Can Be Dangerous

A person's habitual explanatory style can significantly impact his or her ability to resist disease. When a problem crops up or an unfortunate incident occurs, a person with a pessimistic explanatory style immediately internalizes all the blame, then assumes the negative outcome can never be changed, and finally expands the negative effect to everything else. The thought pattern runs: "It's all my fault (internal attribution), will always be this way (stable attribution), and will spoil everything (global attribution)." A healthier causal style, while not absolving oneself of all responsibility, is more realistic and balanced, takes into account external factors—other people, outside circumstances beyond one's control—and recognizes that one negative event does not dictate that all future events will turn out badly.

In research at the University of Pennsylvania, psychologist Martin Seligman and his colleagues were able to predict who among a group of 172 undergraduates would become depressed, sick, or fail at a job, both one month and one year later, simply by evaluating their tendency to make internal-stable-global (ISG) attributions. In a group of 13 patients with malignant melanomas, this pessimistic explanatory style was a more powerful predictor of mortality than even the patient's level of natural killer cell activity.[20]

The mind/body studies consistently show that when we cope effectively with stressful situations, we lessen their power to do us damage. Effective coping consists of: (1) optimistic appraisal (viewing problems with more pragmatism and less pessimism), (2) taking some action to change the external problem, if change is possible, and (3) palliating the problem's physical and mental effects by exercise, relaxation training, or some other health-promoting behavior, such as the mind/body techniques discussed below.

How the Mind Can Heal

Although most of the mind/body research so far has been focused on disease-producing mechanisms, scientists are now beginning to study the alteration in neurotransmitters that occurs when we feel positive thoughts—love, compassion, peace, courage, commitment, faith, hope. Just as angry, hostile thoughts bring about physiological changes, positive thoughts produce corresponding changes via the different composition of neurotransmitters and hormones generated. Negative thoughts suppress the immune system; positive thoughts stimulate it. Hostile, angry thoughts damage the cardiovascular system; peaceful, loving thoughts soothe and strengthen it.

In studies at Harvard, when psychologist David McClelland showed students a film of Mother Theresa, the nun who won the Nobel Peace Prize for her work caring for the poor on the streets of Calcutta, the students' salivary IgA (an antibody that is part of the immune system's first line of defense against colds and upper respiratory infection) increased. Even students who scoffed at Mother Theresa and claimed she was a fake showed enhanced immune function. Conversely, when the students were shown a film of Attila the Hun, their antibody levels dropped. The data supported McClelland's theory that we respond to love and caring on a deep, unconscious level even when our conscious thoughts are neutral or negative. McClelland also found that people with high scores on tests evaluating their capacity for intimacy have generally higher levels of IgA antibodies.[21]

In a five-year prospective study, researchers at Tel Aviv University followed almost 10,000 men diagnosed as being at high risk for heart disease. Researchers in the Israel Ischemic Heart Disease Study were surprised to find that the most predictive factor in the men's risk of developing angina pectoris was neither hypertension nor high cholesterol, but whether they felt loved and supported by their wives. Those whose marital satisfaction was high were nearly two times less likely to develop angina pectoris than the men without such support.[22]

In Roseto, Pennsylvania, a closely knit community of Italian Americans, heart disease rates were dramatically lower than in the rest of the United States—despite their high-fat diet. As the younger generations moved away and ties weakened, however, their heart disease rates quickly escalated to national norms.[23]

Numerous statistics from a nine-year study that tracked the health of thousands of people living in Alameda County, California, suggest that a loving and supportive family and a feeling of belonging to a wider community favorably impact both health and longevity. People in Alameda County with a variety of social ties—marriage, contact with relatives, belonging to religious and other groups—had much lower mortality rates.[24] Middle-aged men with inadequate income but an abundance of social support lived longer than affluent men with few social ties. Socially isolated women had a significantly higher risk of dying of cancer.[25]

When social contact is increased or loneliness reduced, the immune system seems to strengthen. A group of 30 elderly people in retirement homes showed increased immune competence in terms of both natural killer cells and antibodies after being visited three times a week for a month.[26] In a study of 38 married women, researchers at Ohio State University College of Medicine found that a good marriage was significantly associated with better immune function, including the percentage of helper T cells and ratio of helper to suppressor lymphocytes.[27]

Pets as well as people can provide the love and companionship that improves our health. The survival rates of persons who have experienced heart attacks are higher for those who have pets waiting for them at home. Hospitalized patients (including those in mental hospitals) with pets tend to recover faster and go home sooner. In people with hypertension, the presence of a pet has been shown to significantly lower blood pressure.[28]

Accessing the Healing Forces Within

According to James Gordon, M.D., director of the Center for Mind-Body Medicine, Washington, D.C., chair of the Program Advisory Council to NIH's Office of Alternative Medicine:

> Once you have taken seriously the fact that your attitudes do affect your health, the first thing you must do to use your mind as healer is to figure out what's stressing you. It's definitely possible to know what distresses you and why. Some people find keeping a journal effective; others use art, drawing pictures for insight. Others just sit and let the ideas come. For some, dialogue with a therapist is most helpful. In my opinion, such a dialogue is the first job of any physician, using the Socratic method to try to figure out what's going on. If your physician cannot help you find out, look for a doctor who can.[29]

Harmon Bro, Ph.D., formerly of Harvard Divinity School and a practicing Jungian therapist for more than 50 years, also believes a self-inventory is the first step in using the mind to promote not only physical but spiritual health. Bro asks his clients four simple, but very powerful questions in relation to the

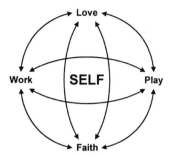

Figure 10-1 Each Aspect of Our Self Is Connected

four primary areas of human life: work, play, love, and faith.[30] As Figure 10-1 indicates, each of the four areas affects each of the others and the development of the self. The health of the mind/body and the spirit is shaped by what you do and how you do it. The four questions to consider in each area are:

1. What are you doing in this area of your life? What actions are you taking?
2. How are you doing it? What is your attitude, your style? Are you driving yourself, filled with anxiety, constantly proving yourself? Or are you acting in this area with confidence, charity, hope, and trust? Are you optimistic or pessimistic?
3. What are your ends, goals, or purposes in this area? What value(s) do you believe each area creates and sustains?
4. How do you see yourself progressing in each area? How is your growth, maturity, independence of self, and feeling of community in relation to each area?

Therapeutic Mind/Body Techniques

Once you have completed a self-inventory and have some idea of what's stressing you, think about how to address it. A significant amount of research shows that it is possible to change our attitudes, our causal styles, and reduce stress. Regular exercise has long been recognized as an excellent stress reducer, and therapeutic techniques such as biofeedback and meditation have been proven effective. Which approach you choose has more to do with who you are and what works for you. For example, workaholics might prefer exercise to meditation, while someone who likes high-tech gadgets might find biofeedback, which uses equipment to monitor bodily responses, most appealing. Carol Goldberg, assistant director of the Center for Mind-Body Medicine, explains, "Everything is not right for everyone. If one approach doesn't work, try another. Also, if meditation appeals to you but you just won't take 20 to 30 minutes twice a day, try just 5 minutes. You'll still receive some benefits and may be encouraged to devote more time later."[31]

Biofeedback

Biofeedback training teaches a person how to consciously influence body functions that are normally unconscious (e.g., breathing, heart rate, blood pressure, muscle tension, and skin temperature). A device is placed on the patient's skin that monitors the bodily function he or she is learning to control and reports its status with sounds or a blinking light. Using techniques such as visualization, meditation, or relaxation, the patient learns to control the function with progress confirmed by changes in the frequency of sounds or flashes. Biofeedback has been found effective in the treatment of stress and stress-related disorders including insomnia, TMJ, migraines, asthma, gastrointestinal disorders, hypertension, muscular dysfunction, and incontinence. Biofeedback has also proved to be a useful stress-reduction therapy for patients with cancer and AIDS. Patricia Norris, Ph.D., clinical director of the Life Sciences Institute of Mind-Body Health in Topeka, Kansas, has used biofeedback to help more than 300 cancer patients with results ranging from increased comfort and reduced stress to complete recovery. Using biofeedback and visualization, her first cancer patient, nine-year-old Garret Porter (now a grown, healthy man), overcame an inoperable brain tumor.[32]

Meditation

Although there are various forms of meditation, the best researched is Transcendental Meditation (TM). TM involves sitting quietly or lying down and thinking a specific sound, called a *mantra*. Mantras have no meaning for the meditator, but are chosen by the meditation teacher for a sound quality that is conducive to producing the deep rest and refined awareness characteristic of TM. Because individuals differ, TM must be taught by personal instruction. The teacher must select a sound that fits the prospective meditator's personality and guide him or her through the basic elements of the technique to ensure that it is learned correctly.

A number of published research studies have shown that during TM the body experiences a much more profound rest than while sleeping. The physiological effects include a drop in metabolic rate to a level significantly lower than that of sleep or eyes-closed rest, suspension of respiration without oxygen deprivation, stabilization of the autonomic nervous system (the part that regulates all involuntary functions including the heart muscle, blood pressure, and digestion), and decreases in plasma lactate (a chemical marker of metabolic activity) and the stress hormone, cortisol. While the rest of the body tunes down, however, the brain tunes up. Blood flow shunts decisively to the brain, and EEG patterns reveal significantly increased interaction between the right and left portions of the brain.[33]

According to Hari Sharma, M.D., of Ohio State University, more than 500 studies have been conducted to analyze the physiological effects of TM in 220 universities and research institutions in 27 countries. Studies examining the effects of TM on the aging process have found that, when compared to normal values established over many years by standardized tests, those who had practiced TM for up to five years had an average biological age five years younger than their chronological age. Those who had meditated over five years had an average biological age 12 years younger. After many years of meditation, many of the subjects' test results showed a biological age younger than the chronological age they were when they first learned to meditate![34]

One of the primary ways in which TM has been found to promote health is by reducing stress. Stress revs up the body's metabolic rate, which, in turn, engenders increasing amounts of free radicals produced as metabolic by-products. Free radicals are thought to be a major contributing factor in aging as well as all the chronic degenerative diseases, including heart disease, strokes, arthritis, osteoporosis, emphysema, cataracts, even cancer. Researchers at Ohio State University collaborated with investigators at Maharishi International University in Fairfield, Iowa, to determine TM's effectiveness in lowering free radical production. Specifically, they checked blood levels of lipid peroxide (a fat oxidized by free radicals) in elderly people who had practiced TM for many years and in non-meditating controls. Tests for lipid peroxide are commonly used to determine overall free radical activity in the body since, if lipids are being damaged, other free radical damage is assumed to be occurring at a similar pace. When the meditators were compared to non-meditating controls consuming a diet with comparable amounts of fat, the 60- to 69-year-old meditators' level of lipid peroxide was 14.5% lower than the controls, but the 70- to 79-year-old meditators lipid peroxide level was even lower: 16.5%. The meditators were actually getting healthier as they aged.[35]

Another way in which TM may promote health and slow the aging process is through preserving higher levels of DHEA-S, a hormone found in abundance in young adults, which typically declines rapidly with age. Relatively high levels of DHEA-S correspond with less atherosclerosis and heart disease in men and less breast cancer and osteoporosis in women. DHEA-S also directs the body to build muscle tissue and counterbalances the breakdown of muscle tissue for energy that is triggered by the stress hormone, cortisol. A recent study compared DHEA-S levels in the blood of 423 people who practiced TM compared to 1,253 healthy controls who did not. Ages ranged from 20 to 81 and results were gathered in five-year age ranges. After factoring out the effects of diet, obesity, and exercise, the researchers found that people who practiced TM had levels of DHEA-S comparable to members of the control group who were five to ten years younger.[36]

TM is taught by qualified TM teachers worldwide (see Appendix C, for a list of resources). Learning the simple technique takes a total of about eight hours over four consecutive days.

Spirituality and Health

A spiritual path may also lead to health in body as well as mind. In research supported by a grant from the National Institutes of Health (NIH), Jeffrey S. Levin, Ph.D., an epidemiologist at Eastern Virginia Medical School whose focus has been the effects of spiritual and religious practices, has uncovered more than 250 empirical studies published in the medical and epidemiological literature in which spiritual or religious practices have been statistically associated with beneficial health outcomes. Positive effects have been found for cardiovascular disease, hypertension, stroke, colitis, enteritis, and almost every type of cancer. More than two dozen studies demonstrate the health-promoting effects of simply attending church or synagogue regularly. The benefits have been consistently found across all divisions of race, age, and religious preference, and have applied to illnesses of all types, from self-limiting acute conditions to fatal chronic diseases.[37] Levin's findings are confirmed by a review of ten years of the Journal of Family Practice by F. C. Craigie and his colleagues. They found that 83% of the studies showed physical health benefits from participation in religious ceremony, social support, prayer, and relationship with God; the remaining 17 percent were neutral, and none showed harm.[38] Prayer and spiritual practices may positively influence physical health in a variety of ways: through fostering a sense of belonging or community; through providing social support; through rituals that engender positive emotions, which, in turn, cause the release of neurochemicals that promote healthful immune and cardiovascular function; and through requiring healthful behaviors of the devout, e.g., precautions regarding diet, alcohol, and hygiene.

In his book, *Healing Words*, Larry Dossey, M.D., pulls together what he describes as "one of the best kept secrets in medical science"—the extensive experimental evidence for the beneficial effects of prayer. Dossey reviews studies that provide evidence for a positive effect of prayer on not only humans but mice, chicks, enzymes, fungi, yeast, bacteria, and cells of various sorts. These experiments lend credence to the belief that prayer may serve as a healing force even for those who do not believe and who do not know they are being prayed for. Dossey emphasizes, "We cannot dismiss these outcomes as being due to suggestion or placebo effects, since these so-called lower forms of life do not think in any conventional sense and are presumably not susceptible to suggestion."[39]

The beneficent effects of prayer on others may remain mysterious, but prayer's effects on the one who prays are not as mysterious, sharing common ground with the placebo effect. Both give the body's self-healing mechanisms permission to turn on. In the numerous instances of spontaneous remissions and cures of various cancers discussed by Dossey in *Healing Words*, the only common thread is a letting go at the deepest level and some variation of the prayer, "Thy will be done."

The magnitude of the placebo response is estimated to be about 35%, meaning that approximately one in three patients will improve without an effective treatment as long as they believe in the effectiveness of the treatment. Factors that contribute to the placebo response include the effects of the doctor's personality, patient involvement with the choice of therapy, and the expense of the therapy or procedure.

Placebos—actually a person's belief in them—have been shown to be at least as powerful as drugs. In one clinical trial, patients were relieved of nausea when given a pill they were told was a powerful anti-nausea drug. In fact, the pill was a powerful nausea-inducing drug.[40] Similarly, in medical circles, it is well-known that newly released drugs are more effective. Blair Justice, Ph.D, professor of psychology at the University of Texas Health Science Center, suggests their effectiveness is due, at least in part, to the beliefs of the medical community: "Typically new drugs are marketed with sensation, hype and fanfare, whipping up enthusiasm among physicians and shaping their effects positively. But when other factors begin to enter the picture, including the beliefs and expectations of patient populations as well as the information about the drug's side effects, negative reports begin to circulate. The community of physician-enthusiasts are thus converted toward a more skeptical stance. As beliefs about the mechanism swing toward the negative, the drug's effectiveness diminishes."[41]

Conclusion

In the disease-treatment model, the placebo effect (the healing power of belief) has been viewed as a nuisance, a confounding variable that must be controlled. In mind/body medicine, the placebo effect is recognized as a marshaling of our self-healing abilities—the life-force within each of us, which naturopathic physicians call the *vis medicatrix naturae*. The real promise that links mind/body medicine, naturopathy, and certainly prayer, is much more than mere physical health. And the key element is not the technique that provokes the insight. It is increased awareness of and access to this teleological force, the healer within, that is the essence of each of us. The real promise is a deepening understanding of and faith in a universe in which the underlying design is one of total wellness.

Keep Track of How Your Behaviors and Health Are Improving

I strongly recommend you track how your behaviors and health are improving. Keep a daily diary of what you are doing and experiencing using a format that is convenient for you. Then, once a week, score yourself using the chart below to summarize your inappropriate behaviors, symptoms, and diseases. Add it all up and see how you've changed. I think you'll be pleased to see how much your health improves once you understand where to put your best energy.

Keeping a record of your improvement is important. People are usually so aware of their discomforts and diseases that they often don't notice how much they have improved. Many times, I've had patients express discouragement and wonder if they are ever going to improve—and even doubt if taking better care of themselves is worth the effort. Using their charts, I then remind them of all their initial symptoms and the severity of their disease(s). We then compare this with their current state of health. It's amazing to see how a simple record of improvements helps patients rededicate themselves to attaining total wellness.

Scoring

Behaviors		Symptoms		Diseases	
Never	0	Never	0	Never	0
Weekly	1	Mild/once a week	1	Mild/once a week	1
Once a day	2	Moderate/once a day	2	Moderate/once a day	2
2+ times a day	3	Severe/almost constant	3	Severe/almost constant	3

Date	Behaviors	Symptoms	Diseases	Total

Date	Behaviors	Symptoms	Diseases	Total

Which Chapters to Study

The tables below can quickly help you identify the chapters you should study first. They list the behaviors that tend to cause one of your healing systems to go out of balance, the symptoms that commonly occur when a system is out of balance, and the diseases associated with or caused by imbalances in these systems. Look through the tables, determine which of your systems seem most out of balance, and then use the advice in the appropriate chapter to help move you along the road to total wellness.

Behaviors or Factors That Increase Your Risk of Going Out of Balance

Behavior	4	5	6	7	8	9	10
Age over 65				✔		✔	
Alcohol use (enough to cause intoxication)	✔	✔		✔	✔	✔	
Antacid use				✔		✔	
Antibiotics: heavy use	✔	✔		✔			
Birth control pills		✔			✔		
Bottle-fed child	✔		✔				
Diet: conventionally-grown rather than organically grown	✔	✔	✔	✔	✔	✔	
Diet: high in food additives		✔	✔			✔	
Diet: high in hydrogenated fats		✔				✔	
Diet: high in meat		✔				✔	
Diet: high in refined foods	✔	✔	✔	✔	✔	✔	
Diet: low in fruits and vegetables	✔	✔	✔	✔		✔	
Diet: low in minerals	✔	✔	✔	✔	✔	✔	
Drugs: prescription, over-the-counter, or recreational		✔				✔	
Eating allergenic foods	✔	✔		✔		✔	
Exercise: excessively	✔						
Exercise: infrequently						✔	✔

Behaviors or Factors That Increase Your Risk of Going Out of Balance (continued)

Behavior	4	5	6	7	8	9	10
Few friends							✔
Food: excessively large meals		✔		✔			
Frequent exposure to infectious agents	✔						
Grapefruit juice: drink more than 4 oz per day		✔					
Over scheduled							✔
Oxidants: high level of exposure	✔	✔				✔	
Personality: Type A					✔		
Severe trauma	✔			✔			
Sleep: inadequate	✔	✔			✔	✔	
Smoking		✔			✔	✔	
Spiritual life: disregarded							✔
Stress: excessive	✔*				✔		✔
Sugar: excessive	✔			✔		✔	
Toxins: high level of exposure (e.g., a painter)	✔	✔	✔	✔	✔	✔	
Work: dislike your job							✔

Refer to chapter (column headings above)

Common Symptoms When You Are Out of Balance

Symptoms	4	5	6	7	8	9	10
Abdominal bloating				✔*			
Bruises easily				✔			
Angers easily							✔
Caffeine-containing drinks and foods keep you awake		✔					
Allergies		✔	✔	✔			
Asparagus causes a strong odor in your urine		✔					
Bad breath		✔		✔			
Bed wetting				✔			
Chest pain				✔			
Chronic diarrhea				✔			
Chronic fatigue	✔	✔*		✔	✔*	✔	✔
Chronic red eyes			✔				

Refer to chapter (column headings above)

* Indicates there is a patient example or explicit discussion of how to treat the disease in the chapter.

Common Symptoms When You Are Out of Balance *(continued)*

Behavior	4	5	6	7	8	9	10
Chronic headaches		✔					
Chronic intestinal infections	✔			✔			
Chronic runny nose			✔				
Chronic swollen glands	✔			✔			
Constipation		✔	✔	✔	✔		
Dark circles under eyes				✔			
Depression					✔	✔	✔
Dry skin, especially behind the ears, and around the nose and eyebrows		✔		✔			
Feel life has little meaning							✔
Feel you have little control over your life							✔
Feeling of toxicity		✔					
Fibrocystic breast disease	✔				✔		
Foul smelling breath or stools	✔	✔					
Fluid retention			✔		✔	✔	
Frequently feel overwhelmed					✔		✔
Garlic makes you sick		✔					
Greasy stools				✔			
Hair and nails of poor quality				✔			
Indigestion		✔		✔*			
Loss of distance focus						✔	
Loss of memory						✔	
Loss of strength and/or agility						✔	
Loss of sexual interest and ability					✔	✔	
Laugh infrequently							✔
Out-of-control blood sugar						✔	
Mental impairment						✔	
Menstrual cycle irregularities					✔		
Mood swings				✔	✔		
Muscle weakness					✔	✔*	
Nonsteroidal anti-inflammatory drugs	✔	✔		✔		✔	
Passing gas				✔			
Pain and stiffness in the morning	✔	✔	✔				
Painful menstruation					✔		
Perfumes and other environmental chemicals make you feel ill		✔					

* Indicates there is a patient example or explicit discussion of how to treat the disease in the chapter.

Common Symptoms When You Are Out of Balance *(continued)*

Behavior	\# *Refer to chapter* 4	5	6	7	8	9	10
Pigmentation spots on the skin						✔	
Premature graying of hair						✔	
Premature aging						✔	
Premenstrual tension			✔		✔		
Puffiness under eyes		✔		✔			
Receding gums				✔		✔	
Rectal itching		✔		✔			
Sensitivity to chemicals		✔					
Sleep poorly				✔	✔		
Sulfites, such as in commercial potato salad or salad bars, make you feel ill		✔					
Swollen ankles			✔				
Toxemia of pregnancy		✔					
Unexplained abdominal pain		✔	✔	✔			
Unexplained itching		✔					
Unexplained weight loss				✔			
Vaginal dryness					✔		
Varicose veins						✔	

Diseases Associated with or Caused by Imbalances in These Systems

Disease	\# *Refer to chapter* 4	5	6	7	8	9	10
Abscess (boils)	✔*						
Acne		✔		✔			
Acute infection	✔*						
AIDS	✔*	✔					
Allergies		✔	✔*				
Amyotrophic lateral sclerosis						✔	
Alzheimer's disease		✔		✔		✔*	
Anemia		✔		✔			
Ankylosing spondylitis		✔					
Angina pectoris						✔	
Asthma		✔	✔*	✔			
Atherosclerosis		✔			✔		
Athlete's foot	✔						
Autoimmune diseases			✔	✔		✔*	

* Indicates there is a patient example or explicit discussion of how to treat the disease in the chapter.

Diseases Associated with or Caused by Imbalances in These Systems (continued)

Disease	4	5	6	7	8	9	10
Benign prostatic hyperplasia						✔*	
Cancer	✔	✔	✔			✔	✔
Candidiasis	✔*			✔			
Canker sores		✔		✔			
Cataracts		✔		✔		✔*	
Celiac disease		✔		✔			
Cellulitis	✔*						
Cervical dysplasia				✔		✔	
Chronic bronchitis			✔*				
Chronic ear infections	✔*						
Chronic Epstein-Barr virus infection	✔						
Chronic fatigue syndrome	✔	✔*					
Chronic infections	✔*						
Chronic inflammatory conditions			✔				
Chronic obstructive pulmonary disease			✔*				
Colic in infants		✔		✔			
Common cold	✔*						
Congestive heart failure						✔*	
Coronary artery spasm				✔*			
Crohn's disease		✔	✔*	✔			
Cystic acne (also called inflammatory acne)	✔		✔				
Cystitis (urinary tract infection)	✔*						
Depression					✔	✔*	✔
Dermatitis		✔	✔	✔			
Dermatitis herpetiformis				✔			
Diabetes		✔	✔	✔*		✔*	
Eczema		✔	✔*	✔			
Emphysema			✔*				
Endometriosis					✔		
Epilepsy		✔					
Failure to thrive in children		✔*		✔			
Food allergies		✔		✔			
Frequent acute infections	✔						
Frequent herpes attacks	✔						

Refer to chapter

* Indicates there is a patient example or explicit discussion of how to treat the disease in the chapter.

Diseases Associated with or Caused by Imbalances in These Systems (continued)

Disease	4	5	6	7	8	9	10
			Refer to chapter				
Fungal fingernail infection	✔*						
Gall stones		✔					
Gilbert's syndrome		✔*					
Hay fever			✔*				
Henock-Schöenlein purpura			✔*				
Hepatitis		✔					
Herpes	✔*						
High blood pressure						✔	✔*
Hives		✔		✔			
Huntington's disease						✔	
Hypoglycemia				✔*		✔	
Hypothyroid					✔*		
Impotence						✔	✔*
Infertility (female)						✔*	✔*
Infertility (male)						✔*	✔*
Inflammatory bowel disease		✔	✔*	✔			
Influenza	✔*						
Insomnia				✔	✔	✔*	✔
Irritable bowel syndrome		✔	✔	✔			✔
Liver disease		✔					
Macular degeneration						✔*	
Menopause (excessive, uncomfortable)					✔*		
Migraine headaches		✔*	✔				
Multiple chemical sensitivity syndrome		✔*					
Multiple sclerosis			✔	✔	✔		
Myasthenia gravis		✔		✔			
Myocardial infarction		✔		✔		✔	
Obesity		✔			✔	✔*	
Osteoarthritis			✔			✔*	
Osteoporosis				✔	✔	✔	
Ovarian cysts		✔			✔		
Pancreatitis		✔					
Parasites	✔			✔*			
Parkinson's disease		✔				✔	
Periodontal disease						✔*	

* Indicates there is a patient example or explicit discussion of how to treat the disease in the chapter.

Diseases Associated with or Caused by Imbalances in These Systems
(continued)

Disease	Refer to chapter						
	4	5	6	7	8	9	10
Pernicious anemia				✔			
Persistent chronic viral activity	✔						
Pre-eclampsia		✔		✔*			
Psoriasis		✔					
Reiter's disease		✔					
Retinitis pigmentosa						✔	
Rheumatoid arthritis		✔*	✔*				
Rosacea				✔			
Schizophrenia		✔					
Scleroderma						✔	
Seborrheic dermatitis			✔				
Senile dementia		✔				✔	
Sick building syndrome		✔*					
Sinusitis	✔*						
Sjogren's syndrome				✔			
Systemic lupus erythematosis		✔	✔	✔	✔*	✔*	
Ulcerative colitis			✔*	✔	✔		
Ulcers				✔*			
Vaginitis, trichomonal or candidal	✔*						
Vitiligo				✔			
Warts	✔*						

* Indicates there is a patient example or explicit discussion of how to treat the disease in the chapter.

Resources

Education

Bastyr University
14500 Juanita Drive, NE
Bothell, WA 98011
(206) 823-1300 / Fax (206) 823-6222

Provides accredited education in naturopathic medicine (N.D.), nutrition (B.S., M.S., R.D.), acupuncture and Chinese medicine (B.S., M.S.), applied behavioral sciences (B.S., M.A.), midwifery (certificate), Chinese herbal medicine (certificate), homeopathy (certificate), and Ayurvedic medicine (certificate).

Organizations

American Association of Naturopathic Physicians
2366 Eastlake Avenue, Suite 322
Seattle, WA 98102

Nationwide directory and referrals of accredited and licensed naturopathic physicians.

The Center for Mind/Body Medicine
5225 Connecticut Avenue, NW, Suite 414
Washington, D.C. 20015
(202) 966-7338 / Fax (202) 966-2589

EarthSave
706 Frederick Street
Santa Cruz, CA 95062
(408) 423-4069

Nonprofit organization providing education programs for adults and children on the impact of dietary choices on our health and that of our planet.

Great Smokies Diagnostic Laboratory
18A Regent Park Boulevard
Asheville, NC 28806
(800) 522-4762
Offers a variety of functional testing.

Herb Research Foundation
1007 Pearl Street, Suite 200
Boulder, CO 80302
(303) 440-2265
Provides research materials for consumers and scientists.

Meridian Valley Clinical Laboratory
24030 132nd Avenue, SE
Kent, WA 98042
(800) 234-6825
Offers a wide variety of functional testing.

Recommended Books and Magazines

Borysenko, J. *Minding the Body, Mending the Mind.* N.Y.: Bantam Books, 1988.

Brown, Don J. *Herbal Prescriptions for Better Health.* Rocklin, California: Prima Publishing, 1996.

Chopra, D. *Perfect Health.* New York: Harmony Books, 1991.

Delicious! New Hope Communications, Boulder, Colorado.

Dossey, L. *Healing Words.* San Francisco: HarperCollins, 1993.

Goleman, D. and J. Gurin. *Mind/Body Medicine: How to Use Your Mind for Better Health.* New York: Consumer Reports Books, 1993.

Haas, E. M. *Staying Healthy with Nutrition.* Berkeley: Celestial Arts, 1992.

Justice, B. *Who Gets Sick?* New York: Tarcher Putnam, 1987.

Lemeron, T. *Seven Keys to Vibrant Health.* Green Bay: Impakt Communications, 1995.

Lonsdorf, N. and M. Lonsdorf. *A Woman's Best Medicine.* New York: Tarcher Putnam, 1993.

Mayell, M. *The Natural Health First-Aid Guide.* New York: Pocket Books, 1994.

McDougall, J. *The McDougall Plan.* Clinton, New Jersey: New Win Publishers, 1983.

Murray, M. *Natural Alternatives to Over-the-Counter Prescription Drugs.* New York: William Morrow, 1994.

Murray, M. and J. Pizzorno. *Encyclopedia of Natural Medicine*. Rocklin, California: Prima Publishing, 1991.

Natural Health Magazine. Boston Common Press, Brookline, Massachusetts.

Quillin, P. *Healing Nutrients*. New York: Vintage, 1987.

Robbins, J. *Diet for a New America*. Walpole, New Hampshire: Stillpoint Publishing, 1987.

Sharma, H. *Freedom from Disease*. Toronto: Veda Publishing, 1993.

Ullman, D. *Discovering Homeopathy: Your Introduction to the Science and Art of Homeopathic Medicine*. Berkeley, California: North Atlantic Books, 1991.

Weil, A. *Spontaneous Healing*. New York: Alfred Knopf, 1995.

Wright, J. *Dr. Wright's Guide to Healing with Nutrition*. New Canaan: Keats, 1990.

Zand, J., R. Walston, and B. Roundtree. *Smart Medicine for a Healthier Child*. Garden City Park, New York: Avery, 1994.

References

Chapter 1
1. Bland, J.: *Functional Medicine: Understanding the Basics*. HealthComm, Gig Harbor, WA, 1995

Chapter 2
1. Clinton, W.: *Health Security: The President's Report to the American People*. The White House, 1993
2. Pelletier, K. R.: A review and analysis of the health and cost-effective outcome studies of comprehensive health promotion and disease prevention programs at the worksite: 1991–1993 update. *Am J Health Promotion* 8:50–61, 1993
3. Geyman, J. P. and Hart, G.: Family practice and the health care system, Primary care at a crossroads: Progress, problems and future projections. *JABFP* 7:60–70, 1994
4. Leape, L. L.: Unnecessary surgery. *Health Serv Res* 24:351–407, 1989
5. Graboys, T. B. et al.: Results of second-opinion trial among patients recommended for coronary angiography. *JAMA* 268:2537–40, 1992
6. American Western Life Insurance Company report, 1993
7. Murray, M. T.: *Natural Alternatives to Over-the-Counter and Prescription Drugs*. Morrow, New York, 1994
8. Beasley, J. D. and Swift, J. J.: *The Kellogg Report: The Impact of Nutrition, Environment and Lifestyle on the Health of Americans*. The Bard College Center, Annandale-on-Hudson, New York 1989, p. 300
9. October 9, 1995, Archives of Internal Medicine
10. Gambert, S. R. et al.: How many drugs does your aged patient need? *Patient Care*, March 30, 1994:61–72
11. Beers, M. H. et al.: Inappropriate medication prescribing in skilled-nursing facilities. *Ann Int Med* 117:684–89, 1992
12. Radetsky, P.: Killer hospitals. *Longevity*, July 1994, p. 18
13. Mullan, F. et al.: Doctors, dollars and determination: Making physician work-force policy. *Health Affairs* 12(suppl):138–51, 1993
14. Curzer, H. J.: Do physicians make too much money? *Theor Med* 13:45–65, 1992
15. Woolhandler, S. and Himmelstein, D. U.: The deteriorating administrative efficiency of the U.S. health care system. *NEJM* 324:1253–58, 1991
16. Leaf, A.: Preventive medicine for our ailing health care system. *JAMA* 269:616–18, 1993
17. Monheit, A. C. and Vistnes, J. P.: Implicit pooling of workers from large and small firms. *Health Affairs* 13:301–14, 1994 (Uses data from 1987 National Medical Expenditure Survey [NMES] of 23,685 persons under age of 65)
18. Verbrugge, L. M. and Patrick, D. L.: Seven chronic conditions: Their impact on U.S. adults' activity levels and use of medical services. *Am J Pub Health* 85:173–82, 1995 for note
19. Raloff, J.: Non-smoking-related cancers on rise. *Sci News* 145:102, 1991

20. Beardsley, T.: A war not won. *Sci Am* 270:130–38, 1994
21. Changes in U.S. life expectancy. *Statistical Bull* 11–17:Jul.–Sept. 1994
22. Robine, J. M. and Ritchie, K.: Healthy life expectancy: Evaluation of global indicator of change in population health. *Br Med J* 302:457–60, 1991
23. Hogan, C.: Physician incomes under an all-payer fee schedule. *Health Affairs* 12:170–75, 1993
24. Salive, M. E.: The practice and earnings of preventive medicine physicians. *Am J Prev Med* 8:257–62, 1992
25. Curzer, H. J.: Do physicians make too much money? *Theor Med* 13:45–65, 1992
26. Goodman, J. C. and Musgrave G. L.: *Patient Power: Solving America's Health Care Crisis.* Cato Inst, 1992, p. 146
27. Farquhar, J. et al.: Effects of community-wide education on cardiovascular risk factors: The Stanford Five-City Project. *JAMA* 264:359–65, 1990
28. Monro, J., Brostoff, J., Carini, C., and Zilkha, K.: Food allergy in migraine. *Lancet* ii:1–4, 1980
29. Mattei, F. M. et al.: Serenoa repens extract in the medical treatment of benign prostatic hypertrophy. *Urologia* 55:547–52, 1988
30. Albina, J. E.: Nutrition and wound healing. *J Parenteral Enteral Nutr* 18:366–67, 1994
31. Delmi, M. et al.: Dietary supplementation in elderly patients with fractured neck of the femur. *Lancet* 335:1013–16, 1990
32. MacBurney, M. et al.: A cost-evaluation of glutamine-supplemented parenteral nutrition in adult bone marrow transplant patients. *J Am Diet Assoc* 94:1263–66, 1994
33. Reuter, H. D.: Paper presented at: Fifth Phytotherapy Congress in Bonn. Zeitschrift fur Phytotherapie 15:17–27, 1994
34. Oojendijk, W. T. et al.: *What is Better? An Investigation into the Use and Satisfaction with Complementary and Official Medicine in the Netherlands.* Netherlands Institute of Preventive Medicine and the Technical Industrial Organization. 1980
35. *The Wall Street Journal*, Sept. 13, 1993
36. Serudla, M. K. et al.: Fruit and vegetable intake among adults in 16 states: Results of a brief telephone survey. *Am J Pub Health* 85:236–39, 1995
37. Hodgson, T.: Cigarette smoking and lifetime medical expenditures. *The Milbank Quarterly* 70:81–87, 1992

Chapter 3

1. Kleinman, A., Eisenberg, L. and Good, B.: Culture, illness, and cure: Clinical lessons from anthropologic and cross-cultural research. *Ann Int Med* 88:251–58, 1978
2. Peterson, W. L., Sturdevant, R. A., Frankl, H. D. et al.: Healing of duodenal ulcer with antacid regimen. *NEJM* 297:341–45, 1977

Chapter 4

1. van Buchen, F. L., Dunk, J. H. and van Hof, M. A.: Therapy of acute otitis media: Myringotomy, antibiotics, or neither? *Lancet* 2:883–87, 1981
2. Diamant, M. and Diamant, B.: Abuse and timing of use of antibiotics in acute otitis media. *Arch Otol* 100:226–32, 1974
3. Breiman, R. F. et al.: Emergence of drug-reistant pneumococcal infections in the United States. *JAMA* 271:1831–35, 1994
4. Epstein, P. R.: Emerging diseases and ecosystem instability: New threats to public health. *Am J Publ Health* 85:168–72, 1995
5. Beck, M. A.: Rapid genomic evolution of a non-virulent coxsackievirus B3 in selenium-deficient mice results in selection of identical virulent isolates. *Nature* Nat Med 1:405–6, 1995
6. Adler, T.: Diet causes viral mutation in mice. *Science News* 147:276, 1995

7. Dale, D. C. and Federman, D. D.: *Scientific American Medicine* 7:Inf Dis:I-2, *Scientific American*, New York, 1995

8. Sanchez, A., Reeser, J., Lau, H. et al.: Role of sugars in human neutrophilic phagocytosis. *Am J Clin Nutr* 26:1180–84, 1973

9. Ringsdorf, W., Cheraskin, E. and Ramsay, R.: Sucrose, neutrophilic phagocytosis and resistance to disease. *Dent Surv* 52:46–48, 1976

10. Bernstein, J., Alpert, S., Nauss, K. and Suskind, R.: Depression of lymphocyte transformation following glucose ingestion. *Am J Clin Nutr* 30:613, 1977

11. Rinkel, H. J., Randolph, T. G. and Zeller, M.: *Food Allergy*. C. C Thomas, Springfield, IL, 1951

12. Pennisi, E.: Food allergies linked to ear infections. *Sci News* 146:231, 1994

13. *Infectious Disease News*: Editorial: Drinking and infections don't mix, December 1992

14. Suskind, R.: "Immunologic Mechanisms and the Role of Nutrition," in Suskind, R.: *Principals and Practices of Environmental Medicine,*" *Plenum Medical Book Company, New York, 1992*

15. Semba, R. et al.: Depressed immune response to tetanus in children with vitamin deficiency. *J Nutr* 122:101–7, 1992

16. Barclay, A. J. et al.: Vitamin A supplements and mortality related to measles: A randomised clinical trial. *BMJ* 294:294–96, 1987

17. *Nutr Res* 9:1017–25, 1989

18. Chandra, R. K.: Nutrition and immunity: Basic considerations, Part 1. *Contemp Nutr* 11:11, 1986

19. Levy, J. A.: "Nutrition and the Immune System," in Sitites, D. P. et al. *Basic and Clinical Immunology*, 4th ed. Lange Medical Publications, Los Altos, CA, 1982

20. Frieden, T. R. et al.: Vitamin A levels and severity of measles. *Am J Dis Child* 146:182–86, 1992

21. Hussey, G. and Klein, M.: The interaction between vitamin A status and measles infection. Beyond deficiency: New views on the function and health of vitamins. *New York Acad Sci Abstract* 17, February 9–12, 1992

22. Beisel, W. R. et al.: Single-nutrient effects on immunological functions. *JAMA* 245:53–58, 1981

23. Halpern, G. M. and Trapp, C. L. Nutrition and immunity: Where are we standing? *Allergy Immunopath* 21:122–26, 1993

24. Prasad, A.: Clinical, biochemical and nutritional spectrum of zinc deficiency in human subjects: An update. *Nutr Rev* 41:197–208, 1983

25. Bondestram, M. et al.: Subclinical trace element deficiency in children with undue susceptibility to infections. *Acta Paediatr Scand* 74:515–20, 1985

26. Fraker. P. J. et al.: Zinc requirement for macrophage function: Effect of zinc deficiency on uptake and killing of a protozoan parasite. *Immunology* 68:114–19, 1989

27. Schrauzer, G. N.: Selenium and the immune response. *Nutr Rep* 10:17–24, 1992

28. Nougouchi, M.: The role of fatty acids in eicosanoid synthesis inhibitors in breast cancer. *Oncology* 52:265–71, 1995

29. Stejskal, J.: Beware of metals: A possible cause of immunological disorders. CFN Symposium: Immunotoxicity and in vitro possibilties. Stockholm, Sweden, September 19–21, 1993

30. Rae, W. J. and Liang, H. C.: Effects of pesticides on the immune system. *J Nutr Med* 2:399–410, 1991

31. Esser, C.: Dioxins and the immune system: Mechanisms of interference. *Int Arch Allergy Immunol* 126:130, 1994

32. Graham, N. M. H.: Adverse effects of aspirin, acetaminophen and ibuprofen on immune function, viral shedding and clinical status in rhinovirus-infected volunteers. *J Inf Dis* 162:1277–82, 1990

33. Dale, D. C. and Federman, D. D.: *Scientific American Medicine* 7:Inf Dis:X-2,3, 1995

34. Campbell, A., Nachman, B. and Vodjani, A.: Suppressed natural killer cell activity in patients with silicone breast implants: Reversal upon explantation. *Toxicol Ind Hlth* 10:144–49, 1994

35. Vodjani, A., Campbell, M. and Brautbar, N.: Immune alteration associated with exposure to toxic chemicals. *Toxicol Ind Hlth* 8:231–46, 1992

36. Baenkler, H. W.: Exercise and the immune system: The impact on diseases. *Rheumatic Diseases Sport Rheumatology* 16:5–21, 1992

37. Eichner, E. R.: Infection, immunity, and exercise: What to tell patients. *Physician Sports Medicine* 21:125–33, 1993

38. Rose, R.: Endocrine responses to stressful psychological events. *Psych Clin N Amer* 3:251–75, 1980

39. Keller, S. E., Weiss, J. M., Schleifer, SJ. et al.: Suppression of immunity by stress: Effects of graded series of stressors on lymphocyte stimulation in the rat. *Science* 213:1397, 1981

40. Herbert, T. B. and Cohen, S.: Stress and immunity in humans: A meta-analytic review. *Psychosom Med* 55:364–79, 1993

41. Zisook, S. et al.: Depression and immune function. *Psychiatry Res* 52:1–10, 1994

42. Spiegel, D.: Mind-body meld may boost immunity. *J Natnl Canc Inst* 86:256–57, 1994

43. *Sci News:* Fail to snooze, immune cells lose. 147:11, 1995

44. Palmblad, J., Hallberg, D. and Rossner, S.: Obesity, plasma lipids and polymorphonuclear (PMN) granulocyte functions. *Scand J Heamatol* 19:293–303, 1977

45. Sweeney, J. F. et al.: Impaired polymorphonuclear leukocyte anticandida function in injured adults with elevated candida antigen titers. *Arch Surg* 128:40–46, 1993

46. Luostarinen, R. et al.: Effect of dietary fish oil supplementation with different doses of vitamin E on neutrophil chemotaxis in healthy volunteers. *Nutr Res2* 12:1419–30, 1992

47. Choen, B. et al.: Reversal of postoperative immunosuppression in man by vitamin A. *Surg Gynecol Obstet* 149:658–62, 1979

48. Cerra, F. B. et al.: Role of nutrition in the management of malnutrition and immune dysfunction of trauma. *J Am Coll Nutr* 11:512–18, 1992

49. Brody, J. A., Overfield, T. and Hammes, L. M.: Depression of the tuberculin reaction by viral vaccines. *NEJM* 271:1294–96, 1964

50. Eibl, M., Mannhalter, J. W. and Zlabinger, G.: Abnormal T-lymphocyte subpopulations in healthy subjects after tetanus booster immunization (letter). *NEJM* 310:198–99, 1984

51. Siegel, R. L., Issekutz, T., Schwaber, J. et al.: Deficiency of T-helper cells in transient hypogammaglobulinemia of infancy. *NEJM* 305:1307–13, 1981

52. Fulginiti, V.: Commentary: Measles immunization. *J Ped* 94: 1019–20, 1979

53. Toraldo, R. et al.: Effect of measles-mumps-rubella vaccination on polymorphonuclear neutrophil functions in children. *ACTA Pediatr* 81:887–90, 1992

54. Bernier, R. H., Frank, J. A., Dondero, T. J. and Turner, P.: Diphtheria-tetanus toxoids-pertussis vaccination and sudden infant death syndrome in Tennessee. *J Ped* 101:419–21, 1982

55. Baraff, L. J.: Possible temporal association between diphtheria-tetanus toxoid-pertussis vaccination and sudden infant death syndrome. *Ped Infec Dis* 2:7–11, 1983

56. Reid, G.M. and Tervit H.: Sudden infant death syndrome (SIDS): immunoglobulins and hypoxia. *Med Hypotheses* 44:202-6, 1995

57. Wilson, G.: *The Hazards of Immunization.* Oxford University Press, New York, 1967

58. Thompson, N. P. et al.: Is measles vaccination a risk factor for inflammatory bowel disease? *Lancet* 345:1071–74, 1995

59. Stratton, K. et al.: Adverse events associated with childhood vaccines other than pertussis and rubella: Summary of a report from the Institute of Medicine. *JAMA* 271:1602–5, 1994

60. Mattman, L. H.: *Cell Wall Deficient Forms: Stealth Pathogens,* 2nd ed. CRC Press, Boca Raton, FL, 1992

61. Chandr, R. K.: Effect of vitamin and trace-element supplementation on immune responses and infection in elderly subjects. *Lancet* 340:1124–7, 1992

62. Demetriou, A., Franco, I., Bark, S. et al.: Effects of vitamin A and beta carotene on intra-abdominal sepsis. *Arch Surg* 119:161–65, 1984

63. Tachibana, K., Sone, S., Tsubura, E. and Kishino, Y.: Stimulation effect of vitamin A on tumoricidal activity of rat alveolar macrophages. *Br J Cancer* 49:343–8, 1984

64. Seifter, E., Rettura, G., Seiter, J. et al.: Thymotrophic action of vitamin A. *Fed Proc* 32:947, 1973

65. Reinhardt, A., Auperin, D. and Sands, J.: Mechanism of viricidal activity of retinoids: Protein removal from bacteriophage 6 envelope. *Antimicrob Agents Chemother* 17:1034–37, 1980

66. Burton, G. and Ingold, K.: Beta-carotene: An unusual type of lipid antioxidant. *Science* 224:569–73, 1984

67. Edes, T. E.: Beta-carotene and vitamin A: Casting separate shadows? *Nutr Rep* 10:9–16, 1992

68. Alexander, M. et al.: Oral beta-carotene can increase the number of OKT4+ cells in human blood. *Immunol Letters* 9:221–24, 1985

69. Murata, T. et al.: Effect of long-term administration of beta-carotene on lymphocyte subsets in humans. *Am J Clin Nutr* 60:597–602, 1994

70. Hemila, H. and Herman, Z. S.: Vitamin C and the common cold: A retrospective analysis of Chalmer's review. *J Am Coll Nutr* 14:116–23, 1995

71. Wilson, C. W. M.: Clinical pharmacological aspects of ascorbic acid. *Ann NY Acad Sci* 258:355–76, 1975

72. Aloe, J. J. and Padh, H.: Inhibition of ascorbic acid uptake by endotoxin: Evidence of mediation by serum factor(s). *Proc Soc Exp Biol Med* 179:128–31, 1985

73. Schwerdt, P. and Schwerdt, C.: Effect of ascorbic acid on rhinovirus replication in WI-38 cells. *Proc Soc Exp Biol Med* 148:1237–43, 1975

74. Fletcher, R., Albers, A., Chen, A. and Albertson, J.: Ascorbic acid inhibition of Campylobacter jejuni growth. *App Env Micro* 45:792–95, 1983

75. Dieter, M.: Further studies on the relationship between vitamin C and thymic hormonal factor. *Proc Soc Exp Biol Med* 136:316–22, 1971

76. Scott, J.: On the biochemical similarities of ascorbic acid and interferon *J Theor Biol* 98:235–38, 1982

77. Hunt, C.: The clinical effects of vitamin C supplementation in elderly hospitalized patients with acute respiratory infection. *Int J Vit Nutr Res* 64:212–19, 1994

78. Meydani, S. N.: Vitamin E supplementation suppresses prostaglandin E1(2) synthesis and enhances the immune response of aged mice. *Mech Aging Dev* Apr. 34:191–201, 1986

79. Nockels, C. F.: Protective effects of supplemental vitamin E against infection. *Fed Proc* 38:2134–38, 1979

80. Meydaini, S. N. et al.: Vitamin E supplementation enhances cell-mediated immunity in healthy elderly subjects. *Am J Clin Nutr* 52:557–63, 1990,

81. Prasad, J. S.: Effect of vitamin E supplementation on leukocyte function. *Am J Clin Nutr* 33:606–8, 1980

82. Duchateau, J. et al.: Influence of oral zinc supplementation on the lymphocyte response to mitogens of normal subjects. *Am J Clin Nutr* 34:88–93, 1981

83. Gershwin, M., Beach, R. and Hurley, L.: Trace metals, aging, and immunity. *J Am Ger Soc* 31:374–78, 1983

84. Chandra, R. K.: Excessive intake of zinc impairs immune responses. *JAMA* 252:1443–46, 1984

85. Kiremidijian-Schumacher, L. et al.: Supplementation with selenium and human immune cell functions, II: Effect on cytotoxic lymphocytes and natural killer cells. *Biol Trace Element Res* 41:115–27, 1994

86. Newman, J.: How breast milk protects newborns. *Sci Am* 273:76–79, 1995

87. Chandra, R. K. and Hamed, A.: Cumulative incidence of atopic disorders in high risk infant whey hydrolysate, soy, and conventional cow milk formulas. *Ann Allergy* 67:129–32, 1991

88. Wacker, A. and Hilbig, W.: Virus-inhibition by *Echinacea purpurea*. *Planta Medica* 33:89–102, 1978

89. Wagner, V., Proksch, A., Riess-Maurer, I. et al.: Immunostimulating polysaccharides (heteroglycanes) of higher plants: Preliminary communications. *Arzneim Forsch* 34:659–60, 1984

90. Mose, J.: Effect of echinacin on phagocytosis and natural killer cells. *Med Welt* 34:1463–67, 1983

91. Vomel, V.: Influence of a non-specific immune stimulant on phagocytosis of erythrocytes and ink by the reticuloendothelial system of isolated perfused rat livers of different ages. *Arzneim Forsch* 34:691–95, 1984

92. Roesler, J., Steinmuller, C., Kiderlen, A. et al.: Application of purified polysaccharides from cell cultures of the plant *Echinacea purpurea* to mice mediates protection against systemic infections with *Listeria monocytogenes* and *Candida albicans*. *Int J Immunopharmac* 13:27–37, 1991

93. Bauer, R., Jurcic, K., Puhlmann, J. and Wagner, H.: Immunological in vivo and in vitro examinations of Echinacea extracts. *Arzneim Forsch* 38:276–81, 1988

94. Erhard, M., Kellner, J. et al.: Effect of Echinacea, Aconitum, Lachesis and Apis extracts, and their combinations on phagocytosis of human granulocytes. *Phytother Res* 8:14–17, 1994

95. Wildfeuer, A. and Meyerhofer, D.: Study of the influence of phytopreparation on the cellular function of bodily defense. *Arzneim Forsch Drug Res* 44:361–66, 1994

96. Bauer, R. and Wagner, H.: Echinacea species as potential immunostimulatory drugs. *Econ Med Plant Res* 5:253–321, 1991

97. Womble, D. and Helderman, J. H.: Enhancement of allo-responsiveness of human lymphocytes by acemannan (Carrisyn). *Int J Immunopharmac* 10:967–74, 1988

98. Hart, L. A., Nibbering, P. H., van den Barselaar, M. T. et al.: Effects of low molecular constituents from Aloe vera gel on oxidative metabolism and cytotoxic and bactericidal activities of human neutrophils. *Int J Immunopharmac* 12:427–34, 1990

99. Zhao, K. S., Mancini, C. and Doria, G.: Enhancement of the immune response in mice by *Astragalus membranaceus*. *Immunopharmacol* 20:225–33, 1990

100. Chu, D.-T. et al.: Immunotherapy with Chinese medicinal herbs, I: Immune restoration of local xenogenic graft-versus-host reaction in cancer patients by fractionated Astragalus membranaceus in vitro. *J Clin Lab Immunol* 25:119–23, 1988

101. Sabir, M. and Bhide, N.: Study of some pharmacologic actions of berberine. *Ind J Physiol Pharm* 15:111–32, 1971

102. Kumazawa, Y., Itagaki, A., Fukumoto, M. et al.: Activation of peritoneal macrophages by berberine alkaloids in terms of induction of cytostatic activity. *Int J Immunopharmac* 6:587–92, 1984

103. Chihara, G., Hamuro, J., Maeda, Y. et al.: Fractionation and purification of the polysaccharides with marked antitumor activity, especially lentinan from *Lentinus edodes* (Berk.) Sing. (an edible mushroom). *Cancer Res* 30:2776–81, 1971

104. Sipka, S., Abel, G., Scongor, J. et al.: Effect of lentinan on the chemiluminescence produced by human neutrophils and the murine cell line C4M. *Int J Immunopharmac* 7:747–51, 1985

105. Fruehauf. J., Bonnard, G. and Herberman, R.: The effect of lentinan on production of interleukin-1 by human monocytes. *Immunopharmacol* 5:65–74, 1982

106. Aoki, T. et al.: Low natural killer syndrome: Clinical and immunological features. *Nat Immunol Cell Growth Regul* 6:116–28, 1987

107. Morioka, N., Morton, D. L. and Irie, R. F.: A protein fraction from aged garlic extract enhances cytotoxicity and proliferation of human lymphocytes mediated by interleukin-2 and conconavalin. *Proc Ann Meet Am Assoc Cancer* 34:A3297, 1993

108. Lau, B. H., Yamasaki, T. and Gridley, D. S.: Garlic compounds modulate macrophage and T-lymphocyte functions. *Mol Biother* 3:103–7, 1991

109. Kandil, O. M. et al.: Garlic and the immune system in humans: Its effect on natural killer cells. *Fed Proc* 46:441, 1987

110. Hirao, Y. et al.: Activation of immunoresponder cells by the protein fraction from aged garlic extract. *Phytotherapy Res* 1:161–64, 1987

111. Adetumbi, M. A. and Lau, B. H.: Allium sativum (garlic): A natural antibiotic. *Med Hypothesis* 12:227–37, 1983

112. Scaglione, F. et al.: Immunomodulatory effects of two extracts of *Panax ginseng* C. A. Meyer. *Drugs Exp Clin Res* 16:537–42, 1990

113. Kenarova, B. et al.: Immunomodulating activity of ginsenoside Rg1 from *Panax ginseng. Jpn J Pharmacol* 54:447–54, 1990

114. Jie, Y. H., Cammisuli, S. and Baggiolini, M.: Immunomodulatory effects of *Panax ginseng* C. A. Meyer in the mouse. *Agents Actions* 15:386–91, 1984

115. Bohn, B., Nebe, C. T. and Birr, C.: Flow-cytometric studies with Elutherococcus senticosus extract as an immunomodulatory agent. *Arzneim-Forsch* 37:1193–96, 1987

116. Rimoldi, R., Ginesu, F. and Giura, R.: The use of bromelain in pneumological therapy. *Drugs Exp Clin Res* 4:55–66, 1978

117. Neubauer, R.: A plant protease for the potentiation of and possible replacement of antibiotics. *Exp Med Surg* 19:143–60, 1961

118. Fiocchi, A. et al.: A double-blind clinical trail for evaluation of the therapeutic effectiveness of a calf thymus derivative (Thymodulin) in children with recurrent respiratory infections. *Thymus* 831–9, 1986

119. Nash, M. S.: Exercise and immunology. *Med Sci Sports Exerc* 26:125–27, 1994

120. Nieman, D. C. and Henson, D. A.: Role of endurance exercise in immune senescence. *Med Sci Sports Exerc* 26:172–81, 1994

121. Hahn, F. E. and Ciak, J.: Berberine. *Antibiotics* 3:577–88, 1976

122. Ghosh, A. K.: Effect of berberine chloride on *Leishmania donovani. Ind J Med Res* 78:407–16, 1983

123. Majahan, V. M., Sharma, A. and Rattan, A.: Antimycotic activity of berberine sulfate: An alkaloid from an Indian medicinal herb. *Sabouraudia* 20:79–81, 1982

124. Subbaiah, T. V. and Amin, A. H.: Effect of berberine sulfate on *Entamoeba histolytica. Nature* 215:527–28, 1967

125. Choudry, V. P., Sabir, M. and Bhide, V. N.: Berberine in giardiasis. *Ind Pediatr* 9:143–46, 1972

126. Amin, A. H., Subbaiah, T. V. and Abbasi, K. M.: Berberine sulfate: Antimicrobial activity, bioassay, and mode of action. *Can J Microbiol* 15:1067–76, 1969

127. Sun, D., Courtney, H. S. and Beachey, E. H.: Berberine sulphate blocks adeherence of Streptococcus pyogenes to epithelial cells, fibronectin and hexadane. *Antimicrobi Agents Chemother* 32:1370–74, 1988

128. Huddleson, I. F. et al.: Antibacterial substances in plants. *J Am Vet Med Assoc* 105:394–97, 1944

129. Cavallito, C. J. and Bailey, J. H.: Allicin, the antibacterial principle of Allium sativum, I: Isolation, physical properties and antibacterial action. *J Am Chem Soc* 66:1950–51, 1944

130. Sharma, V. D. et al.: Antibacterial property of *Allium sativum* Linn.: In vivo and in vitro studies. *Ind J Exp Biol* 15:466–68, 1977

131. Elnima, E. I. et al.: The antimicrobial activity of garlic and onion extracts. *Pharmazie* 38:747–48, 1983

132. Vahora, S. B., Rizwan, M., and Khan, J. A.: Medicinal uses of common Indian vegetables. *Planta Med* 23:381–93, 1973

133. Robson, M. C., Heggers, J. P. and Hagstron, W. J.: Myth, magic, witchcraft, or fact? Aloe vera revisited. *J Burn Care Rehab* 3:157–62, 1982

134. Klein, A. D. and Penneys, N. S.: Aloe vera. *J Am Acad Dermatol* 18:714–9, 1988

135. Mitscher, L, Park, Y., and Clark, D.: Antimicrobial agents from higher plants: Antimicrobial isoflavonoids from *Glycyrrhiza glabra* L. var. typica. *J Nat Products* 43:259–69, 1980

136. Carson, C. F. and Riley, T. V.: The antimicrobial activity of tea tree oil (letter to the editor). *Med J Australis* 160:236, 1994

137. Abe, N., Ebina, T. and Ishida, N.: Interferon induction by glycyrrhizin and glycyrrhetinic acid in mice. *Microbiol Immunol* 26:535–9, 1982

138. Pompei, R., Pani, A., Flore, O., Marcialis, M. and Loddo, B.: Antiviral activity of glycyrrhizic acid. *Experientia* 36:304–5, 1980

139. Kumagai, A., Nanaboshi, M., Asanuma, Y. et al.: Effects of glycyrrhizin on thymolytic and immunosuppressive action of cortisone. *Endocrinol Japon* 14:39–42, 1967

140. Mori, K. et al.: Effects of glycyrrhizin (SNMC: Stronger Neo-Minophagen C) in hemophilia patients with HIV-1 infection. *Tohoku J Exp Med* 162:183–93, 1990

141. Wobling, R. H. and Leonhardt, K.: Local therapy of herpes simplex with dried extract from *Melissa offinalis*. *Phytomedicine* 1:25–31, 1994

142. Kahlon, J. B. et al: In vitro evaluation of the synergistic antiviral efects of acemannan in combination with azidothymidine and acyclovir. *Mol Biother* 3:214–23, 1991

143. McDaniel, H. R. et al.: Extended survival and prognostic criteria for acemannan (ACE-M) treated HIV-1 patients. *Antiviral Res* 13(suppl. 1):117, 1990

144. Sheets, M. A., Unger, B. A., Giggleman, G. F. and Tizard, I. R.: Studies of the effect of acemannan on retrovirus infections: Clinical stabilization of feline leukemia virus-infected cats. *Mol Biother* 3:41–45, 1991

145. Yang, Y. Z. et al.: Effect of Astragalus membranaceus on natural killer cell activty and induction with coxsacke B viral myocarditis. *Chin Med J* 103:304–7, 1990

146. Weber, N. D. et al.: In vitro virucidal effects of *Allium stativum* (garlic) extract and compounds. *Planta Med* 58:417–23, 1992

147. Katz, E. and Margalith, E.: Inhibition of vaccinia virus maturation by zinc chloride. *Antimicrob Agents Chemother* 19:213–7, 1981

148. Eby, G. A., Davis, D. R., and Halcomb, W. W.: Reduction in duration of common colds by zinc gluconate lozenges in a double-blind study. *Antimicrob Agents Chemother* 25:20–24, 1984

149. Brody, I.: Topical treatment of recurrent herpes simplex and post-herpetic erythema multiforme with low concentrations of zinc sulfate solution. *Br J Dermatol* 104:191–213, 1981

150. Belaiche, P.: Treatment of vaginal infections of *Candida albicans* with the essential oil of Melaleuca alternafolia. *Phytotherapie* 15, 1985

151. Adetumbi, M. A. and Lau, B. H.: *Allium sativum* (garlic): Natural antibiotic. *Med Hypotheses* 12:227–37, 1983

152. Davis, L. E., Shen, J. and Royer, R. E.: In vitro syndergism of concentrated Allium sativum extract and amphotericin B against Cyrptoccus neoformans. *Planta Med* 60:546–49, 1994

153. Moore, G S. and Atkins, R. D.: The fungicidal and fungistatic effects of an aqueous garlic extract on medically important yeast-like fungi. *Mycologia* 69:341–48, 1977

154. Sandhu, D. K., Warraich, M. K. and Singh, S.: Sensitivity of yeasts isolated from cases of vaginitis to aqueous extracts of garlic. *Mykosen* 23:691–98, 1980

155. Prasad, G. and Sharma, V. D.: Efficacy of garlic (*Allium sativum*) treatment against experimental candidiasis in chicks. *Br Vet J* 136:448–51, 1980

156. Hunan Hospital: Garlic in cryptococcal meningitis: A preliminary report of 21 cases. *Chinese Med J* 93:123–6, 1980

157. Bastidas, G. J.: Effect of ingested garlic on *Necator americanus* and *Ancylostoma canium*. *Am J Trop Med Hyg* 18:920–23, 1969

158. Kaneda, Y, Torii, M. et al.: In vitro effects of berberine sulfate on the growth of *Entamoeba histolytica*, *Giardia lablia* and *Trichimonas vaginalis*. *Ann Tropical Med Parasitol* 85:417–25, 1991

159. Gupte, S.: Use of berberine in the treatment of giardiasis. *Am J Dis Chil* 129:866, 1975

160. Reuter, H. D.: Fifth Phytotherapy Congress in Bonn. *Zeitschrift fur Phytotherapie* 15:17–27, 1994

161. Ryan, R.: A double-blind clinical evaluation of bromelains in the treatment of acute sinusitis. *Headache* 7:13–17, 1967

162. Avorn, J., Monane, M. et al.: Reduction of bacteruria and pyuria after ingestion of cranberry juice. *JAMA* 271:751–54, 1994

163. Kilbourne, J. P.: Craneberry juice in urinary tract infection. *J Naturopathic Med* 2:45–47, 1991

164. Zafriri, D., Ofek, I. et al.: Inhibitory activity of cranberry juice on adherence of type I and type P fimbriated *Escherichia coli* to eucaryotic cell. *Antimicrob Agents Chemother* 33:92–8, 1989

165. Ofek, I., Goldhar, J. et al.: Anti-escherichia adhesion activity of cranberry and blueberry juices. *NEJM* 324:1599, 1991

166. Braunig, B. et al.: Echinacea *purpurea* radix for strengthening the immune reponse, I: Flu-like infections. *Z Phytother* 13:7–13, 1992 (in German)

167. Schoneberger, D.: The influence of immune-stimulating effects of pressed juice from *Echinacea purpurea* on the course and severity of colds: Results of double-blind study. *J Forum Immunologie* 8:2–12(in German)

168. *Br J Phytotherapy* 2:2, 1991

169. Partridge, M. and Poswillo, D.: Topical carbonoxolone sodium in the management of *Herpes simplex* infection. *Br J Oral Maxillofac Surg* 22:138–45, 1984

170. Csonka, G. and Tyrrell, D.: Treatment of herpes genitalis with carbonoxolone and cicloxolone creams: A double-blind placebo-controlled trial. *Br J Ven Dis* 60:178–81, 1984

171. Buck, D. S., Nidorf, D. M. and Addino, J. G.: Comparison of two topical preparations for the treatment of onychomycosis: *Melaleuca alternafolia* (tea tree) oil and clotrimasole. *J Fam Pract* 38:601–5, 1994

172. Pena, E. O.: Melaleuca alternafolia oil: Uses for trichomonal vaginitis and other vaginal infections. *Obst Gynecol* 19:793–95, 1962

Chapter 5

1. Ames, B. N.: Comparing synthetic to natural chemicals is essential for perception in "risk assessment." *Risk Analysis* 18:1–9, 1993

2. Rea, W. J. and Hsueh-Chia, L.: Effects of pesticides on the immune system. *J Nutr Med* 2:399–410, 1991

3. McKinnon, R. A. and Nebert, D. W.: Possible role of cytochrome P450 in lupus erythematosis and related disorders. *Lupus* 3:473–78, 1994

4. Talska, G. et al.: Genetically based n-acetyltransferase metabolic polymorphism and low-level environmental exposure to carcinogens. *Nature* 369:154–56, 1994

5. Russel, M, W., Brown, T. A., Claflin, J. L. et al.: Immunoglobulin A-mediated hepatobiliary transport constitutes a natural pathway for disposing of bacterial antigens. *Infect Immunity* 42:1041–48, 1983

6. Cantor, H. M. and Dumont, A. E.: Hepatic suppression of sensitization to antigen absorbed into the portal system. *Nature* 215:744–45, 1967

7. Triger, D. R., Alp, M. H. and Wright. R.: Bacterial and dietary antibodies in liver disease. *Lancet* i:60–63, 1972

8. Simopoulos, A. P., Corning, T. and Rerat, A.: Intestinal flora, immunity, nutrition, and health. *World Rev Nutr Diet* 74:123–48, 1993

9. Gallagher, J. E. et al.: Comparison of DNA adduct levels in human placenta from polychlorinated biphenyl exposed women and smokers in which CYP 1A1 levels are similarly elevated. *Terato Carcino Mutagen* 14:183–92, 1994

10. Campbell, M, E. et al.: Biotransformation of caffeine, paraxanthine, theophylline, and theobromine by polycyclic aromatic hydrocarbon-inducable cytochrome P-450 in human liver microsomes. *Drug Metab Disp* 15:237–49, 1987

11. Mansmann, H. C.: Consider magnesium homeostasis, III: Cytochrome P450 enzymes and drug toxicity. *Pediatric Asthma Allergy Immunol* 8:7–28, 1994

12. Beecher, C. W. W.: Cancer preventive properties of varieties of Brassica oleracea: A review. *Am J Clin Nutr* 59(suppl.):1166S–70S, 1994

13. Crowell, P. L. and Gould, M. N.: Chemoprevention and therapy of cancer by d-limonene. *Critical Rev Oncogenesis* 5:1–22, 1994

14. Yee, G. C. et al.: Effect of grapefruit juice on blood cyclosporin concentration. *Lancet* 345:955–56, 1995

15. Nagabhushan, M. and Bhide, S. V.: Curcumin as an inhibitor of cancer. *J Am Coll Nutr* 11:192–98, 1992

16. Elegbede, J. A. et al.: Effects of anticarcinogenic monoterpenes on phase II hepatic metabolizing enzymes. *Carcinogenesis* 14:1221–23, 1993

17. Hagen, T. M. et al.: Fate of dietary glutathione: Disposition in the gastrointestinal tract. *Am J Physiol* 259:G524-9, 1990

18. Ketter, B. et al.: The human glutathione S-transferase supergene family: Its polymorphism, and its effects on susceptibility to lung cancer. *Env Health Persp* 98:87–94, 1992

19. Ghadirian, P. et al.: Food habits and esophageal cancer: An overview. *Cancer Prev Detect* 16:163–68, 1992

20. Azzalis, L. A. et al.: Prooxidant and anitoxidant hepatic factors in rats chronically fed an ethanol regimen and treated with an acute dose of lindane. *Free Rad Biol Med* 19:147–59, 1995

21. White, A. C. et al.: Glutathione deficiency in human disease. *J Nutr Biochem* 5:218–26, 1994

22. Peristeris, P., Clark, B. D., Gatti, S. et al.: N-acetylcysteine and glutathione as inhibitors of tumor necrosis factor production. *Cell Immunol* 140:390–99, 1992

23. Flanagan, R. J. and Meridith, T. J.: Use of N-acetylcysteine in clinical toxicology. *Am J Med* 91(suppl.3C):3C–131S–9S, 1991

24. Burgunder, J. M. and Lautergurg, B. H.: Decreased production of glutathione in patients with cirrhosis. *Eur J Clin Invest* 17:408–14, 1987

25. Smith, C. V.: Will glutathione become a hot new supplement? *Nutr Report* 11:81–88, 1993

26. Richie, J. P.: The role of glutathione in aging and cancer. *Exp Gerontol* 27:615–26, 1992

27. Hagen, T. M., Wierzbicka, G. T., Sillua, A. H. et al.: Bioavailability of dietary glutathione: Effect of plasma concentration. *Am J Physiol* 259:G524–29, 1990

28. Pangborn, J.: *Mechanisms of Detoxification and Procedures for Detoxification*. Bionostics, West Chicago, 1994, pp. 115–18

29. Quick, A. J.: Clinical value of the test for hippuric acid in cases of disease of the liver. *Arch Int Med* 57:544–56, 1936

30. Frezza, M., Pozzato, G., Chiesa, L. et al.: Reversal of intrahepatic cholestasis of pregnancy in women after high dose S-adenosyl-L-methionine (SAMe) administration. *Hepatology* 4:274–78, 1984

31. Gregus, S. et al.: Nutritionally and chemically induced impairment of sulfate activation and sulfation of xenobiotics in vivo. *Chem-Biol Interactions* 92:169–77, 1994

32. Barzatt, R. and Beckman, J. D.: Inhibition of phenol sulfotransferase by pyridoxal phosphate. *Biochem Pharmacol* 47:2087–95, 1994

33. Skvortsova, R. I. et al.: Role of vitamin factor in preventing phenol poisoning. *Vopr Pitan* 2:32–35, 1981

34. *Medical Tribune:* Orange peel oil studied as cancer-fighting agent, May 30, 1991, p.11

35. Birkmayer, J. G. D. and Beyer, W.: Biological and clinical relevance of trace elements. *Arztl Lab* 36:284–87, 1990

36. Jeffrey, E. H. et al.: The role of cytochrome P450IIE1 in bioactivation of acetaminophen in diabetic and acetone treated mice. *Adv Exp Med Biol* 283:249–51, 1991

37. Robbins, S., Cotran, R. and Kumar, V.: *Pathologic Basis of Disease*, W. B. Saunders, Philadelphia, 1984

38. Padova, C., Tritapepe, R., Padova, F. et al.: S-adenosyl-L-methionine antagonizes oral contraceptive-induced bile cholesterol supersaturation in healthy women: Preliminary report of a controlled randomized trial. *Am J Gastroenterol* 79:941–44, 1984

39. Crissinger, K. D., Kvietys, P. R. and Granger, D. N.: Pathophysiology of gastrointestinal mucosal permeability. *J Int Med* 228: 145–54, 1990

40. Madara, J. L.: Pathobiology of the intestinal epithelial barrier. *Am J Pathol* 137: 1273–81, 1990

41. Tagesson, C. et al.: Passage of molecules through the wall of the intestinal tract. *Scan J Gastro* 18:481–6, 1983

42. Roland, N., Nugon-Baudon, L. and Rabot, S.: Interactions between the intestinal flora and xenobiotic metabolizing enzymes and their health consequences. *World Rev Nutr Diet* 74:123–48, 1993

43. Dantsker, D. R.: The gastrointestinal tract: The canary of the body? *JAMA* 270:1247–48, 1993

44. Cummings, J. H.: Fermentation in the human large intestine: Evidence and implications for health. *Lancet* i:1208, 1983

45. Voorhees, J. J.: Polyamines and psoriasis. *Arch Dermatol* 115:943–44, 1979

46. Liehr, H. and Grun, M.: *Progress in Liver Disease: Endotoxins in Liver Disease*. Grune and Straten, New York, 1979, pp. 313–26

47. Chadwick, R. W., George, S. E. and Claxton, L. D.: Role of the gastrointestinal mucosa and microflora in the bioactivation of dietary and environmental mutagens or carcinogens. *Drug Metabol Rev* 24:425–92, 1992

48. Belew, P. W., Rosenberg, E. W., Skinner, R. B. et al.: Endotoxemia in psoriasis. *Arch Dermatol* 118:142–43, 1982

49. Skinner, R. B., Rosenberg, E. W., Belew, P. W. and Marley, W. M.: Improvement of psoriasis with cholestyramine. *Arch Dermatol* 118:144, 1982

50. Thurman, F. M.: The treatment of psoriasis with sarsaparilla compound. *N Eng J Med* 227:128–33, 1942

51. Lahesmaa-Rantala, R., Magnusson, K. E., Granfors, K. et al.: Intestinal permeability in patients with Yersinia triggered reactive arthritis. *Anal Rheumatic Dis* 50: 91–94, 1991

52. Inman, R. D.: Nutrition and rheumatic diseases: Antigens, the gastrointestinal tract, and arthritis. *Rheumatic Dis Clin N Am* 17:309–21, 1991

53. Mielants, H., De Vos, M., Goemaere, S. et al.: Intestinal mucosal permeability in inflammatory rheumatic diseases, II: Role of disease. *J Rheumatol* 18:394–400, 1991

54. Smith, M. D., Gibson, R. A. and Brooks, P. M.: Abnormal bowel permeability in ankylosing spondylitis and rheumatoid arthritis. *J Rheumatol* 12:299–305, 1985

55. LeRoith, D., Shiloach, J., Roth, J. and Lesniak, M.: Insulin or a closely related molecule is native to Escherichia coli. *J Biolchem* 256:6533–36, 1981

56. Soderstrom, T., Hansson, G. and Larson, G.: The Escherichia coli K1 capsule shares antigenic determinants with the human gangliosides GM3 and GD3. *N Eng J Med* 310:11, 726–77, 1984

57. Stephansson, K., Dieperink, M. E., Richman, D. P. et al.: Sharing of antigenic determinants between the nicotinic acetylcholine receptor and proteins in Escherichia coli, Proteus vulgaris, and Klebsiella pneumoniae. *N Eng J Med* 312:221–25, 1985

58. Weiss, M. and Ingbar, S. H.: Demonstration of a saturable binding site for thyrotropin in Yersinia enterocolitica. *Science* 219:1331–35, 1983

59. Ebringer, A., Khalapfour, S. and Wilson, C.: Rheumatoid arthritis and Proteus: A possible aetiological association. *Rheumatol Int* 9: 223–28, 1989

60. Ebringer , A., Cox, N., Abuljadayel, A. I., Ghuloom, M., Khalapfour, S., Ptaszynska, T., Shodjai-Moradi, F. and Wilson, C.: Klebsiella antibodies in ankylosing spondylitis and Proteus antibodies in rheumatoid arthritis. *Bri J of Rheu* 27: 72–85, 1988

61. Madara, J. L., Nash, S., Moore, R. and Atisook, K.: Structure and function of the intestinal epithelial barrier in health and disease. *Gastrointestinal Pathol* 9: 306–24, 1990

62. Paganelli, R. et al.: Intestinal permeability in patients with chronic urticaria-angioedema with and without arthralgia. *Ann Allergy* 66:181–84, 1991

63. Teahon, K. et al.: Intestinal permeability in patients with Crohn's disease and their first degree relatives. *Gut* 33:320–23, 1992

64. Troncone, R. et al.: Increased intestinal sugar permeability after challenge in children with cow's milk allergy or intolerance. *Allergy* 49:142–46, 1994

65. Martinez-Gonzales, O. et al.: Intestinal permeability in patients with ankylosing spondylitis and their healthy relatives. *Br J Rheumatol* 33:644–47, 1994

66. Tepper, R. E. et al.: Intestinal permeability in patients infected with human immunodeficiency virus. *Am J Gastroent* 89:878, 1994

67. Kapembwa, M. S. et al.: Altered small-intestine permeability associated with diarrhea in human-immunodeficiency-virus-infected Caucasians and African subjects. *Clin Sci* 81:327–34, 1991

68. Paganelli, R. et al.: Intestinal permeability in patients with chronic urticaria-angioedema with and without arthralgia. *Ann Allergy* 66:181–84, 1991

69. Olaison, G., Sjodahl, R. and Tagesson, C.: Abnormal intestinal permeability in Crohn's disease. *Scand J Gastroenterol* 25: 321–28, 1990

70. Pearson, A. D. J., Eastham, E. J., Laker, M. F. and Craft, A. W.: Intestinal permeability in children with Crohn's disease and coeliac disease. *Br Med J* 285: 20–21, 1982

71. Shippee, R. L. et al.: Simultaneous determination of lactulose and mannitol in urine of burn patients by gas-liquid chromatography. *Clin Chem* 36:343–45, 1992

72. Sanderson, I. R., Boulton, P., Menzies, I. and Walker-Smith, J. A.: Improvement of abnormal lactulose/rhamnose permeability in active Crohn's disease of the small bowel by an elemental diet. *Gut* 28: 1073–76, 1987

73. Pironi, L., Miglioli, M., Ruggeri, E. et al.: Relationship between intestinal permeability to (51Cr) EDTA and inflammatory activity in asymptomatic patients with Crohn's disease. *Dig Dis Sci* 35:582–88, 1990

74. Wallace, J. L.: Pathogenesis of nonsteroidal anti-inflammatory drug gastropathy: Recent advances. *Eur J Gastro Hepatol* 5:403–7, 1993

75. Crotty, B.: Ulcerative colitis and xenobiotic metabolism. *Lancet* 343:35–38, 1994

76. Paganelli, R., Fagiolo, U., Cancian, M. and Scala, E.: Intestinal permeability in patients with chronic urticaria-angioedema with and without arthralgia. *Ann Allergy* 66:181–84, 1991

77. Dockhorn, R. J. and Smith, T. C.: Use of a chemically defined hypoallergenic diet in the management of patients with suspected food allergy. *Ann Allergy* 47:264–66, 1981 GET-6

78. Bjarnason, I., Ward, K. and Peters, T. J.: The leaky gut of alcoholism: Possible route of entry for toxic compounds. *Lancet* i:179–82, 1984

79. Hollander, D. and Tarnawski, H.: Aging-associated increase in intestinal absorption of macromolecules. *Gerontology* 31:133–37, 1985

80. Isolauri, E., Juntunen, M., Wiren, S. et al.: Intestinal permeability changes in acute gastroenteritis: Effects of clinical factors and nutritional management. *J Ped Gastroenterol Nutr* 8:466–73, 1989

81. O'Dwyer, S. T., Michie, H. R., Ziegler, T. R. et al.: A single dose of endotoxin increases intestinal permeability in healthy humans. *Arch Surg* 123:1459–64, 1988

82. Deitch, E. A.: Intestinal permeability is increased in burn patients shortly after injury. *Surgery* 107:411–16, 1990

83. Jenkins, A. P., Trew, D. R., Crump, B. J. et al.: Do non-steroidal anti-inflammatory drugs increase colonic permeability? *Gut* 32:66–69, 1991

84. Worthington-Roberts, B.: *Contemporary Developments in Nutrition*. C. V. Mosby, St. Louis, MO, 1981

85. Iacono, G. et al.: Chronic constipation as a symptom of cow's milk allergy. *J Pediatr* 126:34–39, 1995

86. Smith, C. V.: "Free Radical Mechanisms in Tissue Injury," in Moslen, M.T. and Smith, C.V. (eds.): *Free Radical Mechanisms of Tissue Injury*. CRC Press, Boca Raton, FL 1992, pp. 2–22

87. Menkes, M. S., Comstock, G. W., Vuilleumier, J. P. et al.: Serum beta-carotene, vitamins A and E, selenium, and the risk of lung cancer. *NEJM* 315:1250–54, 1986

88. Esterbauer, H., Gebick, J., Puhl, H. and Jurgens, G.: The role of lipid peroxidation and antioxidants in oxidative modification of LDL. *Free Radic Biol Med* 13:341–90, 1992

89. Liles, M. R., Newsome, D. A. and Oliver, P. D.: Antioxidant enzymes in the aging human retinal pigment epithelium. *Arch Opthalmal* 109:1285–88, 1991

90. Suryaprabha, P., Das, U. N., Ramesh, G. et al.: Reactive oxygen species, lipid peroxides and essential fatty acids in patients with rheumatoid arthritis and systemic lupus erythematosus. *Prostaglandins Leukot Essent Fatty Acids* 43:251–55, 1991

91. Cross, C. E., van der Vliet, A., O'Neill, C. A. and Eiserich, J. P.: Reactive oxygen species and the lung. *Lancet* 344:930–33, 1994

92. Jenner, P.: Oxidative damage in neurodegenerative disease. *Lancet* 344:796–98, 1994

93. Ames, B. N., Shigenaga, M. K. and Hagen, T. M.: Oxidants, antioxidants, and the degenerative diseases of aging. *Proc Natl Acad Sci USA* 90:7915–22, 1993

94. Olanow, C. W. and Arendash, G. W.: Metals and free radicals in neurodegeneration. *Curr Opin Neurol* 7: 548–58, 1994

95. Halliwell, B.: Free radicals, antioxidants, and human disease: Curiosity, cause or consequence? *Lancet* 344:721–24, 1994

96. Reed, P. J.: "Mechanisms of Chemically Induced Cell Injury and Cellular Protection Mechanisms," in Hodgson, E. and Levi, P.E. (eds.): *Introduction to Biochemical Toxicology*, 2nd ed. Appleton and Lange, Norwalk, CT, 1994, pp. 267–95

97. Corbett, M. D. and Corbett, B. R.: "Bioactivation of Xenobiotics by the Respiratory Burst of Human Granulocytes," in Moslen, M.T. and Smith, C.V. (eds.): *Free Radical Mechanisms of Tissue Injury*. CRC Press, Boca Raton, FL, 1992, pp. 144–51

98. Block, G.: Antioxidant intake in the U.S. *Toxicol Ind Health* 9:295–301, 1993

99. Patterson, B. H., Block, G., Rosenberger, W. F. et al.: Fruits and vegetables in the American diet: Data from NHACVES II survey. *Am J Pub Health* 80:1432–39, 1990

100. Madsen, C.: Prevalence of food additive intolerance. *Human & Exp Toxicol* 13:393–99, 1994

101. Whitcomb, D. C. and Block, G. D.: Association of acetaminophen hepatotoxicity with fasting and alcohol use. *JAMA* 272:1845–50, 1994

102. Rifat, S. L.: Aluminum hypothesis lives. *Lancet* 343:3–4, 1994

103. Rifat, S. L. et al.: Effect of exposure of miners to aluminum powder. *Lancet* 336:1162–65, 1990

104. White, D. M. et al.: Neurologic syndrome in 25 workers from an aluminum smelting plant. *Arch Int Med* 152:1443–48, 1992

105. Knoll, O. et al.: Consequences from eeg findings and aluminum encephalopathy. *Trace Element Med* 8:S18–S20, 1991

106. Nylander, M. et al.: Mercury concentrations in human brain and kidneys in relation to exposure from dental amalgam fillings. *Swed Dent J* 11:179–87, 1987

107. Lorscheider, F. L. et al.: Toxicity assessment of mercury vapor from dental amalgams. *Fundam Appl Tox* 19:319–29, 1992

108. Siblerud, R. L.: The relationship between mercury from dental amalgam and mental health. *Am J Psychother*, October 18:575–87, 1989

109. Landrigan, P. J.: Lead in the modern workplace. *Am J Pub Health* 80:907–8, 1990

110. Holtzman, R. B. and Flcewicz, F. H.: Lead-210 and polmium-210 in tissues of cigarette smokers. *Science* 153:1259–60, 1966

111. Flora, G. J. S. et al.: Therapeutic efficacy of combined meso 2,3-dimercaptosuccinate and calcium sodium edetate treatment during acute lead intoxication in rats. *Human Exp Toxicol* 14:410–13, 1995

112. Werbach, M. R.: *Nutritional Influences on Illness*, 2nd Ed. Third Line Press, Tarzana, CA, 1993, pp 679–80

113. Austin, S. and Soloway, N.: II:Hair analysis. In: Pizzorno, J. E. and Murray, M. T.: *A Textbook of Natural Medicine*. Bastyr University Publ, Seattle, WA, 1995

114. Jamall, I., et al,: Use of hair as an indicator of environmental lead pollution in women of childbearing age in Karachi, Pakistan and Bangladesh. *Bull Envir Contam Toxicol* 44:350–6, 1990

115. Katz, S. A. and Katz, R. B.: Use of hair analysis for evaluating mercury intoxication of the human body: A review. *J Appl Tox* 12:79–84, 1992

116. Hwang, H., Dwyer,J. and Russell, R. M.: Diet, Helicobacter pylori infection, food preservation and gastric cancer risk: Are there new roles for preventive factors? *Nutr Rev* 52:75–83, 1994

117. Correa, P.: How does Helicobacter pylori infection increase risk of gastric cancer? *Eur J Gastro & Hepatol* 6:1117–18, 1994

118. Jones, S. T. M. et al.: Chronic NSAID use: Helicobacter antibodies may predict ulcer risk. *Br J Rheum* 30:16–20, 1991

119. Conway, C.: Truth and consequences of coffee. *Stanford Med* Winter:24–26, 1991

120. Banerjee, S. et al.: Effect of Helicobacter pylori and its eradication on gastric juice ascorbic acid. *Gut* 35:317–22, 1994

121. Al-Somal, N., Coley, K.E. et al.: Susceptibility of Helicobacter pylori to the antibacterial activity of manuka honey. *J Royal Soc Med* 87:9–12, 1994

122. Campbell, A. et al.: Suppressed killer cell activity in patients with silicone breast implants: Reversal upon removal. *Toxicol & Indust Health* 10:149–54, 1994

123. Blair, A.: Herbicides and non-Hodgkin's lymphoma: New evidence from a study of Saskatchewan farmers. *J Ntnl Canc Inst* 82:544–45, 1990

124. Leiss, J. and Savits, D.: Home pesticide use and childhood cancer: A case control study. *Am J Public Health* 85:249–52, 1995

125. Tappel, A. L. and Chen, H.: Protection by vitamin E, selenium, trolox C, ascorbic acid palmitate, acetylcysteine, coenzyme Q, beta-carotene, canthaxanthin and (+)-catechin against oxidative damage to liver slices measured by oxidized heme proteins. *Free Rad Biol Med* 16:437–44, 1994

126. Put, A. et al.: Clinical efficacy of "essential" phospholipids in patients chronically exposed to organic solvents. *J Int Med Res* 21:185–91, 1993

127. Hikino, H., Kiso, Y., Wagner, H. and Fiebig, : Antihepatotoxic actions of flavonolignans from Silybum marianum fruits. *Planta Medica* 50:248–50, 1984

128. Albrecht, M. Frerick, H. et al.: Therapy of toxic liver pathologies with Legalon. *Z Klin Med* 47:87–92, 1992

129. Salmi, H. A. and Sarna, S.: Effect of silymarin on chemical, functional, and morphological alteration of the liver: A double-blind controlled study. *Scand J Gastroenterol* 17:417–21, 1982

130. Vogel, G., Trost, W., Braatz, R. et al.: Studies on pharmacodynamics: Site and mechanism of action of silymarin, the antihepatotoxic principle from Silybum marianum *(L.) Gaert. Arzneim.-Forsch* 25:179–85, 1975

131. Boari, C., Montanari, M., Galleti, G. P. et al.: Occupational toxic liver diseases: Therapeutic effects of silymarin. *Min Med* 72:2679–88, 1985

132. Palasciano, G., Portinacasa, P. et al.: The effect of silymarin on plasma levels of malondialdehyde in patients receiving long-term treatment with psychotropic drugs. *Curr Ther Res* 55:537–45, 1994

133. Scevola, D. et al.: Possible anti-endotoxin activity of (+)-Cyanidanol-3 in experimental hepatitis in the rat. *Hepatogastroenterol* 29:178–82, 1982

134. World, M. et al.: (+)-Cyanidanol-3 for alcoholic liver disease: Results of a six month clinical trial. *Alcohol Alcoholism* 19:23–29, 1984

135. Katiyar, S. K. et al.: Protective effects of green tea polyphenols administered by oral intubation against chemical carcinogen-induced forestomach and pulmonary neoplasia in A/J mice. *Canc Lett* 73:167–72, 1993

136. Gandolfo, G. M. et al.: Hemolytic anemia and thrombocytopenia induced by cyanidanol. *Acta Haematol* 88:96–99, 1992

137. Sachan, D. S., Rhew, T. H. and Ruark, R. A.: Ameliorating effects of carnitine and its precursors on alcohol-induced fatty liver. *Am J Clin Nutr* 39:738–44, 1984

138. Coulter, D. L.: Carnitine, valproate, and toxicity. *J Child Neurol* 6:7–14, 1991

139. Sakuma, T.: Alterations of urinary carnitine profile induced by benzoate administration. *Arch Dis Children* 66:873–75, 1991

140. Leung, A. Y.: *Encyclopedia of Common Natural Ingredients Used in Food, Drugs and Cosmetics.* John Wiley, New York 1980

141. Faber, K.: The dandelion: Taraxacum officinale Weber. *Pharmazie* 13:423–35, 1958

142. Kirchhoff, R., Beckers, C. H. et al.: Increase in choleresis by means of artichoke extract. *Phytomed* 1:107–15, 1994

143. Montini, M., Levoni, P., Angoro, A. and Pagani, G.: Controlled trial of cynarin in the treatment of the hyperlipemic syndrome. *Arzneim-Forsch* 25:1311–14, 1975

144. Kiso, Y., Suzuki, Y., Watanabe, N. et al.: Antihepatotoxic principles of Curcuma longa rhizomes. *Planta Medica* 49:185–87, 1983

145. Rao, D. S. et al.: Effect of curcumin on serum and liver cholesterol levels in the rat. *J Nutr* 100:1307–16, 1970

146. Sanbe, K., Murata, T., Fujisawa, K. et al.: Treatment of liver disease with particular reference to liver hydrolysates. *Jap J Clin Exp Med* 50:2665–76, 1973

147. Fujisawa, K., Suzuki, H., Yamamoto, S. et al.: Therapeutic effects of liver hydrolysate preparation on chronic hepatitis: A double-blind, controlled study. *Asian Med J* 26:497–526, 1984

148. Wagner, H.: "Antihepatotoxic Flavonoids," in Cody, V., Middleton, E. and Harbourne, J. B. (eds.): *Plant Flavonoids in Biology and Medicine: Biochemical, Pharmacological, and Structure-Activity Relationships*, Alan R. Liss, New York, 1986, pp. 545–58

149. Krijgsheld, K. R. et al.: The oxidation of L- and D-cysteine to inorganic sulfate and taurine in the rat. *Biochemica et Biophysica Acta* 677:7–12, 1981

150. Bogaards, J. J. P. et al.: Consumption of brussels sprouts results in elevated (-class glutathione-S-transferase levels in human blood plasma. *Carcinogenesis* 15:1073–75, 1994

151. Wortelboer, H. M. et al.: Acid reaction products of indole-3-carbinol and their effects on cytochrome P450 and Phase II enzymes in rat and monkey hepatocytes. *Biochem Pharmacol* 43:1439–47, 1993

152. Beecher, C. W. W.: Cancer preventive properties of varieties of Brassica oleracea: A review. *Am J Clin Nutr* 59(suppl.):1166S–70S, 1994

153. Gershoff, S. N.: Vitamin C (ascorbic acid): New roles, new requirements? *Nutr Rev* 51:313–26, 1993

154. Tribble, D. L. et al.: Reduced plasma ascorbic acid concentrations in nonsmokers regularly exposed to environmental tobacco smoke. *Am J Clin Nutr* 58:886–90, 1993

155. Harrison, D. F. et al.: Glutathione S-transferases in alcoholic liver disease. *Gut* 31:909–11, 1990

156. Watanbe, A., Obata, T. and Nagashima, H.: Berberine therapy of hypertyraminemia in patients with liver cirrhosis. *Acta Med Okayam* 36: 277–81, 1982

157. Huddleson, I. F. et al.: Antibacterial substances in plants. *J Am Vet Med Assoc* 105:394–97, 1944

158. Cavallito, C. J. and Bailey, J. H.: Allicin, the antibacterial principle of Allium sativum, I: Isolation, physical properties and antibacterial action. *J Am Chem Soc* 66:1950–51, 1944

159. Sharma, V. D. et al.: Antibacterial property of Allium sativum Linn.: In vivo and in vitro studies. *Ind J Exp Biol* 15:466–68, 1977

160. Elnima, E. I. et al.: The antimicrobial activity of garlic and onion extracts. *Pharmazie* 38:747–48, 1983

161. Roberfroid, M. G. and Gibson, G. R.: Dietary modulation of the human colonic microbiota: Introducing the concept of prebiotics. *J Nutr* 125:1401–12, 1995

162. Lee, Y.-K. and Salminen, S.: The coming of age of probiotics. *Trends Food Sci Technol* 6:241–45, 1995

163. Friend, B. A. and Shahani, K. M.: Nutritional and therapeutic aspects of lactobacilli. *J App Nutr* 36:125–36, 1984

164. Hidaka, H. et al.: "The Effects of Undigestible Fructo-Oligosaccharides on Intestinal Micorflora and Various Physiological New Functions in Human Health," in Furda, I. and Brine, C. J. (eds.): *New Developments in Dietary Fiber*. Plenum Press, New York, 1990, pp.105–17

165. Tomomatsu, H.: Health effects of oligosaccharides. *Food Tech*, October 1994:61–65

166. Shah, N., Atallah, T., Mahoney, R. R. and Pellett, P. L.: Effect of dietary fiber components on fecal nitrogen excretion and protein utilization. *J Nutr* 112:658–66, 1982

167. Vahouny, G. and Kritchevsky, D.: *Dietary Fiber in Health and Disease*. Plenum Press, New York, 1982

168. Burkitt, D. P., Walke, A. R. P. and Painter, N. S.: Effects of dietary fiber on stools and transit times and its role in the causation of disease. *Lancet* ii:1408–12, 1972

169. Bengmark, S. and Jeppsson, B.: Gastrointestinal surface protection and mucosa reconditioning. *J Parent Ent Nutr* 19:410–15, 1995

170. Falth-Magnusson, K., Kjellman, N.-I. M., Odelram, H. et al.: Gastrointestinal permeability in children with cow's milk allergy: Effect of milk challenge and sodium cromoglycate as assessed with polyethylenegols (PEG 400 and PEG 1000). *Clin Allergy* 16:543–51, 1986

171. Ci Carlo, G., Mascolo, N. et al.: Effects of quercetin on the gastrointestinal tract in rats and mice. *Phytotherapy Res* 8:42–45, 1994

172. Bjarnason, I., Williams. P., Smethurst, P. et al.: Effect of non-steroidal anti-inflammatory drugs and prostaglandins on the permeability of the human small intestine. *Gut* 27:1292–97, 1986

173. Andre, C. Andre, F. andColin, L.: Effect of allergen ingestion challenge with and without cromoglycate cover on intestinal permeability in atopic dermatitis, urticaria and other symptoms of food allergy. *Allergy* 44:47–51, 1989

174. Saltzman, J. R. et al.: Bacterial overgrowth without clinical malabsorption in elderly hypochlorhydric subjects. *Gastroenterol* 106:615–23, 1994

175. Nakamura, T. et al.: Short-chain carboxylic acid in the feces in patients with pancreatic insufficiency. *Acta Gastrointerol Belg* 56:326–31, 1993

176. Cummings, J. H.: Short chain fatty acids in the human colon. *Gut* 22:763–79, 1981

177. Scoba, W. W.: Glutamine: A key substrate for the splanchnic bed. *Ann Rev Nutr* 11:285–308, 1991

178. Klimberg, V. S., Salloum, R. M., Kasper, M. et al.: Oral glutamine accelerates healing of the small intestine and improves outcome after whole abdominal radiation. *Arch Surg* 125:1040–45, 1990

179. Klimberg, V. S. et al.: Prophylactic glutamine protects the intestinal mucosa from radiation injury. *Cancer* 66:62–68, 1990

180. Weir, C. D. et al.: Glutamine enhanced elemental diet modifies colonic damage in a hapten induced model of colitis. *Gastroenterol* 102,Part II:A711, 1992

181. Skoldstam, L. and Magnusson, K.-E.: Fasting, intestinal permeability, and rheumatoid arthritis. *Rheum Dis Clin N Amer* 17:363–71, 1991

182. Mergens, W.J., Kammi, J. J. and Newark, H. L.: "Alpha tocopherol: Uses in Preventing Nitrosoamine Formation, " in Walker, E. A., Castegnaro, M., Gricute, L., and Lyle, R. E. (eds.): *Environmental Aspects of N-Nitroso Compounds*, IARC Scientific Publications, Lyon, 1978, pp. 190–212

183. Steiner, M.: Influences of vitamin E on platelet function in humans. *J Am Coll Nutr* 10:466–73, 1991

184. Horwilt, M. K.: Supplementation with Vitamin E. *Am J Clin Nutr* 47:1088–89, 1988

185. Chan, A. C.: Partners in defense: Vitamin C and Vitamin E. *Canad J Physiol Pharm* 71:725–31, 1993

186. Beyer, R. E.: The role of ascorbate in antioxidant protection of biomembranes: Interaction with vitamin E and coenzyme Q. *J Bioenerg & Biomemb* 26:349–57, 1994

187. Trevithick, J. R., et al.: Topical tocopherol acetate reduces post-UVB, sunburn associated erythema, edema, and skin sensitivity in mice. *Arch Biochem Biophys* 296:575–82, 1992

188. Frei, B., England, L. and Ames, B. N.: Ascorbate is an outstanding antioxidant in human blood plasma. *Proc Natl Acad Sci* 86:6377–81, 1989

189. Chandra, D. B., Varma, R., Ahmad, S. and Varma, S. D.: Vitamin C in the aqueous humor and cataracts. *Int J Vit Nutr Res* 56:165–68, 1986

190. Jakob, R. A., Kelly, D. S., Piamalto, F. S. et al.: Immunocompetence and antioxidant defense during ascorbate depletion of healthy men. *Am J Clin Nutr* 54: (6 Suppl):1302S–9S, 1991

191. Calabrese, E.J., Stoddard, A., Leonard, D. A. and Dinardi, S. R.: The effect of vitamin C supplementation on blood and hair levels of cadmium, iron and mercury. *Ann NY Acad Sci* 498:347–53, 1987

192. Tannenbaum, S. R. and Wishnor, J. S.: Inhibition of nitrosamine formation by ascorbic acid. *Ann NY Acad Sci* 498:354–63, 1987

193. Stahelin, H. B., Grey, K.F., Eichholzer, M. et al.: Plasma antioxidant vitamins and subsequent cancer mortality in the 12-year follow up of the prospective basal study. *Am J Epidemiol* 133:766–75, 1991

194. Yasukawa, M. et al.: Radiation-induced neoplastic formation of C3H102 cells suppressed by ascorbic acid. *Radiation Res* 120:456–67, 1989

195. Rose, R. C.: Ascorbic acid metabolism in protection against free radicals: A radiation model. *Biochem Biophys Res Com* 169:430–36, 1990

196. Parker, R. S.: "Analysis of Carotenoids in Human Plasma and Tissue," in Packer, L. (ed.): Carotenoids. Part B: Metabolism, genetics and biosynthesis. Methods in Enzymology vol. 124, Academic Press, San Diego, 1993, pp. 86–93

197. Bendich, A. and Olson, J. A.: Biological action of carotenoids. *FASEB J* 3:1927–32, 1989

198. Vile, G. F. and Winterbourin, C. C.: Inhibition of adriamycin promoted microsomal lipid peroxidation by beta carotene, alpha-tocopherol and retinal at high and low oxygen partial pressure. *FEBS Lett* 238:353–56, 1988

199. Block, G.: The data support a role of antioxidants in reducing cancer risk. *Nutr Rev* 50:207–13, 1992

200. The alpha-tocopherol, beta carotene cancer prevention study group: the effect of vitamin E and beta carotene on the incidence of lung cancer and other cancers in male smokers. *NEJM* 330:1029–35, 1994

201. Jialal, I., Norju, E. P., Cristol, L. and Grundy, S. M.: Beta-carotene inhibits the oxidative modification of low-density lipoprotein. *Biochem Biophys Acta* 1086:134–8, 1991

202. Morris, D. L., Kritchevsky, S. B. and Davis, C. E.: Serum carotenoids and coronary heart disease. *JAMA* 272:1439–41, 1994

203. Seddon, J. M., Ajani, U. A., Sperduto, R. D. et al.: Dietary carotenoids, vitamins A, C and E, and advanced age-related macular degeneration. *JAMA* 272:1413–20, 1994

204. Kandaswami, C., Perkins, E., Soloniuk, D. S. et al.: Ascorbic acid-enhanced antiproliferative effect of flavonoids on squamous cell carcinoma in vitro. *Anti Cancer Drugs* 4:91–96, 1993

205. Robak, J. and Gryglewski, R. J.: Flavonoids are scavengers of superoxide. *Biochem Pharmacol* 37:837–41, 1988

206. DeWhalley, C. V., Rankin, S., Hoult, J. R. S. et al.: Flavonoids inhibit the oxidation modification of low density lipoproteins by macrophages. *Biochem Pharmacol* 39:1743–50, 1990

207. Monboissi, J. C., Braquet, P., Pandoux, A. and Borel, J. B.: Nonenzymatic degradation of acid soluble calf skin collagen by superoxide ion: Protective effect of flavonoids. *Biochem Pharmacol* 32:53–58, 1983

208. Afanasev, J. B., Dorozhko, A. I., Brodskii, A. V. et al.: Chelating and free radical scavenging mechanism of inhibition action of rutin and quercitin in lipid peroxidation. *Biochem Pharmacol* 38:1763–69, 1989

209. Stavric, B. and Matula, T. I.: "Flavonoids in Foods: Their Significance for Nutrition and Health," in Ong, A. S. H. and Packer, L. (eds.): *Lipid-Soluble Antioxidants: Biochemistry and Chemical Applications*, Birkhauser Verlag, Basel, Switzerland, 1992, pp. 274–94

210. Visner, G. A., Dougall W. C., Wilson, J. M. et al.: Regulation of manganese superoxide dismutase by lipopolysaccharide, interleukin-1, and tumor necrosis factor. *J Biol Chem* 265:2856–64, 1990

211. Giri, S. N. and Misra, H. P.: Fate of superoxide dismutase in mice following oral route of administration. *Med Biol* 62:285–89, 1984

212. Niwa, Y., Sominya, K., Michelson, A. M. and Puget, F.: Effect of liposomal encapsulated superoxide dismutase on active oxygen-related human disorders. *Free Radical Res Commun* 1:137–53, 1985

213. Rhee, P., Waxman, K., Clark, L. et al.: Superoxide dismutase polyethylene glycol improves survival in hemorrhagic shock. *Am Surg* 57:747–50, 1991

214. Nayak, M. S., Kita, M. and Marmor, M. F.: Protection of rabbit retina from ischemic injury by superoxide dismutase and catalase. *Invest Ophthalmol Vis Sci* 34:2018–22, 1993

215. Kohen, R., Kakunda, A. and Rubinstein, A.: The role of cationized catalase and cationized glucose oxidase in mucosal oxidative damage induced in the rat jejunum. *J Biol Chem* 267:21349–54, 1992

216. Jones, J. B., Cramer, H. M., Inch, W. R. and Lamps, H. B.: Radioprotective effect of free radical scavenging enzymes. *J Otolaryngol* 19:299–306, 1990

217. Newsome, D., et al.: Trace element and antioxidant economy of the human macula: Can dietary supplementation influence the course of macular degeneration? *J Am Coll Nutr* 10:536/Abs 12, 1991

218. Reddy, V. K., Kumar, C. T., Prasad, M. and Reddanna, P.: Exercise-induced oxidant stress in the lung tissue: Role of dietary supplementation of vitamin E and selenium. *Biochem Int* 26:863–71, 1992

219. Akerboom, T. P. M. and Sies, H.: "Assay of Glutathione, Glutathione Disulfide and Glutathione Mixed Disulfides," in Jakopy, W. (ed.): *Detoxification and Drug Metabolism: Conjugation and Related Systems: Methods in Enzymology*, vol. 77, Academic Press, New York, 1981, pp. 373–82

220. Maguire, J. J., Kagan, V., Ackrell, B. A. and Packer, L.: Succinate-ubiquinone reductase linked recycling of alpha-tocopherol in reconstituted systems and mitochondria: Requirement for reduced ubiquinone. *Arch Biochem Biophys* 292:47–53, 1992

221. Gaby, A.: "Coenzyme Q10," in Pizzorno, J. E. and Murray, M. A.: *Textbook of Natural Medicine*. Bastyr University Publications, Seattle, WA, 1995

222. Stocker, R., Bowry, V. W. and Frei, B.: Ubiquinol-10 protects human low density lipoproteins more efficiently against lipid peroxidation than does alpha tocopherol. *Proc Natl Acad Sci USA* 88:1646–50, 1991

223. Harmon, D.: Free radicals in aging. *Mol Cell Biochem* 84:154–66, 1988

224. Reimund, E.: The free radical flux theory of sleep. *Medical Hypothesis* 43:231–33, 1994

225. Poeggeler, B. et al.: Melatonin, hydroxyl radical-mediated oxidative damage, and aging: A hypothesis. *J Pineal Res* 14:151–68, 1993

226. Chen, H. and Tappel, A. L.: Protection by vitamin E, selenium, Trolox c, ascorbic acid palmitate, acetylcysteine, coenzyme Q, beta-carotene, canthaxanthin, and (+)-catechin against oxidative damage to liver slices measured by oxidized heme proteins. *Free Rad Biol Med* 16:437–44, 1994

227. Martin, D. S., et al.: N-acetylcysteine in the treatment of human arsenic poisoning. *J Am Board Fam Pract* 3:293–6, 1990

228. Tandon, S. K., et al.: Influence of selenium during chelation of lead in rats. *Ind J Physiol Pharmacol* 36:201–4, 1992

229. Baulici, S. and Chirila, M.: Zinc supplementation of chelation therapy in saturnism. Preliminary study. *Rom J Int Med* 30:211–5, 1992

230. Whanger, P.D.: Selenium in the treatment of heavy metal poisoning and chemical carcinogenesis. *J Trace Elem Electrolytes Health Dis* 6:209–21, 1992

231. Gooneratne, R. and Olkowski, A.: Lead toxicity chelation therapy: New findings. *J Advanc Med* 6:225–231, 1993

232. Herkovits, J. and Perez-Coll, C. S.: Zinc protection against delayed development produced by cadmium. *Biol Trace Elem Res* 24:217–21, 1990

233. Koch, H. P. and Lawson, D. L.: *Garlic*. Williams Wilkins, Baltimore, MD, 1996, pp 205-6

234. Trakhtenberg, I. M., et al.: The prophylactic use of pectin in chronic lead exposure in industry. *Vrach Delo* 1:132–6, 1995

235. Shakman, R. A.: Nutritional influences on the toxicity of environmental pollutants: A review. *Arch Env Health* 28:105–33, 1974

236. Goodhart, R. S. and Shils, M. E.: *Modern Nutrition in Health and Disease*, 6th ed. Lea & Febiger, Philadelphia, 1980, pp. 738, 826, 983–86, 1086

237. Young, V. R. and Scrimshaw, N. S.: The physiology of starvation. *Sci Am* 225:4:14–21, 1971

238. Reinmuth, O. M., Scheinberg, P. and Bourne, B.: Total cerebral blood flow and metabolism. *Arch Neurol* 12:49–66, 1965

239. Saudek, C. and Felig, P.: The metabolic events of starvation. *Am J Med* 60:117–26, 1976

240. Cahill, G. F. Jr., Owen, O. E. and Morgan, A. P.: The consumption of fuels during prolonged starvation. *Adv Enzyme Regul* 6:143–50, 1968

241. Uden, A. M., Trang, L., Venizelos, N. and Palmblad, J.: Neutrophil function and clinical performances after total fasting in patients with rheumatoid arthritis. *Ann Rheum Dis* 42:45–51, 1983

242. Palmblad, J., Cantell, K., Holm, G. et al.: Acute energy deprivation in man: Effect on serum immunoglobulins, antibody response, complement factors 3 & 4, acute phase reactants and interferon producing capacity of blood lymphocytes. *Clin Exp Immunol* 30:50–55, 1977

243. Darlington, L. G. and Ramsey, N. W.: Diets for rheumatoid arthritis. *Lancet* 338: 1209, 1991

244. Wall, K. et al.: Food restriction increases detoxification of polycyclic aromatic hydrocarbons in the rat. *Carcinogenesis* 13:519–23, 1992

245. Lithell, H., Bruce, A., Gustafsson, I. B. et al.: A fasting and vegetarian diet treatment trial on chronic inflammatory disorders. *Acta Derm Venereol* 63:397–403, 1983

246. Skoldstam, L., Lindstrom, F. D. and Lindblom, B.: Impaired con A suppressor cell activity in patients with rheumatoid arthritis shows normalization during fasting. *Scand J Rheumatol* 12:4:369–73, 1983

247. Brod, J., Pavkova, L., Fencl, V. et al.: Influence of fasting on the immunological reactions and course of acute glomerulonephritis. *Lancet* i:760–63, 1958

248. Gresham, G. A.: Is atheroma a reversible lesion? *Atherosclerosis* 23:379–91, 1976

249. Allen, F. M.: Prolonged fasting in diabetes. *Am J Med Sci* 150:480–85, 1915

250. Vessby, B., Boberg, M., Karlstrom, B. et al.: Improved metabolic control after supplemented fasting in overweight type 2 diabetic patients. *Acta Med Scand* 216:67–74, 1984

251. Lennox, W. G. and Cobb, S.: Studies in epilepsy. *Arch Neurol Psych* 20:711–79, 1928

252. Sundquist, T., Lindstrom, F., Magnusson, K. and Skoldstam, L.: Influence of fasting on intestinal permeability and disease activity in patients with rheumatoid arthritis shows normalization during fasting. *Scand J Rheumatol* 11:33–38, 1982

253. Folin, O. and Denis, W.: On starvation and obesity with special reference to acidosis. *J Biol Chem* 21:183–92, 1915

254. Stewart, W. K. and Fleming, L. W.: Features of a successful therapeutic fast of 382 days' duration. *Postgrad Med J* 49:203–9, 1973

255. Navarro, S., Rose, E., Aused, R. et al.: Comparison of fasting, nasogastric suction and cimetidine in the treatment of acute pancreatitis. *Digestion* 30:224–30, 1984

256. Imamura, M. and Tung, T.: A trial of fasting cure for PCB poisoned patients in Taiwan. *Am J Ind Med* 5:147–53, 1984

257. Keys, A., Brozek, J., Henschel, A. et al.: *The Biology of Human Starvation,* vols. 1 and 2. University of Minnesota Press, Minneapolis, MN, 1950

258. Young, V. R. and Scrimshaw, N. S.: The physiology of starvation. *Sci Am* 225:4:14–21, 1971

259. Kilburn, K. et al.: Neurobehavioral dysfunction in firemen exposed to polychlorinated biphenyls (PCBs): Possible improvement after detoxification. *Arch Envir Health* 44:345–50, 1989

260. Press, E.: The health hazards of saunas and spas and how to minimize them. *Am J Publ Health* 81:1034–37, 1991

261. Petersdorf, R.: *Harrison's Principles of Internal Medicine.* McGraw-Hill, New York, 1983

262. De Morais, S. M. F., Uetrecht, J. P. and Wells, P. G.: Decreased glucuronidation and increased bioactivation of acetaminophen in Gilbert's syndrome. *Gastronent* 102:577–86, 1992

263. Londsdale, D.: Gilbert's disease: Symptomatic response to nutritional supplementation in patients. *J Nutr Med* 3:319–24, 1992

264. Lee, J. R.: Fluoride linked to Gilbert's syndrome. *Cortlandt Forum* 101:31–33, 1990

265. Bombardieri, G., Milani, A., Bernardi, L. and Rossi, L.: Effects of S-adenosyl-methionine (SAMe) in the treatment of Gilbert's syndrome. *Curr Ther Res* 37:580–85, 1985

266. Buchwald, D. et al.: Chronic fatigue and the chronic fatigue syndrome: Prevalence in a Pacific Northwest health care system. *Ann Int Med* 123:81–88, 1995

267. Bland, J. S. et al.: A medical food-supplemented detoxification program in the management of chronic health problems. *Alt Therapies* 1:62–71, 1995

268. Bell, D. S.: Chronic fatigue syndrome update. *Postgrad Med* 96:73–81, 1994

269. Terr, A. I.: Multiple chemical sensitivities. *J Allergy Clin Immuno* 94/Part II:362–5, 1991

270. Rogers, S.: Chemical sensitivity: Breaking the paralyzing paradigm, Parts 1 and 2. *Int Med World Rep* February, March, 1992

271. Buchwald, D. and Garrity, D.: Comparison of patients with chronic fatigue syndrome, fibromyalgia, and multiple chemical sensitivities. *Arch Int Med* 154:2049–53, 1994

272. Apter, A., et al: Epidemiology of sick building syndrome. *J Allergy Clin Immunol* 94:277–88, 1994

273. Katzung, B. G.: *Basic and Clinical Pharmacology.* Appelton &Lange, Norwalk, CT, 1995

274. Egger, J., Carter, C. M., Wilson, J. et al.: Is migraine food allergy? *Lancet* ii:865–9, 1983

275. Monro, J, Brostoff, J., Carini, C. and Zilkha, K.: Food allergy in migraine. *Lancet* ii:1–4, 1980

Chapter 6

1. Siguel, E. N., Maclure, M.: Relative enzyme activity of unsaturated fatty acid metabolic pathways in humans. *Metabolism* 36:664–69, 1987

2. Whelan, J., Kinsella, J. E. et al.: Dietary arachidonate enhances tissue arachidonate levels and eicosanoid production in Syrian hamsters. *J Nutr* 123:2174–85, 1993

3. Fat: If you can't bear to pare it. *Science News* 149:108, 1996

4. Stenson, W. F. et al.: Dietary supplementation with fish oil in ulcerative colitis. *Ann Int Med* 11:609–14, 1992

5. Siguel, E. N.: *Essential Fatty Acids in Health and Disease.* Nutrek Press, Brookline, MA, 1994

6. Trans-fatty acids: The new enemy. *Harvard Heart Letter* 4:1–3, 1994

7. Siguel, E. N., Lerman, R. H.: Trans-fatty acid patterns in patients with angiographically documented coronary artery disease. *Am J Card* 71:916–20, 1993

8. Michels, K. and Sacks, F.: Trans-fatty acids in European margarines. *NEJM* 332:541–42, 1995

9. Aschero, A., Willett, W. et al.: Trans-fatty acids intake and risk of cardiovascular disease. *Circulation* 89:94–101, 1994

10. Thomas, L. H.: Ischaemic heart disease and consumption of hydrogenated marine oils in England and Wales. *J Epidemiol Community Health* 46:78–82, 1992

11. Manku, M., Horrobin, D., Morse, N. et al.: Reduced levels of prostaglandin precursors in the blood of atopic patients: Defective delta-6-desaturase function as a biochemical basis for atopy. *Prostaglandins, Leukotrienes and Medicine* 9:615–28, 1982

12. Horrobin, D. F.: Review article: Medical uses of essential fatty Acids (EFAs). *Vet Dermatol* 4:161–66, 1993

13. Burton, G. and Ingold, K.: Beta-carotene: An unusual type of antioxidant. *Science* 224:569–73, 1984

14. Cutler, R. G.: Carotenoids and retinol: Their possible importance in determining longevity of primate species. *Proc Natl Acad Sci* 81:7627–31, 1984

15. Cody, V., Middleton, E. and Harborne, J. B.: *Plant Flavonoids in Biology and Medicine: Biochemical, Pharmacological, and Structure-Activity Relationships.* Alan R. Liss, New York, 1986

16. Bunce, G. E.: Nutrition and eye disease of the elderly. *J Nutr Biochem* 5:66–76, 1994

17. Tarlo, S. M. and Sussman, G. L.: Asthma and anaphylactoid reaction to food additives. *Can Fam Phys* 39:1119–23, 1993

18. Smith, J. M.: Adverse reactions to food and drug additives. *Eur J Clin Nutr* 45:17–21, 1991

19. Lucas, P. and Power, L.: Dietary fat aggravates active rheumatoid arthritis. *Clinical Research* 29:754A, 1981

20. Lindahl, O., Lindwall, L., Spangberg, A. et al.: Vegan diet regimen with reduced medication in the treatment of bronchial asthma. *J Asthma* 22:45–55, 1985

21. Rivers, J. P. W., Frankel, T. L.: Essential fatty acid deficiency. *Br Med Bull* 37:59–64, 1981

22. Levine, M.: New concepts in the biology and biochemistry of ascorbic acid. *NEJM* 314:892–902, 1986

23. Mullen, A. and Wilson, C. W. M.: The metabolism of ascorbic acid in rheumatoid arthritis. *Proc Nutr Sci* 35:8A–9A, 1976

24. Johnston, C. S. et al.: Antihistamine effects and complications of supplemental vitamin C. *J Am Dietetic Assoc* 92:988–89, 1992

25. Panganamala, R. V. and Cornwell, D. G.: The effects of vitamin E on arachidonic acid metabolism. *Ann NY Acad Sci* 393:376–91, 1982

26. Trevithick, J. R. et al.: Topical tocopherol acetate reduces post-UVB sunburn-associated erythema, edema, and skin sensitivity in hairless mice. *Arch Biochem Biophys* 296:575–82, 1992

27. Middleton, E. and Drzewieki, G.: Flavonoid inhibition of human basophil histamine release stimulated by various agents. *Biochem Pharmacol* 33:3333–38, 1984

28. Busse, W. W., Kopp, D. E. and Middleton, E.: Flavonoid modulation of human neutrophil function. *J Allergy Clin Immunol* 73:801–9, 1984

29. Yoshimoto, T., Furukawa, M., Yamamoto, S. et al.: Flavonoids: Potent inhibitors of arachidonate 5-lipoxygenase. *Biochem Biophys Res Common* 116:612–18, 1983

30. Ford-Hutchinson, A. W.: Leukotriene involvement in pathological processes. *J Allergy Clin Immunol* 74:437–40, 1984

31. Leventhal LJ, Boyce EG and Zurier RB: Treatment of rheumatoid arthritis with gammalinolenic acid. Ann Int Med 119:867-73, 1993

32. Leventhal, L. J. et al.: Treatment of rheumatoid arthritis with black currant seed oil. *Br J Rheum* 33:847–52, 1994

33. Knapp, H. R.: Omega-3 fatty acids in respiratory diseases. *J Am Coll Nutr* 14:18–23, 1995

34. Berth-Jones, J. et al.: Evening primrose oil and atopic eczema. *Lancet* 345:520, 1995

35. Engler, M. M. and Engler, M. B.: The antihypertensive effect of dietary borage oil. *FASB J* abstract 6:A1681, 1992

36. Lee, T., Hoover, R., Williams, J. et al.: Effect of dietary enrichment with eicosapentaenoic and docosahexanoic acids on in vitro neutrophil and monocyte leukotriene generation and neutrophil generation. *NEJM* 312:1217–24, 1985

37. Strasser, T., Fischer, S. and Weber, P.: Leukotriene B5 is formed in human neutrophils after dietary supplementation with eicosapentaenoic acid. *Proc Natl Acad Sci* 82:1540–3, 1985

38. Kremer, J., Michaelek, A. V., Lininger, L. et al.: Effects of manipulation of dietary fatty acids on clinical manifestation of rheumatoid arthritis. *Lancet* i:184–87, 1985

39. Kremer, J. M., Lawrence, D. A., Jubiz, W. et al.: Dietary fish oil and olive oil supplementation in patients with rheumatoid arthritis. *Arth Rheum* 33:810–20, 1990

40. Bruch, C. A. and Johnson, E. T.: A new dietary regimen for arthritis, value of cod liver oil on a fasting stomach. *J Natl Med Assoc* 51:266–70, 1959

41. Peretz, A. M. et al.: Selenium in rheumatic diseases. *Seminars Arth Rheum* 20:305–16, 1991

42. Laux, P. and Oschmann, R.: Witch hazel: Hamamelis virginiana L. *Zeitschrift fur Phytother* 14:155–66, 1993

43. Korting, H. C., Schafer-Korting, M. et al.: Anti-inflammatory activity of Hamamelis distillate applied topically to the skin. *Eur J Clin Pharmacol* 44:315–18, 1993 GET-4

44. Arora, R., Basu, N., Kapoor, V. and Jain, A.: Anti-inflammatory studies on Curcuma longa (turmeric). *Ind J Med Res* 59:1289–95, 1971

45. Srivastava, R.: Inhibition of neutrophil response by curcumin. *Agents Actions* 28:298–303, 1989

46. Srimal, R. and Dhawan, B.: Pharmacology of diferuloyl methane (curcumin), a non-steroidal anti-inflammatory agent. *J Pharm Pharmac* 25:447–52, 1973

47. Srivastava, R. and Srimal, R. C.: Modifications of certain inflammation-induced biochemical changes by curcumin. *Ind J Med Res* 8:215–23, 1985

48. Taussig, S: The mechanism of the physiological action of bromelain. *Med Hypothesis* 6:99–104, 1980

49. Tassman, G., Zafran, J. and Zayon, G.: A double-blind crossover study of a plant proteolytic enzyme in oral surgery. *J Dent Med* 20:51–54, 1965

50. Heptinstall, S., White, A., Williamson, L. and Mitchell, J. R. A.: Extracts of feverfew inhibit granule secretion in blood platelets and polymorphonuclear leukocytes. *Lancet* i:1071–74, 1985

51. Johnson, E. S., Kadam, N. P., Hylands, D. M., and Hylands, P. J.: Efficacy of feverfew as prophylactic treatment of migraine. *Br Med J* 291:569–73, 1985

52. Cyong, J.: A pharmacological study of the anti-inflammatory activity of Chinese herbs: A review. *Acupunct Electro-Ther* 7:173–202, 1982

53. Okimasa, E., Moromizato, Y., Watanabe, S. et al.: Inhibition of phospholipase A2 by glycyrrhizin, an anti-inflammatory drug. *Acta Med Okayama* 37:385–91, 1983

54. Ohuchi, K., Kamada, Y., Levine, L. and Tsurufuji, S.: Glycyrrhizin inhibits prostaglandin E2 formation by activated peritoneal macrophages from rats. *Prostagland Med* 7:457–63, 1981

55. Panush, R. S.: Delayed reactions to foods: Food allergy and rheumatic disease. *Ann Allergy* 56:500–3, 1986

56. Sundquist, T., Lindstrom, F., Magnusson, K.and Skoldstam, L.: Influence of fasting on intestinal permeability and disease activity in patients with rheumatoid arthritis shows normalization during fasting. *Scand J Rheumatol* 11:33–38, 1982

57. De Witte, T. J., Geerdink, P. J., Lamers, C. B. et al.: Hypochlorhydria and hypergastrinemia in rheumatoid arthritis. *Ann Rheum Dis* 38:14–17, 1979

58. Terano, T., Salmon, J. A., Higgs, G. A. and Moncada, S.: Eicosapentaenoic acid as a modulator of inflammation: Effect on prostaglandin and leukotriene synthesis. *Biochem Pharmac* 35:779–85, 1986

59. Kremer, J. M. et al.: Fish-oil fatty acid supplementation in active rheumatoid arthritis. *Ann Int Med* 106:497–503, 1987

60. Lee, T. H. and Arm, J. P.: Prospects for modifying the allergic response by fish oil diets. *Clinical Allergy* 16:89–100, 1986

61. Bray, G. W.: The hypochlorhydria of asthma in childhood. *Quart J Med* 24:181–97, 1931

62. Dry, J. and Vincent, D.: Effect of fish oil diet on asthma: Results of a one-year double-blind study. *Int Arch Allergy Immunol* 95:156–7, 1991

63. Vanderhoek, J., Makheja, A. and Bailey, J.: Inhibition of fatty acid lipoxygenases by onion and garlic oils: Evidence for the mechanism by which these oils inhibit platelet aggregation. *Biochem Pharmac* 29:3169–73, 1980

64. Dorsch, W. and Weber, J.: Prevention of allergen-induced bronchial constriction in sensitized guinea pigs by crude alcohol onion extract. *Agents Actions* 14:626–30, 1984

65. Kreutner, W. et al.: Bronchodilatory and antiallergy activity of forskolin. *European J Pharmacology* 111:1–8, 1985

66. Lichey, J., Friedrich, T., Priesnitz, M. et al.: Effect of forskolin on methacholine-induced bronchoconstriction in extrinsic asthmatics. *Lancet* ii:167, 1984

67. Marone, G. et al.: Forskolin inhibits the release of histamine from human basophils and mast cells. *Agents Actions* 18:96–99, 1986

68. Bauer, K. et al.: Pharmacodynamic effects of inhaled dry powder formulations of fenoterol and colforsin in asthma. *Clin Pharmacol Ther* 53:76–83, 1993

69. Shahar, E. et al.: Dietary n-3 polyunsaturated fatty acids and smoking-related chronic obstructive pulmonary disease. *NEJM* 331:228–33, 1994

70. Hansen, A. E.: Study of iodine number of serum fatty acids in infantile eczema. *Proc Soc Exp Biol Med* 1198–99, 1933

71. Galli, E. et al.: Analysis of polyunsaturated fatty acids in newborn sera: A screening tool for atopic disease? *Br J Dermatol* 130:752–56, 1994

72. Kerscher, M. J. and Korting, H. C.: Treatment of atopic eczema with evening primrose oil: Rationale and clinical results. *Clin Investig* 70:167–71, 1992

73. Isseroff, R. R.: Fish again for dinner! The role of fish and other dietary oils in the therapy of skin disease. *J Am Acad Dermatol* 19:1073–80, 1988

74. Campbell, K. L.: Clinical use of fatty acid supplements in dogs. *Vet Dermatol* 4:167–73, 1993

75. van de Merwe, J. P.: The human faecal flora and Crohn's disease. *Ant van Leeuwenhoek* 50:691–700, 1984

76. Stenson, W. F. et al.: Dietary supplementation with fish oil in ulcerative colitis. *Ann Int Med* 116:609–14, 1992

Chapter 7

1. Bray, G. W.: The hypochlorhydria of asthma in childhood. *Br Med J* 24:181–97, 1931

2. Hampton, E. M. et al: Intravenous magnesium therapy in acute myocardial infarction. *Ann Pharmacotherapy* 28:212–19, 1994

3. Smith, B.: Organic foods versus supermarket foods: Element levels. *J Appl Nutr* 45:35–39, 1993

4. *Med World News*: Nutritional therapy saves lives, costs. Feb. 24, 1986, p. 99

5. Elsborg, L. et al.: The intake of vitamins and minerals by the elderly at home. *Int J Vit Nutr Res* 53:321–29, 1983

6. Werbach, M. R.: *Nutritional Influences on Illness*, v. I and II. Third Line Press, Tarzana, CA, 1987, 1993

7. Brown, M. L., ed.: *Present Knowledge in Nutrition*, 6th ed. ILSI, Nutrition Foundation, Washington, DC, 1990

8. Schauss, A.: "Suggested Optimal Daily Nutritional Allowances," in Pizzorno, J. E. and Murray, M. T.: *A Textbook of Natural Medicine*. Bastyr University Publications, Seattle, WA, 1995

9. Pizzorno, J. E. and Murray, M. T.: "Vitamin Toxicities and Therapeutic Monitoring," in Pizzorno and Murray: *A Textbook of Natural Medicine*. Bastyr University Publications, Seattle, WA, 1995

10. Russell, R.: Changes in gastrointestinal function attributed to aging. *Am J Clin Nutr* 55:1203s–7s, 1992

11. Doe, W. F.: An overview of intestinal immunity and malabsorption. *Am J Med* 67:1077, 1979

12. Hoverstad, T.: *The normal microflora and short chain fatty acids*. Paper presented at 5th Bengt E. Gustafsson Symposium, Stockholm, June 1 to 4, 1988

13. Savage, D.: Microbial ecology of the gastrointestinal tract. *Ann Rev Microbiol* 31:107–33, 1977

14. *Am J Gastroent* (editorial): Soluble dietary fiber and short chain fatty acids: An advance in understanding the human bacterial flora. 85(10): 1313–14, 1990

15. Grubb, R., Midtevt, T. and Norin, E.: *The regulatory and protective role of the normal microflora*. Paper presented at the 5th Bengt E. Gustafsson Symposium.Stockholm June 1 to 4, 1988

16. Jeejeebhoy, K. N., Royall, D., Wolever, T. M. S.: Clinical significance of colonic fermentation. *Am J Gastroent* 85(10): 1307–12, 1990

17. Latella, C. R.: Metabolism of the large bowel mucosa in health and disease. *Int J Colorectal Dis* (Germany) 6: 127–32, 1991

18. Barrie, S. A.: "Heidelberg pH Capsule Gastric Analysis," in Pizzorno, J. E. and Murray, M. T.: *A Textbook of Natural Medicine*. Bastyr University Publications, Seattle, WA, 1995

19. Vellas, B., Belas, D. and Albarede, J. L.: Effects of aging process on digestive functions. *Comprehensive Therapy* 17:46–52, 1991

20. Baker, H., Frank, O. and Jaslow, S. P.: Oral versus intramuscular vitamin supplementation for hypovitaminosis in the elderly. *J Am Geriat Soc* 48:42–45, 1980

21. Russel, R. M.: Changes in gastrointestinal function attributed to aging. *Am J Clin Nutr* 55:1203s–7s, 1992

22. Adams, F.: *The Genuine Works of Hippocrates*. Williams & Williams, Baltimore, MD, 1939

23. *Eur J Clin Microbiol Infect Dis* (editorial): Evidence of immunoregulation of the composition of intestinal microflora and its practical consequences, Feb. 1988: 103–6

24. Crook, W. G.: *The Yeast Connection: A Medical Breakthrough*. Professional Books, Jackson, TN, 1986

25. Odds, F. C.: *Candida and Candidiasis*, 2nd edition. Bailliere-Tindall, Philadelphia, 1991

26. Casseli. M., Trevisani, L., Bighi, S. et al.: Dead fecal yeast and chronic diarrhea. *Digestion* 41:142–49, 1988

27. Nesheim, M. C.: Human nutrition needs and parasitic infections. *Parasitology* 107:S7–S18, 1993

28. Galland, L.: Persistent GI upset a signal of hidden giardiasis. *Cortlandt Forum* 120–21, 1990

29. Galland, L. et al.: Giardia lamblia infection as a cause of chronic fatigue. *J Nutr Med* 1:27–31, 1990

30. Results of testing for intestinal parasites by state diagnostic laboratories, United States, 1987. *Morbid Mortal Weekly Rep* 40(SS-4):25–30, 1992

31. Cho, C. H.: Zinc: Absorption and role in gastrointestinal metabolism and disorders. *Digestive Diseases* 9:49–60, 1991

32. Prasap, A. S.: Therapeutic role of zinc in disease states. *Nutrition and the M.D.* 17:1–2, 1991

33. Schneider, M. U. et al.: Pancreatic enzyme replacement therapy: Comparative effects of conventional and enteric-coated microspheric pancreatin and acid-stable fungal enzyme preparations on steatorrhea in chronic pancreatitis. *Hepatogastroenterol* 32:97–102, 1985

34. Roberts, J. M.: Magnesium for preeclampsia and eclampsia. *NEJM* 333:250–51, 1995

35. Lucas, M. J. et al.: A comparison of magnesium sulfate with phennytoin for prevention of eclampsia. *NEJM* 333:201–5, 1995

36. Role of magnesium in acute myocardial infarction. *Br Med J* 303:1499, 1991

37. Chernow, B. et al.: Magnesium administration and dysrhythmias after cardiac surgery. JAMA 268:2395–402, 1992

38. Evans, G. W. et al.: The effect of chromium picolinate on serum cholesterol and apolipoprotein fractions in human subjects. Western J Med 152:41–45, 1990

39. Anderson, R. L.: Chromium, glucose tolerance and diabetes. Biol Trace Min Res 32:19–24, 1992

40. Gargas, M. L. et al.: Urinary excretion of chromium by humans following ingestion of chromium picolinate. Drug Metab Disp 22:522–9, 1994

41. Kulpers, E. J. et al.: Long-term sequelae of Helicobacter pylori gastritis. Lancet 345:1525–28, 1995

42. Blaster, M. J.: The bacteria behind ulcers. Sci Am 274:104–7, 1996

43. Cheney, G.: Rapid healing of peptic ulcers in patients receiving fresh cabbage juice. Cal Med 70:10–14, 1949

44. Shive, W., Snider, R. N., DuBiler, B. et al.: Glutamine in treatment of peptic ulcer. Tex J Med 53:840–43, 1957

45. Balakrishnan, V., Pillai, M. V., Raveendran, P. M. and Nair, C. S.: Deglycyrrhizinated liquorice in the treatment of chronic duodenal ulcer. J Asso Phys Ind 26:811–14, 1978

46. Morgan, A., McAdam, W., Pacsoo, C. and Darnboraoug, A.: Comparison between cimetidine and Caved-S in the treatment of gastric ulceration, and subsequent maintenance therapy. Gut 23:545, 1982

47. Marle, J., Aarsen, P., Lind, A. and Van Weeren-Kramer, J.: Deglycyrrhizinised liquorice (DGL) and the renewal of rat stomach epithelium. Eur J Pharm 72:219, 1981

Chapter 8

1. Bemben, D. A. et al.: Thyroid disease in the elderly, Part 1: Prevalence of undiagnosed hypothyroidism. J Fam Pract 38:577–82, 1994

2. Gaspari, A. A. et al.: Prevalence of thyroid abnormalities in patients with dermatitis herpetiformis and in control subjects with HLA-B8/-DR3. Am J Med 88:145–50, 1990

3. Modified from Golan, R.: Optimal Wellness. Ballantine, New York, 1995, pp. 382–83

4. Newberne, P. M.: "Naturally Occurring Food-Borne Toxicants," in Shils, M. E. and Young, V. R.: Modern Nutrition in Health and Disease. Lea & Febiger, Philadelphia, 1988

5. Nishiyama, S. et al.: Zinc supplementation alters thyroid hormone metabolism in disabled patients with zinc deficiency. J Am Coll Nutr 13:62–7, 1994

6. Toro, T.: Selenium's role in thyroid found. New Scientist 129:27, 1991

7. Meinhold, H. et al.: Effects of selenium and iodine deficiency on iodothyronine deiodinases in brain, thyroid and peripheral tissue. AMA 19:8–12, 1992

8. Berry, M. J. and Larsen, P. R.: The role of selenium in thyroid hormone action. Endocrine Rev 13:207–20, 1992

9. Beard, J. L. et al.: Impaired thermoregulation and thyroid function in iron-deficiency anemia. Am J Clin Nutr 52:813–19, 1990

10. Lenon, D. et al.: Diet and exercise training effects on resting metabolic rate. Int J Obesity, 9:39–47, 1985

11. Mulder, J.W. et al.: Dehydroepiandrosterone as predictor for progression to aids in asymptomatic human immunodeficiency virus type-infected men. J Immunodefic 165:413–18, 1992

12. Gordon, G. B. et al.: Serum levels of dehydroepiandrosterone and its sulfate and the risk of developing bladder cancer. Cancer Res 51:1366–69, 1991

13. Aksoy, I. A. et al.: Human liver dehydroepiandrosterone sulfotransferase: Nature and extent of individual variation. Clin Pharmacol Therapeutics 54:498–506, 1993 GET-6

14. Barbieri, R. L. et al.: Contine and nicotine inhibit human fetal adrenal 11-beta-hydroxylase. J Clin Endocrinol Metab 69:1221–24, 1989 GET-6

15. Labbate, L. A. et al.: Physical fitness and perceived stress: Relationships with coronary artery disease factors. Psychosomatics 36:555–60, 1995

16. Raglin, J. S. and Morgan, W. P.: Influence of vigorous exercise on mood state. *Behav Ther* 8: 179–83, 1985
17. Blumenthal, J. A. et al.: Aerobic exercise reduces levels of cardiovascular and sympathoadrenal responses to mental stress in subjects without prior evidence of myocardial ischemia. *Am J Cardiol* 65:93, 1990
18. Glaser, J. L. et al.: Elevated serum dehydroepiandrosterone sulfate levels in practitioners of transcendental meditation and TM-Sidhi programs. *J Behav Med* 15:327–41, 1992
19. Littman, A. B. et al.: Physiologic benefits of a stress reduction program for healthy middle-aged Army officers. *J Psychosom Res* 37:345–54, 1993
20. Satterlee, D. G. et al.: Vitamin C amelioration of the adrenal stress response in broiler chickens being prepared for slaughter. *Comp Biochem Thysiol* 94A:569–s74, 1989
21. Seelig, M. S.: Adverse stress reactions and magnesium deficiency: Preventive and therapeutic implications. *J Am Coll Nutr* 11:609/Abstract 40, 1992
22. Bhattacharya, S. K. and Mitra, S K.: Anxiolytic activity of Panax ginseng roots: An experimental study. *J Ethnopharmacol* 34:87–92, 1991
23. Brekhman II and Dardymov IV: Pharmacological investigation of glycosides from ginseng and Eleutherococcus. *Lloydia* 32:46-51, 1969
24. Regelson, W. and Kalimi, M. Y.: "Dehydroepiandrosterone (DHEA)—A Pleiotropic Steroid: How Can One Steroid Do So Much?" in Klatz, R. M.: *Advances in Anti-Aging Medicine*, vol 1. Mary Ann Liebert Publications, Larchmont, NY, 1996
25. Morales, A. et al.: Effects of replacement dose of dehydroepiandrosterone in men and women of advancing age. *J Clin Endocrin Metab* 78:1360–67, 1994
26. Friess, E. et al.: DHEA administration increases rapid eye movement sleep and EEG power and sigma frequency range. *Am J Physiol* 268:E107–13, 1995
27. Van Vollenhoven, R.: An open study of dehydroepiandrosterone in systemic lupus erythematosus. *Arth Rheum* 37:1305–10, 1994
28. Conference: Dehydroepiandrosterone (DHEA) and aging. *NY Acad Scie* June 17–19, 1995
29. Fackelmann, K. A.: Does testosterone fight artery disease? *Sci News*, May 28:340, 1994
30. Jackson, J. et al.: Testosterone deficiency as a risk factor for hip fracture in men: A case-controlled study. *Am J Med Sci* 304:4–8, 1992
31. Nillson, P. M., Moller, L. and Solstad, K.: Adverse effects of psychosocial stress on gonadal function and insulin levels in middle-aged adults. *J Int Med* 237:479–86, 1995
32. Yeh, J. and Friedman, A. J.: Nicotine and cotinine inhibit rat testes androgen biosynthesis in vivo. *J Steroid Biochem* 33:627–30, 1989
33. Michnovicz, J.: Environmental modulation of oestrogen metabolism in humans. *Intl Clin Nutr Rev* 7:169–73, 1987
34. Diamond, F. et al.: Effects of drug and alcohol abuse upon pituitary-testicular function in adolescent males. *J Adolesc Health Care* 7:28–33, 1986
35. Ralof, J.: Beyond estrogens: Why unmasking hormone-mimicking pollutants proves so challenging. *Sci News* 148:44–46, 1995
36. Newest estrogen mimics the commonest? *Sci News:* 148:47, 1995
37. Brown, S. J.: Environmental doctors take up pollution prevention cause. *Family Practice News*, Jan. 1:6, 1995
38. Prasad, A. S.: Therapeutic role of zinc in disease states. *Nutrition and the M.D.* 17:1–2, 1991
39. Hunt, C. D. et al.: Effects of dietary zinc depletion on seminal volume and zinc loss: Serum testosterone concentrations and sperm morphology in young men. *Am J Clin Nutr* 56:148–57, 1992
40. Bedwal, R.: Zinc, copper and selenium in reproduction. *Experientia* 50:626–40, 1994
41. Krsnjavi, H. et al.: Selenium and fertility in men. *Trace Elem Med* 9:107–8, 1992
42. Meikle, A. W. et al.: Effects of a fat-containing meal on sex hormones in men. *Metabolism* 39:943–46, 1990

43. Hoffman, R.: "Endocrine Aspects of Aging," in Klatz, R. M.: *Advances in Anti-Aging Medicine*. Mary Ann Liebert Publications, Larchmont, NY, 1996

44. Kim, C., Choi, H., Kim, C. C. et al.: Influence of ginseng on mating behavior of male rats. *Am J Chinese Med* 4:163–68, 1976

45. Fahim, W. S., Harman, J. M., Clevenger, T. E. et al.: Effect of Panax ginseng on testosterone level and prostate in male rats. *Arch Androl* 8:261–63, 1982

46. Albert-Puleo, M.: Fennel and anise as estrogenic agents. *J Ethnopharmacol* 2:337–44, 1980

47. Liu, H. et al.: Indole (3,2-b)carbazole: A dietary-derived factor that exhibits both antiestrogenic and estrogenic activity. *J Natl Canc Inst* 86:158–62, 1994 GET-1

48. Golding, B. R.: Nonsteroidal estrogens and estrogen antagonists: Mechanism of action and health implications. *J Natl Canc Inst* 86:1741–42, 1994 GET-1

49. Messina, M. and Barnes, S.: The roles of soy products in reducing risk of cancer. *J Natl Cancer Inst* 83:541–46, 1991

50. Farnsworth, N. et al.: Potential value of plants as sources of antifertility drugs, II. *J Pharmaceut Sci* 64:717–45, 1975 GET-3

51. Aldercreutz, H. C. et al.: Phytoestrogens: Epidemiology and a possible role in cancer protection. *Environ Health Perspect* 103(suppl. 7):103–12, 1995

52. Woods, M. N.: Low-fat, high fiber diet and serum estrone sulfate in premenopausal women. *Am J Clin Nutr* 49:1179–83, 1989

53. Aldercreutz, H. C. et al.: Western diet and Western diseases: Some hormonal and biochemical mechanisms and associations. *Scand J Clin Lab Invest* 50 (suppl. 201):3-23 1990

54. Bernstein, L. et al.: Physical exercise and reduced risk of breast cancer in young women. *J Natl Cancer Inst* 86:1403–7, 1994

55. Aganoff, J. and Boyle, G.: Aerobic exercise, mood states and menstrual cycle symptoms. *J Psychosom Res* 38:183–92, 1994

56. Brown, D. J.: Vitex agnus castus clinical monograph. *Qrtrly Rev Nat Med* Summer:111–21, 1994

57. Schedlowski, M. et al.: Acute psychological stress increases plasma levels of cortisol, prolactin and TSH. *Life Sciences* 50:1201–5, 1992

58. Mendleson, J. H.: Alcohol effects on reproductive function in women. *Psychiatric Letter* 4:35–38, 1986

59. Teelucksingh, S. et al.: Hypothalamic syndrome and central sleep apnea associated with toluene exposure. *Qrtrly J Med* 286:185–90, 1991

60. *The Medical Letter:* Drugs that cause sexual dysfunction: An update. 34(issue 876), 1992

61. Fackelmann, K. A. et al.: PMS: Hints of a link to lunch time and zinc. *Science News* 138:263, 1990

62. Baghurst, P. A. et al.: Diet, prolactin and breast cancer. *Am J Clin Nutr* 56:943–9, 1992

63. Zinc sandwich. *Lancet* 337:273–4, 1991

64. Panth, M. et al.: Effect of vitamin A supplementation on plasma progesterone and estradiol levels during pregnancy. *Int J Vit Nutr Res* 61, 1991

65. Luck, M. R. et al.: Ascorbic acid and fertility. *Biol Reproduc* 52:262–66, 1995

66. Kumagai, A., Nishino, K., Shimomura, A., Kin, T. and Yamamura, Y.: Effect of glycyrrhizin on estrogen action. *Endocrinol Japan* 14:34–38, 1967

67. Hammar, M., Berg, G. and Lindgren, R.: Does physical exercise influence the frequency of postmenopausal hot flushes? *Acta Obstet Gynecol Scand* 69:409–12, 1990

68. Midgette, A. S. and Baron, J. A.: Cigarette smoking and the risk of natural menopause. *Epidemiology* 1:474–80, 1990

69. Finkler, R. S.: The effect of vitamin E in the menopause. *J Clin Endocrinol Metab* 9:89–94, 1949

70. Christy, C. J.: Vitamin E in menopause. *Am J Ob Gyn* 50:84–87, 1945

71. McLaren, H. C.: Vitamin E in the menopause. *Br Med J* ii:1378–81, 1949

72. Smith, C. J.: Non-hormonal control of vasomotor flushing in menopausal patients. *Chic Med* 67:193–95, 1964

73. Murase, Y. and Iishima, H.: Clinical studies of oral administration of gamma-oryzanol on climacteric complaints and its syndrome. *Obstet Gynecol Prac* 12:147–49, 1963

74. Ishihara, M.: Effect of gamma-oryzanol on serum lipid peroxide levels and climacteric disturbances. *Asia Oceania J Obstet Gynecol* 10:317, 1984

75. Yoshino, G., Kazumi, T., Amano, M. et al.: Effects of gamma-oryzanol on hyperlipidemic subjects. *Current Ther Res* 45:543–52, 1989

76. Thastrup, O., Fjalland, B. and Lemmich, J.: Coronary vasodilatory, spasmolytic and cAMP-phosphodiesterase inhibitory properties of dihydropyranocoumarins and dihydrofuranocoumarins. *Acta Pharmacol et Toxicol* 52:246–53, 1983

77. Duker, E. M., Kopanski, L., Jarry, H. and Wuttke, W.: Effects of extracts from Cimicifuga racemosa on gonatropin release in menopausal women and ovariectomized rats. *Planta Medica* 57:420–24, 1991

78. Kleijnen, J. and Knipschild, P.: Drug profiles: Ginkgo biloba. *Lancet* 340:1136–39, 1993

79. Bauer, U.: Six-month double-blind randomized clinical trial of Ginkgo biloba extract versus placebo in two parallel groups in patients suffering from peripheral arterial insufficiency. *Arzneim Forsch* 34:716–21, 1984

80. Rudofsky, V. G.: The effect of Ginkgo biloba extract in cases of arterial occlusive disease: A randomized placebo controlled double-blind cross-over study. *Fortschr Med* 105:397–400, 1987

81. Abraham GE: Nutritional factors in the etiology of the premenstrual tension syndromes. *J Repro Med* 28:446-64, 1983

82. Jones D. V: Influence of dietary fat on self-reported menstrual symptoms. *Physiol Behav* 40:483–7, 1987

83. Goei G. S. and Abraham G. E: Effect of nutritional supplement, Optivite, on symptoms of premenstrual tension. *J Repro Med* 28:527–31, 1983

84. Kleijnen, J. et al.: Vitamin B_6 in the treatment of premenstrual syndrome—a review. *Br J Obstet Gyn* 97:847–52, 1990

85. Barr W.: Pyridoxine supplements in the premenstrual syndrome. *Practitioner* 228:425–7, 1984

86. Sherwood, R. A., et al.: Magnesium and the premenstrual syndrome. *Ann Clin Biochem* 23:667–70, 1986

87. Piesse J. W.: Nutritional factors in the premenstrual syndrome. *Int Clin Nutr Rev* 4:54–81, 1984

88. Weiss, R. F.: *Herbal Medicine*. Ab Arctum, Stockholm, Sweden, 1988

89. Sliutz, G. et al.: *Agnus castus* extracts inhibit prolactin secretion of rat pituitary cells. *Horm Metab Res* 25:253–55, 1993

90. Peters-Welte, C. and Albrecht, M.: Menstrual abnormalities and PMS: Vitex agnus-castus. *TW Gynekologie* 7:49–52, 1994

91. Neumann, P. J., et al.: Cost of a successful delivery with in vitro fertilization. *NEJM* 331:239–43, 1994

92. Domar, A. D., et al.: The mind-body program for infertility: A new behavioral treatment approach for women with infertility. *Fertil Steril* 53:246–9, 1990

93. Mueller, B. A., et al.: Recreational drug use and the risk of primary infertility. *Epidemiology* 1:195–200, 1990

94. Rosevear, S. K., et al.: Smoking and decreased fertilization rates in vitro. *Lancet* 340:1195–6, 1992

95. Grodstein, F. et al.: Infertility in women and moderate alcohol use. *Am J Pub Health* 84:1429–32, 1994

96. Wilcox, A. J. and Weinberg, C. R.: Tea and fertility. *Lancet* 337:1159–60, 1991

97. John, E. M., et al.: Spontaneous abortions among cosmetologists. *Epidemiology* 5:147–55, 1994

98. Bedwal, R.: Zinc, copper and selenium in reproduction. *Experientia* 50:626–40, 1994

99. Sharpe, R. M. and Skakkebaek, N. E.: Are oestrogens involved in falling sperm counts and disorders of the male reproduction tract? *Lancet* 341:1392–95, 1993

100. Field, B., Selub, M. and Hughes, C. L.: Reproductive effects of environmental agents. *Semen Reprod Endocrinol* 8:44–54, 1990

101. Ibeh, I.N., et al.: Dietary Exposure to Aflatoxin in Human Male Infertility in Benin City, Nigeria. *Int J Infertil* 39:208–14, 1994

102. Yamasaki, T., et al.: Effects of allixin, a phytoalexin produced by garlic, on mutagenesis, DNA-binding and metabolism of aflatoxin B1. *Cancer Letters* 59:89–94, 1991

103. Aitken, R. J.: The role of free oxygen radicals and sperm function. *Int J Androl* 12:95–97, 1989

104. Zini, A., De Lamirande, E. and Gagnon, C.: Reactive oxygen species in semen of infertile patients: Levels of superoxide dismutase- and catalase-like activities in seminal plasma and spermatozoa. *Int J Androl* 16:183–88, 1993

105. Kaur, S.: Effect of environmental pollutants on human semen. *Bull Environ Contam Toxicol* 40:102–4, 1988

106. Kulikauskas, V. D., Blaustein, D. and Ablin, D.: Cigarette smoking and its possible effects on sperm. *Fertil Steril* 44:526–28, 1985

107. Fraga, C. et al.: Ascorbic acid protects against endogenous oxidative DNA damage in human sperm. *Proc Natl Acad Sci* 88:11003–6, 1991

108. Dawson, E. B. et al.: Effect of ascorbic acid on male fertility. *Ann NY Acad Sci* 498:312–23, 1987

109. Netter, A. et al.: Effect of zinc administration on plasma testosterone, dihydrotestosterone and sperm count. *Arch Androl* 7:69–73, 1981

110. Sandler, B. and Faragher, B.: Treatment of oligospermia with vitamin B_{12}. *Infertility* 7:133–38, 1984

Chapter 9

1. Kaufman W.: The Common Form of Joint Dysfunction: Its Incidence and Treatment. *EL* Hildreth Co, Brattleboro, VT, 1949

2. Bilger, B.: Forever young. *The Sciences* 35:26–30, 1995

3. Harman, D.: Aging: A theory based on free radical and radiation chemistry. *J. Gerontol* 11:288–300, 1956

4. Ames, B. N. Shigenaga, M. K. and Hagen, T. M.: Oxidants, antioxidants, and the degenerative diseases of aging. *Proc Natl Acad Sci USA* 90:7915–22, 1993

5. Orr, W. C. and Sohal, R. S.: Extension of lifespan by over-expression of superoxide dismutase and catalase in Drosophilia melanogaster. *Science* 263:1128–30, 1994

6. Ronzio, B.: "Antioxidants," in Pizzorno, J. E. and Murray, M. T.: A *Textbook of Medicine*. Bastyr University Publications, Seattle, WA, 1995

7. Schneider, E. L. and Reed, J. D.: Life extension. *NEJM* 312:1159–68, 1985

8. Brooks, P. M., Potter, S. R. and Buchanan, W. W.: NSAID and osteoarthritis: Help or hindrance. *J Rheumatol* 9:3–5, 1982

9. Joosten, E., van den Berg, A., Riezler, R. et al.: Metabolic evidence that deficiencies of vitamin B_{12} (cobalamin), folate, and vitamin B_6 occur more commonly in elderly people. *Am J Clin Nutr* 58:468–76, 1993

10. Voelker, R.: Ames agrees with Mom's advice: Eat your fruits and vegetables. *JAMA* 273:1077–78, 1995

11. Serdula, M. K. et al.: Fruit and vegetable intake among adults in 16 states: Results of a brief telephone survey. *Am J Publ Health* 85:236–39, 1995

12. Ryan, A. S., Craig, L. D. and Finn, S. C.: Nutrient intakes and dietary patterns of older Americans: A national study. *J Gerontol* 47:M145–50, 1992

13. Russell, R. M. and Suter, P. M.: Vitamin requirements of elderly people: An update. *Am J Clin Nut* 58:4–14, 1993

14. Abell, A. et al.: High sperm density among members of organic farmers' association. *Lancet* 343:1498, 1994

15. Chandra, R. K.: Effect of vitamin and trace-element supplementation on immune responses and infection in elderly subjects. *Lancet* 340:1140–47, 1992

16. Levin, B., faculty at Bastyr University, personal communication

17. Gullestad, L. et al.: Magnesium status in healthy, free-living elderly Norwegians. *J Am Coll Nutr* 13:45–50, 1994

18. Deans, S. G. et al.: Promotional effects of plant volatile oils on the polunsaturated fatty acid status during aging. *Age* 16:71–74, 1993

19. Imai, K. and Nakachi, K.: Cross sectional study of effects of drinking green tea on cardiovascular and liver diseases. *Br Med J* 310:693–96, 1995

20. Pizzorno, J. E. and Murray, M. T.: "Eleutherococcus senticosus," in Pizzorno and Murray: *A Textbook of Natural Medicine.* Bastyr University Publications, Seattle, WA, 1995

21. Farnsworth, N. R., Kinghorn, A. D., Soejarto, D. and Waller, D. P.: Siberian ginseng (Eleutherococcus senticosus): Current status as an adaptogen. *Econ Med Plant Res* 1:156–215, 1985

22. D'Angelo, L., Grimaldi, R., Caravaggi, M. et al.: A double-blind, placebo controlled clinical study on the effect of a standardized ginseng extract on psychomotor performance in healthy volunteers. *J Ethnopharmacol* 16:15–22, 1986

23. Pizzorno, J. E. and Murray, M. T.: "Panax ginseng," in Pizzorno and Murray: *A Textbook of Natural Medicine.* Bastyr University Publications, Seattle, WA, 1995

24. Bahrke, M. S. and Morgan, W. P.: Evaluation of the ergogenic properties of ginseng. *Sports Medicine* 18:229–48, 1994

25. Brekhman, I. I. and Dardymov, I. V.: Pharmacological investigation of glycosides from ginseng and Eleutherococcus. *Lloydia* 32:46–51, 1969

26. Grabowski, R.: Nutritional considerations in wound healing. *Quarterly Rev Nat Med:* 329–34, 1994

27. Boiteau, P. and Ratsimamnga, A. R.: Asiaticoside extracted from Centella asiatica: Its therapeutic uses in the healing of experimental or refractory wounds, leprosy, skin tuberculosis, and lupus. *Therapie* 11:125–49, 1956

28. Bonte, F., Dumas, M. et al.: Influence of asiatic acid, madecassic acid and asiaticoside on human collagen I synthesis. *Planta Med* 60:133–35, 1994

29. Monograph: Centella asiatica. Indena S.p.A., Milan, Italy, 1987

30. Kartnig, T.: Clinical applications of Centella asiatica (L.) Urb. *Herbs Spices Med Plants* 3:146–73, 1988

31. Ippolito, F.: Medical treatment of keloids. *G Ital Dermatol* 112:377–81, 1977

32. Bosse, J. P., Papillon, J., Frenette, G. et al.: Clinical study of a new anti-keloid drug. *Ann Plast Surg* 3:13–21, 1979

33. Sasaki S, Shinkai H, Akashi Y and Kishihara Y: Studies on the mechanism of action of asiaticoside (Madecassol) on experimental granulation tissue and cultured fibroblasts and its clinical application in systemic scleroderma. *Acta Diabetol Lat* 52:141-50, 1972

34. Gravel JA: Oxygen dressings and asiaticoside in the treatment of burns. *Laval Med* 36:413–15, 1965

35. Pointel, J. P., Boccalon, H,.Cloarec, M. et al. Titrated extract of Centella asiatica (TECA) in the treatment of venous insufficiency of the lower limbs. *Angiology* 38:46–50, 1987

36. Prevalence of sedentary lifestyle—Behavioral Risk Factor Surveillance System, United States, 1991. *Morbidity and Mortality Weekly Report* 29:576, 1993

37. Lee, I.-M. et al.: Body weight and mortality. *JAMA* 270:2823–81, 1993

38. Nicklas, T. A.: Dietary studies of children: The Bogalusa Heart Study experience. *J Am Dietetic Assoc* 95:1127–33, 1995

39. Evans, W. J.: Exercise, nutrition and aging. *J Nutrition* 122:796–801, 1992

40. Evans, W. J.: Body building for the nineties. *Nutrition Action Health Letter* 5:5–6, 1992

41. Welbourne, T. C. et al.: Increased plasma bicarbonate and growth hormone after an oral glutamine load. *Am J Clin Nut* 61:1058–61, 1995

42. Reimund, E.: The free radical flux theory of sleep. *Med Hypoth* 43:231–33, 1994

43. Jan, J. E. and Espezel, H.: Melatonin treatment of chronic sleep disorders. *Devel Med Child Neurol* 37:279–80, 1995

44. Leathwood P., Chauffard F., Heck E., and Munoz-Box R.: Aqueous extract of valerian root (*Valeriana officinalis* L.) improves sleep quality in man. *Pharmacol Biochem Behavior* 17:65–71, 1982

45. Lindhal O. and Lindwall L.: Double-blind study of a valerian preparation. *Pharmacol Biochem Behav* 32:19065–6, 1989

46. Gotz, M. E., et al: Oxidative stress: free radical production and neural degeneration. *Pharmacol Ther* 63:37–122, 1994

47. Peristeris, P., Clark, B. D., Gatti, S. et al.: N-acetylcysteine and glutathione as inhibitors of tumor necrosis factor production. *Cell Immunol* 140:390–99, 1992

48. Burgunder, J. M. and Lautergurg, B. H.: Decreased production of glutathione in patients with cirrhosis. *Eur J Clin Invest* 17:408–14, 1987

49. Flanagan, R. J. and Meridith, T. J.: Use of N-acetylcysteine in clinical toxicology. *Am J Med* 91(suppl.):3C-131S-9S, 1991

50. Ji, L.: Oxidative stress during exercise: Implication of antioxidant nutrients. *Free Rad Biol Med* 18:1079–86, 1995

51. Ornish, D. et al.: Can lifestyle changes reverse coronary heart disease? *Lancet* 336:129–33, 1990

52. Committee of Principle Investigators: World Health Organization Clofibrate Trial: A cooperative trial in the primary prevention of ischemic heart disease using clofibrate. *Br Heart J* 40:1069–118, 1978

53. Wagner, H. et al.: Inhibition of cholesterol synthesis in vitro by extracts and isolated compounds prepared from garlic and wild garlic. *Athero* 94:79–85, 1992

54. Kiesewetter, H. et al.: Effects of garlic coated tablets in peripheral arterial occlusive disease. *Clin Investig* 71:383–86, 1993

55. Orekhov, A. N. et al.: Direct anti-atherosclerosis-related effects of garlic. *Ann Med* 27:63–65, 1995

56. Cohen, A. F. et al.: A placebo-controlled parallel study of the effect of two types of coffee oil on serum lipids and transaminases: Identification of chemical substances involved in the cholesterol-raising effect of coffee. *Am J Clin Nut* 61:1277–83, 1995

57. Canner, P L. et al.: Fifteen year mortality in Coronary Drug Project patients: Long-term benefit with niacin. *J Am Coll Cardiol* 8:1245–55, 1986

58. El-Enein, A. M. A. et al.: The role of nicotinic acid and inositol hexaniacinate as anticholesterolemic and antilipemic agents. *Nutr Rep Intl* 28:899–911, 1983

59. Arvill, A. and Bodin, L.: Effect of short-term ingestion of konjac glucomannan on serum cholesterol of healthy men. *Am J Clin Nut* 61:585–89, 1995

60. Bishayee, A. and Chatterjee, M.: Hypolipdaemic and antiatheroscerlotic effects of oral Gymnema sylvestre R. br. leaf extract in albino rats fed a high fat diet. *Phytother Res* 8:118–20, 1994

61. Salenius, S. A.and Riekkinen, H. et al.: Long-term effects of guar gum on lipid metabolism after arotic endarterectomy. *Br Med J* 310:95–96, 1995

62. Jialal, I., Fuller, C. J. and Huet, B. A.: The effect of α-tocopherol supplementation on LDL oxidation. *Atheroscler Thromb Vasc Biol* 15:190–98, 1995

63. Hodis, H. N. et al.: Serial coronary angiographic evidence that antioxidant vitamin intake reduces progression of coronary artery atherosclerosis. *JAMA* 273:1849–54, 1995

64. Kritchevsky, S. B. et al.: Serum carotenoids and coronary heart disease. *JAMA* 272:1439–41, 1994

65. Steinberg, D.: Clinical trials of antioxidants in atherosclerosis. *Lancet* 346:36–38, 1995

66. Paolisso, G. et al.: Chronic intake of pharmacological doses of vitamin E might be useful in the therapy of elderly patients with coronary heart disease. *Am J Clin Nut* 61:848–52, 1995

67. Tappel, A. L. and Chen, H.: Protection of vitamin E, selenium, trolox C, ascorbic acid, palmitate, acetylcysteine, coenzyme Q0, coenzyme Q_{10}, beta-carotene, canthaxathin, and (+)-catechin against oxidative damage to rat blood and tissues in vivo. *Free Rad Biol Med* 18:949–53, 1995

68. Phelps, S. and Harris, W. S.: Garlic supplementation and lipoprotein oxidation susceptibility. *Lipids* 28:475–77, 1993

69. Kokkinos, P. F. et al.: Miles run per week and high-density lipoprotein cholesterol levels in healthy middle-aged men: A dose-response relationship. *Arch Int Med* 155:415–20, 1995

70. Pearson, T. A.: What to advise patients about drinking alcohol. *JAMA* 272:967–68, 1994

71. Hein, H. O., Sorensen, H., Suadicani, P. and Gyntelberg, F.: Alcohol consumption, Lewis phenotypes, and risk of ischaemic heart disease. *Lancet* 341:392–96, 1993

72. Folts, J. D. et al.: Administration of wine and grape juice inhibits in vivo platelet activity and thrombosis in stenosed canine coronary arteries. *Circulation* 91:1182–88, 1995

73. Wojcicki, J., Samochowiec, L. et al.: Ginkgo biloba extract inhibits the development of experimental atherosclerosis in rabbits. *Phytomedicine* 1:33–38, 1994

74. Mouren, X., Caillard, P. H. et al.: Study of the anti-ischemic action of Egb 761 in the treatment of peripheral arterial occlusive diseae by TcPO2 determination. *Angiology* 45:413–17, 1994

75. Kromhout, D., Bosscheiter, E. B. and De Lezenne-Coulander, C.: Inverse relation between fish oil consumption and 20 year mortality from coronary heart disease. *NEJM* 312:1205–9, 1985

76. Seidelin, K. N., Myrup, B. and Fischer-Hansen, B.: N-3 fatty acids in adipose tissue and coronary artery disease are inversely correlated. *Am J Clin Nut* 55:1117–19, 1992

77. de Loreril, M. et al.: Mediterranean alpha-linolenic acid-rich diet in secondary prevention of heart disease. *Lancet* 343:1454–59, 1994

78. Cobias, L. et al.: Lipid, lipoprotein, and hemostatic effects of fish vs. fish oil α-3 fatty acids in mildly hyperlidemic males. *Am J Clin Nut* 53:1210–16, 1991

79. Pernigotti, L. M. et al.: "Effect of Meoglycan on Clotting, Fibrinolysis and Platelet Aggregation in Normal Subjects and Hyperaggregating Arteriosclerosis," in Widhalm, K. and Sinzinger, H., eds: *Current Aspects of Atherosclerosis. Lipids, Lipoproteins, Platelets, Prostaglandins, and Experimental Findings.* Verlag Wilhelm, Madrich, 1983, pp. 64–75

80. Mansi, D. et al.: Open trial of mesoglycan in the treatment of cerebrovascular ischemic disease. *Acta Neurologica* 10:108–12, 1988

81. Yamasawa, I., Nohara, Y., Konno, S. et al.: "Experimental Studies on Effects of Coenzyme Q_{10} on Ischemic Myocardium," in Yamamura, Y., Folkers, K. and Ito, Y., eds: *Biomedical and Clinical Aspects of Coenzyme Q*, vol 2. Elsevier/North-Holland Biomedical Press, Amsterdam, 1980, pp. 333–47

82. Kishimoto, C., Tamaki, S., Matsumori, A. et al.: The protection of coenzyme Q_{10} against experimental viral myocarditis in mice. *Jpn Circ J* 48:1358, 1984

83. Folkers, K., Littarru, G. P., Ho, L. et al.: Evidence for a deficiency of coenzyme Q_{10} in human heart disease. *Int J Vit Res* 40:380, 1970

84. Kamikawa, T., Kobayashi, A., Yamashita, T. et al.: Effects of coenzyme Q_{10} on exercise tolerance in chronic stable angina pectoris. *Am J Cardiol* 56:247, 1985

85. Ishiyama, T., Morita, Y. Toyama, S. et al.: A clinical study of the effect of coenzyme Q on congestive heart failure. *Jpn Heart J* 17:32, 1976

86. Vanfraechem, J. H. P., Picalausa, C. and Folkers, K.: "Coenzyme Q_{10} and Physical Performance in Myocardial Failure," in Folkers, K., Yamamura, Y., eds: *Biomedical and Clinical Aspects of Coenzyme Q*, vol 4. Elsevier Science Publ, Amsterdam, 1984, pp. 281–90

87. Folkers, K., Vadhanavikit, S. and Mortensen, S. A.: Biochemical rationale and myocardial tissue data on the effective therapy of cardiomyopathy with coenzyme Q_{10}. *Proc Natl Acad Sci* 82:901, 1985

88. Langsjoen, P. H., Vadhanavikit, S. and Folkers, K.: Response of patients in classes III and IV of cardiomyopathy to therapy in a blind and crossover trial with coenzyme Q_{10}. *Proc Natl Acad Sci* 82:4240, 1985

89. Oda, T. and Hamamoto, K.: Effect of coenzyme Q_{10} on the stress-induced decrease of cardiac performance in pediatric patients with mitral valve prolapse. *Jpn Circ J* 48:1387, 1984

90. Yamagami, T., Shibata, N. and Folkers, K.: Bioenergetics in clinical medicine: Studies on coenzyme Q_{10} and essential hypertension. *Res Commun Chem Pathol Pharmacol* 11:273, 1975

91. Folkers, K. et al.: Bioenergetics in clinical medicine, XVI: Reduction of hypertension in patients by therapy with coenzyme Q_{10}. *Res Commun Chem Pathol Pharmacol* 31:129, 1981

92. Igarashi, T., Kobayashi, M. and Ohtake, S.: Effect of coenzyme Q_{10} on the sodium retaining action of aldosterone in rats. *Jpn J Pharmacol* 23(suppl):121, 1973

93. Reuter, H. D.: Crataegus (hawthorn): A botanical cardiac agent. *Zeits Phytotherapie* 15:73–81, 1994

94. Schmidt, U., Kuhn, U. et al.: Efficacy of the hawthorn (Crataegus) preparation LI 132 in 78 patients with chronic congestive heart failure defined as NYHA functional class II. *Phytomedicine* 1:17–24, 1994

95. Tauchert, M., Ploch, M. and Hubner, W. D.: Effectiveness of hawthorn extract LI 132 compared with the ACE inhibitor Captopril: Multicenter double-blind study with 132 NYHA stage II. *Munch Med* 136(suppl.)1:S27–33, 1994

96. Clostre, F.: "From the Body to the Cellular Membranes: The Different Levels of Pharmacological Action of Ginkgo Biloba Extract," in Funfgeld, E. W., ed.: *Rokan (Ginkgo Biloba): Recent Results in Pharmacology and Clinic.* Springer-Verlag, New York, 1988, pp. 80–98

97. Chatterjee, S. S. and Gabard, B.: Studies on the mechanism of action of an extract of Ginkgo biloba, a drug for the treatment of ischemic vascular diseases. *Naunyn-Schmiedeberg's Arch Pharmacol* 320: R52, 1982

98. Huguet, F., Drieu, K. and Piriou, A.: Decreased cerebral 5-HT1A receptors during aging: Reversal by Ginkgo biloba extract (EGb 761). *J Pharm Pharmacol* 46:316–8, 1994 GET-4

99. Pizzorno, J. E. and Murray, M. T.: *A Textbook of Natural Medicine.* Bastyr University Publications, 1995

100. Hindmarch, I. and Subhan, Z.: The psychopharmacological effects of Ginkgo biloba extract in normal healthy volunteers. *Int J Clin Pharmacol Res* 4:89–93, 1984

101. Modified from Bland, J.: Psychoneuro-nutritional medicine: An advancing paradigm. *Alt Ther* 1:22–27, 1995

102. Joosten, E. et al.: Metabolic evidence that deficiencies of vitamin B_{12} (cobalamin), folate, and vitamin B_6 occurr commonly in elderly people. *Am J Clin Nut* 58:468–76, 1993

103. Arnold, S. E. and Kramer, A.: Reversable dementias. *Med Clin Na* 77:215–30, 1993

104. Lindenbaum, J. et al.: Neuropsychiatric disorders caused by cobalamin deficiency in the absence of anemia or macrocytosis. *NEJM* 318:1720, 1988

105. Rafsky, H. A. and Weingarten, M.: A study of the gastric secretory response in the aged. *Gastroent* May:348–52, 1946

106. Milss, D. E. et al.: Dietary fatty acid supplementation alters stress reactivity and performance in man. *J Hum Hyperten* 3:111–16, 1989

107. Stordy, B. J.: Benefit of docosahexaenoic acid supplements to dark adaptation in dyslexics. *Lancet* 346:385, 1995

108. Streit, W. J. and Kincaid-Colton, C. A.: The brain's immune system. *Sci Am* 273:54–61, 1995

109. Hirata, F. and Axelrod, J.: Phospholipid methylation and biological signal transmission. *Science* 209:1082–90, 1990

110. Uitti, R. J. et al.: Parkinsonism induced by solvent abuse. *Ann Neurol* 35:616–19, 1994

111. Pezzoli, G. et al.: N-hexane-induced Parkinsonism: Pathogenic hypotheses. *Movement Dis* 10:279–82, 1995

112. Shahi, G. S. et al.: Parkinson's disease and cytochorome P450: A possible link? *Med Hypoth* 32:277–82, 1990

113. Beal, M. F.: Aging, energy, and oxidative stress in neurodegenerative disease. *Ann Neurol* 38:357–66, 1995

114. Fisher. L. J. and Gage, F. H.: Radical directions in Parkinson's disease. *Nature Med* 1:201–2, 1995

115. Muller, D. P. R.: Vitamin E and neurological function. *Redox Rep* 1:239–45, 1995

116. Boris, M. and Mandel, F. S.: Foods and additives are common causes of attention deficit disorder in children. *Ann Allergy* 72:462–68, 1994

117. Egger, J., Carter, C. M. et al.: Controlled trial of oligoantigenic treatment in the hyperkinetic syndrome. *Lancet* I:540–45, 1985

118. Dickey, L. D.: *Clinical Ecology.* CC Thomas, Springfield, IL, 1976

119. Pocock, N. A., Eisman, J. A., Yeates, M. G. et al.: Physical fitness is the major determinant of femoral neck and lumbar spine density. *J Clin Invest* 78:618–21, 1986

120. Yeater, R. and Martin, R.: Senile osteoporosis: The effects of exercise. *Postgrad Med* 75:147–49, 1984

121. Donaldson, C., Hulley, S., Vogel, J. et al.: Effect of prolonged bed rest on bone mineral. *Metabolism* 19:1071–84, 1970

122. Lee, C. J., Lawler, G. S. and Johnson, G. H.: Effects of supplementation of the diets with calcium and calcium-rich foods on bone density of elderly females with osteoporosis. *Am J Clin Nut* 34:819–23, 1981

123. Recker, R.: Calcium absorption and achlorhydria. *NEJM* 313:70–73, 1985

124. Nicar, M. J. and Pak, C. Y. C.: Calcium bioavailability from calcium carbonate and calcium citrate. *J Clin Endocrinol Metabol* 61:391–93, 1985

125. Meacham, S. L. et al.: Effect of boron supplementation on blood and urinary calcium, magnesium, and phosphorous, and urinary boron in athletic and sedentary women. *Am J Clin Nut* 61:341–45, 1994

126. Sojka, J. E. and Weaver, C. M.: Magnesium supplementation and osteoporosis. *Nutr Rev* 53:71–80, 1995

127. Bitensky, L., Hart, J. P., Catterall, A. et al.: Circulating vitamin K levels in patients with fractures. *J Bone Joint Surg* 70-B:663–64, 1988

128. Aloia, J. F., Cohn, S. H., Vaswani, A. et al.: Risk factors for postmenopausal osteoporosis. *Am J Med* 78:95–100, 1985

129. Malmivaara, A. et al.: The treatment of acute back pain: Bed rest, exercises, or ordinary activity? *NEJM* 332:351–55, 1995

130. Twomey, L. and Taylor, J.: Spine update: Exercise and spinal manipulation in the treatment of low back pain. *Spine* 20:615–19, 1995

131. Katz, M. L., Parker, K. R., Hadelman, G. et al.: Effects of antioxidant nutrient deficiency on the retina and retinal pigment of albino rats: A light and electron microscopic study. *Exp Eye Res* 34:339–69, 1982

132. West, S., Vitale, S., Hallfrisch, J. et al.: Are anti-oxidants or supplements protective of age-related macular degeneration? *Arch Ophthalmol* 111:104–9, 1994

133. Eye Disease Case-Controlled Study Group: Antioxidant status and neovascular age-related macular degeneration. *Arch Ophthalmol* 111:104–9, 1994

134. Goldberg, J., Flowerdew, G.Smith, E. et al.: Factors associated with age-related macular degeneration. *Am J Epidemiol* 128:700–10, 1988

135. Bendich, A.: The safety of β-carotene. *Nutr Cancer* 11:207–14, 1988

136. Seddon, J. M. et al.: Dietary carotenoids, vitamins A, C, and E, and advanced age-related macular degeneration. *JAMA* 272:1413–20, 1994

137. Newsome, D. A., Swartz, M., Leone, N. C. et al.: Oral zinc in macular degeneration. *Arch Ophthalmol* 106:192–98, 1988

138. Ferrandini, C., Droy-Lefaix, M. T. and Christen, Y., eds.: *Ginkgo Biloba (EGB 761) as a Free-Radical Scavenger.* Elsevier, Paris, 1993

139. Frentzel-Beyme, R. and Chang-Claude, J.: Vegetarian diets and colon cancer: The German experience. *Am J Clin Nut* 59(Suppl. 1):1143S–52S, 1995

140. Steinmetz, K. A. and Potter, J. D.: Vegetables, fruit and cancer, I: Epidemiology. *Cancer Causes Control* 2:325–57, 1991

141. Block, G. et al.: Fruit, vegetables, and cancer prevention: A review of the epidemiologic evidence. *Nutr Cancer* 18:1–29, 1992

142. Steinmetz, K. and Potter, J. D.: Vegetables, fruit and cancer, II: Mechanisms. *Cancer Causes Control* 2:427–42, 1991

143. Aldercreutz, C. H. T. et al.: Soybean phytoestrogen intake and cancer risk. *J Nutr* 125:757S–70S, 1995

144. Aldercreutz, H.: Phytoestrogens: Epidemiology and a possible role in cancer protection. *Environ Health Prospect* 103:103–12, 1995

145. Chihara, G.: Recent progress in immunopharmacology and therapeutic effects of polysaccharides. *Develop Biol Standard* 77:191–97, 1992

146. Steinmetz, K.A., Kushi, L.H. et al.: Vegetables, fruit, and colon cancer in the Iowa women's health study. *Am J Epidemiol* 139:1–5, 1994

147. Ip, C., Lisk, J. and Stoewsand, G. Q.: Mammary cancer prevention by regular garlic and selenium-enhanced garlic. *Nutr Cancer* 17:279–86, 1992

148. Dwivedi, C., Rohlfs, S. et al.: Chemoprotection of chemically induced skin tumor development by disulfide and diallyl disulfide. *Pharmac Res* 9:1669–70, 1992

149. Gao, Y. T. et al.: Reduced risk of esophageal cancer associated with green tea consumption. *J Natl Canc Inst* 86:855–58, 1994

150. Mukhtar, H. et al.: Green tea and skin: Anticarcinogenic effects. *J Invest Dermatol* 102:5–7, 1994

151. Wang, Z. Y., Huang, M.-T. et al.: Inhibitory effects of black tea, green tea, decaffeinated black tea, and decaffeinated green tea on ultraviolet B light-induced skin carcinogenesis in 7,12,-dimethyl-benz[a]anthracene-initiated SKH-mice. *Cancer Res* 54:3428–35, 1994

152. Javitt, N. B. et al.: Breast-gut connection: Origin of chenodeoxycholic acid in breast cyst fluid. *Lancet* 343:633–35, 1994

153. Ling, W. H. et al.: Lactobacillus strain GG supplementation decreases colonic hydrolytic and reductive enzyme activities in healthy female adults. *J Nutr* 124:18–23, 1994

154. Zapatero, M. D. et al.: Serum aluminum levels in Alzheimer's disease and other senile dementias. *Biol Trace Element Res* 47:235–40, 1995

155. Frolich, L. and Riederer, P.: Free radical mechanisms in dementia of the Alzheimer's type and the potential for antioxidative treatment. *Drug Res* 45:443–46, 1995

156. Kambova, L. et al.: Aluminum overload influences cognitive function in patients on dialysis. University Hospital Sofia, Bulgaria, 1994

157. Walton, J. et al.: Uptake of trace amounts of aluminum into the brain from drinking water. *Neurotoxicology* 16:187–90, 1995

158. Nolan, C. R. et al.: Aluminum and lead absorption from dietary sources in women ingesting calcium citrate. *Southern Med J* 87:894–98, 1994

159. Ed: Aluminum in food. *Food Chem Tox* 32:391–2, 1994

160. Martin, R. B.: Aluminum: A neurotoxic product of acid rain. *Accounts Chem Res* 27:204–10, 1994

161. Glick, J. L.: Dementias: The role of magnesium deficiency and hypothesis concerning the pathogenesis of Alzheimer's disease. *Med Hypoth* 31:211–25, 1990

162. Hofferberth, B.: The efficacy of EGb 761 in patients with senile dementia of the Alzheimer type, a double-blind, placebo-controlled study on different levels of investigation. *Human Psychopharmacol* 9:215–22, 1994

163. Jaakaola, K., Lahteenmaki, P. et al.: Treatment with antioxidant and other nutrients in combination with chemotherapy and irradiation in patients with small-lung cancer. *Anticancer Res* 12:599–606, 1992

164. Robertson, J. M.: Cataract prevention: time for a clinical trial? *Br J Clin Pract* 44:475–6, 1990

165. Spector, A.: "The Lens and Oxidative Stress," in *Oxidative Stress: Oxidants and Antioxidants, The Lens and Oxidative Stress*. College of Physicians and Surgeons of Columbia University, New York, NY, 1991, pp. 529–58

166. Hankinson, S. E., Stampfer, M. J., Seddon, J. M. et al.: Nutrient intake and cataract extraction in women: A prospective study. *Br Med J* 305:335–39, 1992 GET-3

167. Bravetti, G.: Preventive medical treatment of senile cataract with vitamin E and anthocyanosides: Clinical evaluation. *Ann Ophthalmol Clin Ocul* 115:109, 1989

168. Willett, W. C. et al.: Mediterranean diet pyramid. *Am J Clin Nut* 61(suppl):1042S–46S, 1995

169. Anderson, R. A.: Chromium, glucose tolerance, and diabetes. *Biol Trace Element Res* 32:19–24, 1992

170. Riales, R. and Albrink, M.: Effect of chromium chloride supplementation on the glucose tolerance and serum lipids, including HDL, of adult men. *Am J Clin Nut* 34:2670–78, 1981

171. JAMAl, G A.: "A New Model for Diabetic Neuropathy and a Pilot-Controlled Trial of Gamma-Linolenic Acid," in Horrobin, D., ed.: *Treatment of Diabetic Neruoathy: A New Approach.* Churchill Livingston, Edinburgh, pp. 21–39, 1992 GET-3

172. Julu, P. O.: "Responses of Peripheral Nerves Conduction Velocities to Treatment with Essential Fatty Acids in Diabetic Rats: Possible Mechanisms of Action," in Horrobin, D., ed: *Treatment of Diabetic Neuropathy: A New Approach.* Churchill Livingston, Edinburgh, pp. 41–61, 1992

173. JAMAl, G. A. and Carmichael, H.: The effect of gamma-linolenic acid on human diabetic peripheral neuropathy: A double-blind placebo-controlled trial. *Diabetic Med* 7:319–23, 1990

174. Paolisso, G. et al.: Metabolic benefits derived from chronic vitamin C supplementation in aged non-insulin dependent diabetes. *J Am Coll Nutr* 14:387–92, 1995

175. Raghuram, T. C., Sharma, R. D. et al.: Effect of fenugreek seed on intravenous glucose disposition in non-insulin dependent diabetic patients. *Phytotherapy Res* 8:83–86, 1994

176. Ghannam, N.: The anti-diabetic activity of aloes: Preliminary clinical and experimental observations. *Hormone Res* 24:288–94, 1986

177. Bever, B. O. and Zahnd, G. R.: Plants with oral hypoglycemic action. *Qtrly J Cruce Drug Res* 17:139–96, 1979

178. Sharma, K. K. et al.: Antihyperglycemic effect of onion: Effect on fasting blood sugar and induced hyperglycemia in man. *Ind J Med Res* 65:422–29, 1977

179. Setnikar, I. et al.: Pharmacokinetics of glucosamine in man. *Arzneim Forsch* 43:1109–13, 1993

180. Lopez, V. A.: Double-blind clinical evaluation of the relative efficacy of ibuprofen and glucosamine sulfate in the management of osteoarthritis of the knee in out-patients. *Curr Med Res Opin* 8:145–49, 1982

181. Harrer, G. and Sommer, H.: Treatment of mild/moderate depressions with Hypericum. *Phytomedicine* 1:3–8, 1994

182. Reuter, H. D.: Fifth Phytotherapy Congress in Bonn. *Zeitschrift fur Phytotherapie* 15:17–27, 1994

183. Schubert, H. and Halama, P.: Depressive episode primarily unresponsive to therapy in elderly patients: Efficacy of Ginkgo biloba extract (Egb 761) in combination with antidepressants. *Geriatr Forsch* 3:45–53, 1993

184. Christen, Y., Constentin, J. and Lacour, M., eds.: *Effects of Ginkgo Biloba (Egb 761) on the Central Nervous System.* Elsevier, Paris, 1992

185. Mancini, M., Agozzino, B. and Bompani, R.: Clinical and therapeutic effects of Ginkgo biloba extract (GBE) versus placebo in the treatment of psychorganic senile dementia of arteriosclerotic origin. *Gazetta Med Italiana* 152:69–80, 1993

186. NIH Consensus Conference on Impotence: Impotence. *JAMA* 270:83–90, 1993

187. Sohn, M. and Sikora, R.: Ginkgo biloba extract in the therapy of erectile dysfunction. *J Sex Educ Ther* 17:53–61, 1991

188. Sikora, R. et al.: Ginkgo biloba extract in the therapy of erectile dysfunction. *U Urol* 141:188A, 1989

189. Fahim, M., Fahim, Z., Der, R. and Harman, J.: Zinc treatment for the reduction of hyperplasia of the prostate. *Fed Proc* 35:361, 1976

190. Leake, A., Chisholm, G. D., and Habib, F. K.: The effect of zinc on the 5-alpha-reduction of testosterone by the hyperplastic human prostate gland. *J Steroid Biochem* 20:651–55, 1984

191. Hart, J. P. and Cooper, W. L.: *Vitamin F in the Treatment of Prostatic Hyperplasia: Report Number 1.* Lee Foundation for Nutr Res, Milwaukee, WI, 1941

192. Scott, W. W.: The lipids of the prostatic fluid, seminal plasma and enlarged prostate gland of man. *J Urol* 53:712–18, 1945

193. Rugendorff, E. W., Weidner, W. et al.: Results of treatment with pollen extract (Cernilton) in chronic prostatitis and prostatodynia. *Br J Urol* 71:433–38, 1993

194. Braekman, J.: The extract of Serenoa repens in the treatment of benign prostatic hyperplasia: A multicenter open study. *Curr Ther Res* 55:776–86, 1994

195. Bereges RR, Windeler J, et al: Randomized, placebo-controlled, double-blind clinical trial of β-sitosterol in patients with benign prostatic hyperplasia. *Lancet* 345:1529-32, 1995

Chapter 10

1. Kabat-Zinn, J.: "Meditation," in Moyers, B.: *Healing and the Mind*, Doubleday, New York, 1993, p. 130

2. Pert, C.: "The Chemical Communicators," in ibid, pp. 177–93

3. Kemeny, M.: "Emotions and the Immune System," in ibid, pp. 195–211

4. Kemeny, M.: Psychological and immunological predictions of recurrence in Herpes simplex II. *Psychosomatic Med* 51:195–208, 1989

5. Felten, D.: "The Brain and the Immune System," in Moyers, B.: *Healing and the Mind*, Doubleday, New York, 1993, pp. 213–36

6. Ader, R. and Cohen, N.: Behaviorally-conditioned immuno-suppression and murine systemic lupus erythematosus. *Science* 215:1534–36 1982

7. Spivak, L. and Wormser, G.: AIDS virus: Infection up? *Science News*, Nov. 23, 1985:325

8. Mason, J. W.: A historical view of the stress field:II. *J Human Stress* 1:35, 1975

9. Selye, S: *The Stress of Life*. McGraw-Hill, New York, 1976, p. 301

10. Hinkle, L. E. and Wolff, H. G.: Ecologic investigations of the relationship between illness, life experiences and the social environment. *Ann Int Med* 49:1373–88, 1958

11. Christenson, W. N. and Hinkle, L. E.: Differences in illness and prognostic signs in two groups of young men. *JAMA* 177:247–53, 1961

12. Selye, S.: loc. cit.

13. Kobasa, S. C.: Stressful life events, personality and health: An inquiry into hardiness. *J Personal Soc Psychol* 37:1–111, 1979; Kobasa, S. C., Maddi, S. R. and Courrington, S.: Personality and constitution as mediators in the stress-illness relationship. *J Health Soc Behav* 22:368, 1981; Maddi, S. R. and Kobasa, S. C.: *The Hardy Executive: Health Under Stress*. Dow Jones-Irwin, Homewood, IL, 1984

14. Rahe, R. H. and Arthur, R. J.: Life change and illness studies: Past history and future directions. *J Hum Stress* 5:3–15, 1978

15. Phone interview to discuss Jenkins's interview in *Clinical Pearls*, Oct. 1994

16. Williams, R. B., Haney, T. L., Lee, K. L. et al.: Type A behavior, hostility, and coronary atherosclerosis. *Psychosom Med* 42:539–49, 1980

17. Barefoot, J. C., Dahlstrom, W. G. and Williams, R. B.: Hostility, coronary heart disease incidence, and total mortality: A 25-year follow-up study of 255 physicians. *Psychosom Med* 45:59–63, 1983

18. Kiecolt-Glaser, J. K., Stephens, R. E., Lipetz, P. D. et al.: Distress and DNA repair in human lymphocytes. *J Behav Med* 8:311–19, 1985 Glaser, R., Thorn, B. E., Tarr, K. L., et al.: Effects of stress on methyltransferase synthesis: An important DNA repair enzyme. *Health Psychol* 4:403–12, 1985

19. Weisburg, S.: Food for mind and mood. *Science News*, Apr. 7, 1984:216–19

20. Seligman, M. E. P.: Helplessness and explanatory style: Risk factors for depression and disease. Paper presented at the annual meeting of the Society of Behavioral Medicine, San Francisco, March 1986

21. McClelland, D. C.: Motivation and immune function in health and disease. Paper presented at the annual meeting of the Society of Behavioral Medicine, New Orleans, March 1985

22. Medalie, J. H. and Goldbourt, U.: Angina pectoris among 10,000 men, II: Psychosocial and other risk factors. *Am J Med* 60:910–21, 1976

23. Bruhn, J. G.: An epidemiological study of myocardial infarctions in an Italian-American community. *J Chr Dis* 18:353–65, 1965 Bruhn, J. G., Chandler, B., Miller, C. et al.: Social aspects of coronary heart disease in two adjacent ethnically different communities. *Am J Pub Health* 56:1493–506, 1966

24. Berkman, L. F. and Syme, S. L.: Social networks, host resistance, and mortality: A nine-year follow-up study of Alameda County residents. *Am J Epidem* 109:186–204, 1979

25. Reynolds, P. and Kaplan, G. A.: Social connections and cancer: A prospective study of Alameda County residents. Paper presented at the annual meeting of the Society of Behavioral Medicine, San Francisco, March 1986

26. Kiecolt-Glaser, J., Glaser, R., Williger, D. et al.: The enhancement of immune competence by relaxation and social contact. Paper presented at the annual meeting of the Society of Behavioral Medicine, Philadelphia, May 1984

27. Kiecolt-Glaser, J.: Clinical psychoneuroimmunology in health and disease: Effects of marital quality and disruption. Paper presented at the annual meeting of the Society of Behavioral Medicine, San Francisco, March 1986

28. Messini, P.: Panel on pets as social support. Meeting of the Pacific division of the American Association for the Advancement of Science San Francisco, June 1984. Phone interview with James Gordon, January 17, 1995

30. Phone interview with Harmon Bro, March 29, 1996

31. Phone interview with Carol Goldberg, January 17, 1995

32. Phone interview with Patricia Norris, March 29, 1996. Norris, P. and Porter, G. *Why Me? Harnessing the Healing Power of the Human Spirit*. Stillpoint Publishing, Walpole, NH, 1985

33. Wallace, R. K.: Physiological effects of transcendental meditation. *Science* 167:1751–54, 1970; Badawi, K. et al.: Electrophysiologic characteristics of respiratory suspension periods occuring during the practice of the transcendental meditation program. *Psychosomatic Med* 46 no. 3:267–76, 1984; Dillbeck, M. C., Orme-Johnson, D. W.: Physiological differences between transcendental meditation and rest. *American Physiologist* 92: 879–81, 1987; Jevning, R. et al.: The physiology of meditation, A review: A wakeful hypometabolic integrated response. *Neuroscience and Biobehavioral Reviews* 16: 415–24, 199234. Wallace, R. K. et al.: *Int J Neurosci* 16:53–58, 1982

35. Sharma, H.: *Freedom from Disease*. Veda Publishing, Toronto, 1993, pp. 187–88

36. Glaser, J. et al.: Elevated serum dehydroepiandrosterone sulfate levels in practitioners of the transcendental meditation (tm) and tm-sidhi programs. *J Behav Med* 15:327–41, 1992

37. Levin, J. S. and Vanderpool, H. Y.: Is frequent religious attendance really conducive to better health? Toward an epidemiology of religion. *Soc Sci Med* 24:589–600, 1987

38. Craigie, F. C., Larson, D. B. and Liu, I. Y.: References to religion in the Journal of Family Practice: Dimensions and valence of spirituality. *J Fam Prac* 30:477–80, 1990

39. Dossey, L.: *Healing Words*. Harper, San Francisco, 1993, p. 167. Studies listed in Appendix 1, pp. 231–35

40. Wolf, S. and Goodell, H.: *Behavioral Science in Clinical Medicine*. Charles C. Thomas, Springfield, IL, 1976

41. Justice, B.: *Who Gets Sick?* G. P. Putnam's, New York, 1987, p. 136

Glossary

Acemannan (acetylated mannose) a potent immunostimulant extracted from aloe vera

Acetylation one of the phase II detoxification pathways

Adaptogen a substance that increases the body's ability to handle stress and that has a normalizing or balancing effect on body processes

Adenocarcinoma a malignant growth arising from a glandular organ

Adrenocorticotropin a pituitary hormone that activates the adrenal gland

Aldosterone a hormone secreted by the adrenals to increase water and salt retention by the kidneys

Allicin a biologically active compound found in garlic

Allopathy the conventional method of medicine which combats a disease by using substances and techniques specifically against that disease

Alpha-linolenic acid an essential fatty acid of the omega-3 group; best sources are flax seed oil, borage oil, evening primrose oil

Amenorrhea the absence of menstrual periods

Amino acid conjugation one of the phase II detoxification pathways

Amyloid proteins degenerative form of protein that is secreted to wall off damage in certain pathological states and that is associated with a variety of chronic diseases, e.g. tuberculosis, carcinoma, Alzheimer's disease

Androgens male sex hormones produced by the testes, including testosterone, dihydrotestosterone, and androstenedione

Angina pectoris the heart pain that comes when there is an inadequate supply of blood to meet the needs of the heart

Anthocyanidins the antioxidant flavonoids responsible for the red to blue colors of blueberries, blackberries, cherries, grapes, hawthorn berries, and many flowers

Antigen any substance (e.g., pieces of bacteria, toxins, foreign proteins) that, when introduced into the body, provokes an immune response resulting in the formation of antibodies

Antioxidants substances that neutralize free radicals

Antipyretic reducing fever

Arachidonic acid an essential fatty acid from which the body produces the pro-inflammatory series 2 prostaglandins; arachidonic acid is found only in land-animal fats

Arachidonic acid cascade a series of inflammatory chemical reactions induced as a response to free radical damage or injury

Arginine an essential amino acid

Articular tissue joint tissue

Astragalus a traditional Chinese medicinal herb used for viral infections

ATP adenosine triphosphate, the energy currency of the cell

Atrophic vaginitis the loss of vaginal elasticity and mucus secretion associated with menopause

Autoimmune diseases diseases that result when the immune system develops antibodies against the body's own tissues

Autolysis the body's digestion or removal of a severely damaged cell

Autonomic nervous system the bodily system that regulates involuntary functions such as heart rate, blood pressure, and digestion

Benzoate clearance test a test that evaluates the function of one of the phase II pathways, amino acid conjugation, by measuring the rate at which the body detoxifies benzoate by conjugating it with glycine to form hippuric acid which is excreted by the kidneys

Bilirubin the orange or yellowish breakdown product of hemoglobin that is found in the bile

Blood/brain barrier prevents the passage of substances from the blood to the brain

B-lymphocytes special white cells that produce specific antibodies to pathogens with which they come in contact

Brassica family of vegetables the crucifers, i.e., cabbage, broccoli and brussels sprouts

Bromelain a protein-digesting enzyme extracted from the stem of the pineapple plant

Carcinogens substances that can cause cancer

Cardiomyopathy a degenerative condition of the heart

Carotene the yellow pigment in carrots and other orange fruits and vegetables which, besides being converted into vitamin A, functions as an antioxidant

Carotenoids the most widespread group of naturally occurring pigments in nature-more than 600 types have been identified; carotenoids or carotenes are very potent quenchers of free radicals

Catabolism the destructive phase of metabolism during which complex substances are converted into simpler substances, usually with the release of energy

Catecholamines the fight or flight hormones released by the adrenal glands

Catalases antioxidant enzymes that require iron for proper function

Cell-mediated immunity also called non-specific defenses, the immune system's first strike forces; involves special white cells (typically T cell lymphocytes and neutrophils) that immediately attack an invader. Cell-mediated immunity is especially important in the body's ability to resist infection by yeasts (such as *Candida albicans*), fungi (such as athlete's foot), parasites (worms), and viruses (such as *Herpes simplex* and Epstein-Barr). Cell-mediated immunity is also critical in protecting against the development of cancer and is commonly involved in allergic reactions

Cellular respiration the production of energy in the cells from oxygen and fuel

Cervical dysplasia proliferation of precancerous cells in the cervix

Chelating agent an chemical that binds to minerals

Chemotactic factors a class of chemicals, including lymphokines, leukotrienes and pro-inflammatory prostaglandins, that attract white cells to a damaged area and stimulate them to digest and remove the damaged tissues

Cholagogues agents that stimulate the gall bladder to contraction and excrete bile into the intestines

Choleretic agents that stimulate the liver to secrete bile into the gall bladder

Cholestasis the accumulation of bile in the gall bladder

Circadian rhythms physiological phenomena that cycle at approximately 24-hour intervals, i.e., our biological clock

Collagen the protein that is the main component of connective tissue

Complement a group of proteins found in the blood that aid in the destruction of invading pathogens

Conjugation a process in which various enzymes in the liver attach small chemicals to a toxin, either neutralizing it or making it more easily excreted through the urine or bile

Corticosteroids hormones released by the adrenal glands during stress

Cortisol an adrenal hormone secreted in response to stress

Cortisone a stress-induced hormone that prepares the body for the flight or fight response

Coxsackievirus a type of virus that is usually benign but attacks the heart in susceptible people

Cutaneous pertaining to the skin

Cyclosporin a drug used to suppress the immune system after organ transplants

Cytochrome P450   a collective name for a group of enzymes used in phase I detoxification of environmental toxins, also called the "mixed function oxidative enzymes"

Cytotoxic test   a test for food allergies that evaluates food sensitivity and allergy by mixing some of a person's white cells with extracts of suspected foods. The white cells sensitized to specific foods are destroyed by the digestive enzymes released when the white cells engulf the extracts of those foods

Daidzein   a phytoestrogen found in high concentrations in soy foods

DHEA   a hormone found in abundance in young adults that typically declines with age

Dihydrotestosterone   an inflammatory form of testosterone

Double-blind, placebo-controlled study   one in which neither the participants nor those conducting the study know who is receiving the substance studied or placebo; the current scientific gold standard

Dysmenorrhea   painful menstrual periods

Edema   excessive fluid retention

Eicosapentaenoic acid (EPA)   an essential fatty acid from which the series 3 prostaglandins are made. EPA comes to us in our diet from fish oils or is synthesized from linolenic acid

Ejection fraction   the amount of blood the heart pumps per beat

Endogenous   any substance produced internally

Endometriosis   a proliferation of the uterine lining in inappropriate places, like the fallopian tubes

Endotoxins   toxins produced internally from gut bacteria or from incomplete breakdown of various metabolic compounds

Enterodiol   a lignin found in rye that is converted by health-promoting bacteria in the intestines to phytoestrogens which help lower the risk of several cancers

Epidemiological studies   studies of disease as it affects a particular population

Epidemiologist   a scientist who conducts epidemiological research

Epithelial cancer   cancer of the lungs, gastrointestinal tract, genitourinary tract, and skin

Epithelium   the cells that cover the surface of the body and line most of the internal organs

Essential fatty acids   labeled "essential" because the body can't synthesize them, these fatty acids are required for the production of prostaglandins

Estrogen   female hormone, produced by the ovaries during reproductive years, responsible for female sexual characteristics

Etiology   cause

Eustachian tubes   little tubes that connect the ear to the throat—what you pop when changing elevation in an airplane

Flavonoid   a group of antioxidant plant pigments (4,000 have now been identified) largely responsible for the colors of fruits and flowers

Food allergy   an inflammatory reaction to foods mediated by antibodies

Food intolerance   a reaction to a food that is not mediated by antibodies

Fructooligosaccharides   short-chain carbohydrates, essentially indigestible by humans, that are the preferred food of health-promoting intestinal bacteria, *Bifidobacteria* and lactobacilli

Functional medicine   a philosophy of health care focused on improving the function of the body's systems

Gastric atrophy   a condition in which the cells and glands of the stomach have degenerated, and the stomach is no longer able to produce adequate amounts of stomach acid or of intrinsic factor, a special compound used to ensure absorption of vitamin B_{12}

Genistein   a phytoestrogen found in highest amounts in soy foods

Ginsenosides   biologically active components in ginseng

Glucocorticoids   a class of drug commonly used to suppress inflammatory reactions, e.g. cortisone, which also suppresses the immune system

Gluconeogenesis   the process by which the liver converts amino acids to glucose when the body is fasting

Glucose tolerance factor   a body chemical that works with insulin to facilitate the entry of glucose into cells

Glucuronidation   one of the phase II detoxification pathways

Glutamine   an amino acid

Glutathione   the antioxidant most important for neutralizing the free radicals produced as byproducts in phase I detoxification, and also required for one of the phase II detoxification processes, glutathione conjugation

Glutathione conjugation   one of the phase II detoxification pathways

Glutathione peroxidase   a selenium-dependent enzyme that neutralizes free radicals

Gluten   the primary protein in wheat

Gluten-sensitive enteropathy   a severe allergy to wheat, also known as celiac disease

Glycine   an amino acid that is used in phase II amino acid detoxification

Glycyrrhiza glabra   licorice root, an antiviral herb that works by both supporting the immune system and by directly inhibiting various viruses

Glycyrrhizin and glycyrrhetinic acid   two active constituents of licorice root

Goitrogens   foods which, if eaten raw in large amounts, can induce an iodine deficiency by combining with iodine and making it unavailable to the thyroid; these foods include brassica family foods (turnips, cabbage, rutabagas, mustard greens, radishes, horseradishes), cassava root, soybeans, peanuts, pine nuts, and millet

Ground substance   the material that occupies the intercellular spaces in fibrous connective tissue, cartilage, and bone

Healthspan   the years of life we enjoy free of disabling disease

Hepatocytes   liver cells

Hirsutism   abnormal hair growth

Histamine   one of the special chemicals secreted by cells to alert the immune system

Humoral immunity   also called "specific defense," is the immune system's secondary line of defense, and involves sensitized white cells and antibodies formed to uniquely match the surface of invaders

Hyaluronic acid   compound that provides lubrication for the joints

Hyaluronidase   enzyme secreted by bacteria to break through the body's first line of defense, the protective membranes like the skin or mucous membranes, so the organism can enter the body

Hydrastis canadensis **(goldenseal)**   an herb primarily used for its direct antibacterial properties, but which has also shown remarkable immune system-enhancing activity

Hydrogenation   the process used to make margarine and shortening out of vegetable oils, which transforms some fatty acids to what are called the "trans" and other abnormal forms. Trans-fatty acids have their hydrogens on opposite sides which makes them appear to the body the be the same as saturated fatty acids

Hypercarotenemia   when the skin turns yellow because the body is overly saturated with carotenes

Hypertensive heart disease   heart disease resulting from high blood pressure

Hypochlorhydria   insufficient stomach acid

Hypoglycemia   low blood sugar

Hypoxia   poor blood supply

Immunoglobulins   antibodies produced by B-lymphocytes in response to contact with foreign proteins or antigens. The body produces five types of immunoglobulins: sIgA, IgD, IgE, IgG, and IgM

Indole-3-carbinol   a chemical compound found in brassica family or cruciferous vegetables that stimulates both phase I and phase II detoxification enzymes

Insulin   a hormone secreted by the pancreas that facilitates the entry of glucose into the cells

Interferon   a special chemical secreted by cells when they become infected with viruses that alerts natural killer cells to increase their activity and helps other cells better resist viral penetration

Intestinal dysbiosis   the most common type of toxicity in which the bowel contains excessive levels of unhealthy toxin-producing bacteria and inadequate amounts of normal health-promoting bacteria

In vitro   in a test tube, in the laboratory

In vivo   in a living subject

Ischemia   low blood supply

Ischemic heart disease   heart disease resulting from too little blood supply to the heart

Isoflavone   a type of flavonoid

Ketones   the end products of fat metabolism

Krebs cycle   the series of chemical processes in the mitochondria that produce energy for the cells to function

Kupffer cell   a special type of macrophage found in the liver

Lactose   a sugar (disaccharide) present in cow's milk

Lactulose/mannitol absorption test   a procedure that measures the permeability of the gastrointestinal tract by measuring the rate of absorption of lactulose, a molecule so large that it normally does not enter the body in any appreciable amount

Leaky gut   a condition in which damage to the intestinal barrier allows both normal and toxic bowel constituents to leak into the body

Lentinan   a polysaccharide that is the active component in shiitake mushrooms and powerfully stimulates the immune system, suppresses chemical and viral carcinogens, directly attacks cancers, and prevents cancer recurrence or metastasis after surgery

Lentinus edodes (shiitake mushroom)   a mushroom used for centuries in traditional Chinese medicine to increase resistance to infection

Leukotrienes   a group of chemical mediators of inflammation produced by the arachidonic acid cascade, leukotrienes play an important role in asthma because they stimulate contraction of bronchial muscles

Lignin   polysaccharides, found in the cell walls of plants, some of which impact human health

Limonene   a phytochemical found in oranges and tangerines (as well as in the seeds of caraway and dill) that has been found to prevent and even treat cancer in animal models. Limonene's protective effects are probably because it is a strong inducer of both phase I and phase II detoxification enzymes that neutralize carcinogens

Linoleic acid   an essential fatty acid from which the body derives anti-inflammatory series 1 prostaglandins, linoleic acid is found in evening primrose, borage, black currant, safflower, sunflower, and corn oils

Linolenic acid (ALA)   an essential fat obtained in our diet principally from flaxseed (linseed) oil and black currant seed oil

Lipid peroxidation   the damaging of lipids, or fats, by free radicals

Lipid peroxide   a fat oxidized by free radicals

Lipotropic   a nutrient that protects the liver from fat buildup

Livotrit   an Ayurvedic herbal formula for the liver

Lutein   a carotene found in tomatoes and dark green, leafy vegetables, especially spinach and kale, that concentrates in the retina, thus offering significant protection against macular degeneration

Luteinizing hormone   the enzyme secreted by the pituitary gland that, in men, stimulates the testes to secrete testosterone, and, in women, causes the ripe ovum to be released from the cell surrounding it

Lycopene   a red pigment from tomatoes that is prevalent in testes, prostate, and human plasma

Lymphatic system   an extensive network of very thin vein-like tubes that run parallel to our blood vessels throughout the body. It has many functions, including draining the fluid filling the spaces between the cells, draining waste products from the tissues, and transporting the lymph to lymph nodes where macrophages filter out debris and toxins

Lymphocyte   a family of white cells that accounts for 20–40% of the white cells in the blood and includes T cells, B cells, natural killer cells, and others

Lysosome   a special organ within the cell, which, when the cell is traumatized, ruptures, releasing enzymes to digest the damaged parts of the cell

Macrophages   the body's garbage collectors, which are located throughout the body where they are most likely to encounter pathogenic agents. In the liver, they are called Kupffer cells, and in the brain, they are called microglia

Mast cells   white cells that secrete histamine, a chemical that alerts the immune system to the presence of pathogens

Matairesinol   a lignin found in rye that is converted by health-promoting bacteria in the intestines to phytoestrogens that help lower the risk of some cancers

Melaleuca alternafolia (tea tree oil)   a tree, primarily grown in Australia, the oil of which is an excellent anti-fungal

Mercaptate   a water-soluble form of a toxin

Metabolism   a collective term for all the chemical processes that take place in the body

Metabolite   a product of a chemical reaction

Methionine   an essential amino acid that contains sulfur and is a component of s-adenosylmethionine (SAM), a compound used in the phase II detoxification pathway, methylation

Methylation   one of the phase II detoxification pathways

Microglial cells   cells in the brain that monitor the health of surrounding cells and destroy pathogens or injured cells

Microgram (µg, mcg)   1,000 micrograms equals one milligram (mg)

Microvilli   the minuscule folds in the intestines that greatly increase the absorptive surface area of the intestines

Mitochondria   the cell's energy production plants

Mitral valve prolapse   a condition characterized by collapse of one of the valves in the heart

Monoamine oxidase (MAO)   An enzyme responsible for breaking down the brain chemicals serotonin and norepinephrine

Monocyte   a type of white cell that cleans up cellular debris after an infection

Mucus   a sticky substance secreted by the cells of the mucous membranes that traps pathogens and moves them off the membranes, e.g., out the nose or into the intestines where they are destroyed by stomach acid

Myopathy   any disease of the muscles

Myricetin   a flavonoid that scavenges superoxide and blocks LDL oxidation

Myringotomy   a surgical procedure that involves cutting a small hole in the eardrum and inserting ear tubes to allow drainage

N-acetylcysteine (NAC)   a substance that helps increase the synthesis of glutathione, an important antioxidant used in phase II detoxification

Natural killer cells   a type of white cell that does not need to be sensitized to detect and attack pathogens; NK cells are the body's first attack force against cancer cells

Naturopathic medicine   family physicians who help people understand why they get sick and how to become healthy. Naturopaths emphasize the promotion of health rather than the simple treatment of symptoms and disease

Neurons   brain cells

Neuropathy   any disease of the nerves

Neutrophil   the most numerous type of white cell, neutrophils migrate to the area of pathogenic invasion and attack the invaders

Nitrosamines   carcinogenic substances formed in the stomach

Non-steroidal anti-inflammatory drugs (NSAIDS)   drugs used to lessen inflammatory processes including aspirin, acetaminophen, ibuprofen, which also, unfortunately, disrupt the intestinal barrier function and cause increased permeability, allowing inflammatory toxins to leak into the body

Nosocomial infections   infections acquired in the hospital

Nystatin   a drug frequently prescribed for fungal infections

Organic solvents   a class of common chemical toxins that can damage brain health and are found in paint, paint thinner, cleaning fluids, gasoline, kerosene, lighter fluid

Otitis media   infection of the middle ear

Oxidation   when a substance either combines with oxygen or loses an electron

Parasympathetic nervous system   the portion of the autonomic nervous system responsible for bodily functions during periods of rest, relaxation, visualization, meditation, and sleep

Pathogen   disease-producing microorganism

Pathological detoxifiers   individuals with an overactive phase I detoxification pathway, which results in the production of more harmful intermediate products than phase II can disarm quickly, so these people suffer more severe toxic reactions to environmental poisons

Pectin   a fiber found in fruit and also available as a supplement that increases the secretion of digestive enzyme (trypsin, chymotrypsin, lipase, and amylase), prevents absorption of toxic molecules in the bowel, and decreases transit time, thus decreasing the opportunity for absorption of harmful compounds

Phagocytes   the immune cells that surround and destroy undesirable cells and substances

Phagocytic index   a test that evaluates how effectively the non-specific defense system is working by measuring how rapidly phagocytes ingest foreign materials

Phagocytosis   the ingestion and digestion of bacteria or other pathogens by immune cells

Phase I   a liver detoxification pathway that essentially involves oxidizing the toxin, often resulting in the creation of even more toxic activated intermediates which are sent to phase II

Phase II   a liver detoxification pathway that typically involves a process called conjugation, in which various enzymes in the liver attach small chemicals to the xenobiotic. This either neutralizes the toxin or makes it more easily excreted through the urine or bile. There are essentially six major phase II detoxification pathways: glutathione conjugation, amino acid conjugation, methylation, sulfation, acetylation, and glucuronidation

Phthalates   compounds commonly used to make plastics flexible and the most common industrial contaminants in the environment. Two phthalates, butyl benzyl phthalate (BBP) and di-n-butyl phytate (DBP) are estrogenic, causing problems for male gonadal function and stimulating the growth of breast cells in culture, which may be of especial significance in breast cancer. Phthalates are found in butter, margarine, and the food preservative BHA

Phytoestrogens   literally, plant estrogens. Chemicals found in some foods and herbs with weak estrogenic activity

Picnogenols   flavonoid antioxidants

Plasma   the fluid that makes up the non-cellular part of the blood

Polyphenols   a type of phytochemical

Phospholipids   kind of fat found in cell membranes that , in the liver, offers protection from chronic exposure to organic solvents. The phospholipids that protect the liver include phosphatidylcholine, phosphatidylethanolamine, and phosphatidylserine

Postprandial   after a meal

Prebiotics   indigestible substances that help the healthy bacteria in the intestines grow

Proanthocyanidins   the antioxidant flavonoids responsible for the red to blue colors of blueberries, blackberries, cherries, grapes, hawthorn berries, and many flowers

Probiotics   the bacteria found in the healthy intestines; the primary health-promoting intestinal bacteria are *lactobacilli* and *bifidobacteria*

Prophylaxis   to guard against, as a preventive measure

Prostaglandins   hormone like molecules that control inflammatory processes in the body

Proteases   protein-splitting enzymes

Protein carbonyls   oxidized proteins that are carcinogenic

Purines   DNA components

Quercetin   a flavonoid that scavenges superoxide and blocks LDL oxidation

Reactive oxygen species (ROS)   an inclusive term describing the various forms of reactive oxidizing agents, whether or not they are free radicals. All of these various oxidizing molecules are referred to in this book by the term free radicals as it is in more common usage

Renin   an enzyme involved in the regulation of blood pressure

Reperfusion   reestablishment of blood supply after ischemia, the loss of blood supply

Retinol   a form of vitamin A present in animal tissue

Rutin   a flavonoid that scavenges superoxide and blocks LDL oxidation of defense against colds and upper respiratory infection

SCFAS   short chain fatty acids (acetate, propionate, butyrate, and valerate) produced by colonic bacteria's fermentation of carbohydrates. In the healthy intestine, these SCFAS provide much of the energy for lining cells

Secretory IgA   an antibody secreted into the mucus that is part of the immune system's first line

Sepsis   severe infections in the blood

Serenoa repens (saw palmetto)   an herb used in the treatment of benign prostatic hyperplasia (a common problem of men as they age)

Serotonin   a neurotransmitter made from tryptophan

Singlet oxygen   a particularly destructive free radical

Spermatogenesis   sperm production

Spleen   an organ in the left side of the abdomen that stores white cells and processes red cells

Stealth pathogens   cell wall-deficient forms of bacteria that are essentially invisible to most immune cells

Steroid hormones   estrogen, testosterone, cortisone

Sulfation   one of the phase II detoxification pathways

Superoxide   a highly reactive form of oxygen, i.e., a potent free radical

Superoxide dismutase   antioxidant enzyme that requires copper, zinc, or manganese to function

Sympathetic nervous system   the part of the nervous system responsible for the fight or flight response

Syndrome   a group of signs and symptoms that occur together in a pattern characteristic of a particular disease or abnormal condition

Synovial tissue   the tissues that surround the joint

T cells   lymphocytes that come from the thymus and are the major components of cell-mediated immunity

Thymosin, thymopoeitin, and serum thymic factor   hormones produced by the thymus that regulate immune functions. Low levels of these hormones in the blood is associated with depressed immunity and increased susceptibility to infection

Thymus   the major gland of the immune system

Tincture   alcohol extract of an herb

Toluene   a solvent

Triglycerides   the body's storage form of fat

Urticaria   a skin reaction, usually caused by an allergic reaction, characterized by hives and itching

Vasoactive amines   nitrogen-containing compounds that affect blood vessels, e.g. histamine, tyramine, putrescine, and cadaverine, all of which contribute to increased intestinal permeability

Vis medicatrix naturae   the healing power of nature, i.e., the innate drive of the body towards health

Xanthophylls   a type of carotenoid that constitutes most of the carotenoids in green leafy vegetables

Xenobiotic   a general term for all types of toxins

Zeaxanthin   a carotene found in tomatoes and dark green, leafy vegetables, especially spinach and kale, that offers significant protection against macular degeneration

Index